Second Edition

HARRISON'S
Rheumatology

Derived from Harrison's Principles of Internal Medicine, 17th Edition

Editors

ANTHONY S. FAUCI, MD

Chief, Laboratory of Immunoregulation;
Director, National Institute of Allergy and Infectious Diseases,
National Institutes of Health, Bethesda

DENNIS L. KASPER, MD

William Ellery Channing Professor of Medicine,
Professor of Microbiology and Molecular Genetics,
Harvard Medical School; Director, Channing Laboratory,
Department of Medicine,
Brigham and Women's Hospital, Boston

DAN L. LONGO, MD

Scientific Director, National Institute on Aging,
National Institutes of Health, Bethesda and Baltimore

EUGENE BRAUNWALD, MD

Distinguished Hersey Professor of Medicine,
Harvard Medical School; Chairman, TIMI Study Group,
Brigham and Women's Hospital, Boston

STEPHEN L. HAUSER, MD

Robert A. Fishman Distinguished Professor and Chairman,
Department of Neurology,
University of California, San Francisco

J. LARRY JAMESON, MD, PhD

Professor of Medicine; Vice President for Medical
Affairs and Lewis Landsberg Dean,
Northwestern University Feinberg
School of Medicine, Chicago

JOSEPH LOSCALZO, MD, PhD

Hersey Professor of Theory and Practice of Medicine,
Harvard Medical School; Chairman, Department of Medicine;
Physician-in-Chief, Brigham and Women's Hospital, Boston

Second Edition

HARRISON'S
Rheumatology

Editor

Anthony S. Fauci, MD

Chief, Laboratory of Immunoregulation;
Director, National Institute of Allergy and Infectious Diseases,
National Institutes of Health, Bethesda

Associate Editor

Carol A. Langford, MD, MHS

Associate Professor of Medicine;
Director, Center for Vasculitis Care and Research,
Department of Rheumatic and Immunologic Diseases,
Cleveland Clinic, Cleveland

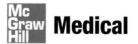 **Medical**

New York   Chicago   San Francisco   Lisbon   London   Madrid   Mexico City
Milan   New Delhi   San Juan   Seoul   Singapore   Sydney   Toronto

1 2 3 4 5 6 7 8 9 0   CTP/CTP   14 13 12 11 10

ISBN 978-0-07-174143-9
MHID 0-07-174143-7

This book was set in Bembo by Glyph International. The editors were James Shanahan and Kim J. Davis. The production supervisor was Catherine H. Saggese. Project management was provided by Arushi Chawla of Glyph International. The cover design was by Thomas DePierro. Cover illustration and illustrations for section and chapter openers © MedicalRF.com. All rights reserved.

China Translation & Printing Services Ltd. was the printer and binder was the printer and binder.

Library of Congress Cataloging-in Publication Data

Harrison's rheumatology / editor, Anthony S. Fauci ; associate
editor, Carol A. Langford. — 2nd ed.
    p. ; cm.
  Includes bibliographical references and index.
  ISBN-13: 978-0-07-174143-9 (pbk. : alk. paper)
  ISBN-10: 0-07-174143-7 (pbk. : alk. paper)
  1. Rheumatology. 2. Rheumatism. 3. Arthritis. 4. Joints—Diseases.
I. Fauci, Anthony S., 1940-   II. Langford, Carol A.   III. Harrison, Tinsley Randolph,
1900-1978. Principles of internal medicine.   IV. Title: Rheumatology.
  [DNLM: 1. Rheumatic Diseases—physiopathology. 2. Arthritis—physiopathology.
3. Rheumatic Diseases—immunology. WE 544 H323   2010]
RC927.H376   2010
616.7'23—dc22
                                                              2009046347

CONTENTS

CONTRIBUTORS

Numbers in brackets refer to the chapter(s) written or co-written by the contributor.

ROBERT P. BAUGHMAN, MD
Professor of Medicine, Cincinnati [13]

GERALD BLOOMFIELD, MD, MPH
Department of Internal Medicine, The Johns Hopkins University School of Medicine, Baltimore [Review and Self-Assessment]

CYNTHIA D. BROWN, MD
Department of Internal Medicine, The Johns Hopkins University School of Medicine, Baltimore [Review and Self-Assessment]

JONATHAN R. CARAPETIS, MBBS, PhD
Director, Menzies School of Health Research; Professor, Charles Darwin University, Australia [6]

LAN X. CHEN, MD
Clinical Assistant Professor of Medicine, University of Pennsylvania, Penn Presbyterian Medical Center and Philadelphia Veteran Affairs Medical Center, Philadelphia [19]

JOHN J. CUSH, MD
Director of Clinical Rheumatology, Baylor Research Institute; Professor of Medicine and Rheumatology, Baylor University Medical Center, Dallas [17]

MARINOS C. DALAKAS, MD
Professor of Neurology; Chief, Neuromuscular Diseases Section, NINDS, National Institute of Health, Bethesda [16]

BETTY DIAMOND, MD
Chief, Autoimmune Disease Center, The Feinstein Institute for Medical Research, New York [3]

ANTHONY S. FAUCI, MD, DSC (Hon), DM&S (Hon), DHL (Hon), DPS (Hon), DLM (Hon), DMS (Hon)
Chief, Laboratory of Immunoregulation; Director, National Institute of Allergy and Infectious Diseases, National Institutes of Health, Bethesda [1, 10]

DAVID T. FELSON, MD, MPH
Professor of Medicine and Epidemiology; Chief, Clinical Epidemiology Unit, Boston University, Boston [18]

DANIEL J. FINK,† MD, MPH
Associate Professor of Clinical Pathology, College of Physicians and Surgeons, Columbia University, New York [Appendix]

BRUCE C. GILLILAND,† MD
Professor of Medicine and Laboratory Medicine, University of Washington School of Medicine, Seattle [12, 21, 22, 23]

BEVRA HANNAHS HAHN, MD
Professor of Medicine; Chief of Rheumatology; Vice Chair, Department of Medicine, David Geffen School of Medicine at UCLA, Los Angeles [4]

BARTON F. HAYNES, MD
Frederic M. Hanes Professor of Medicine and Immunology, Departments of Medicine and Immunology; Director, Duke Human Vaccine Institute, Duke University School of Medicine, Durham [1]

DANIEL KASTNER, MD, PhD
Chief, Genetics and Genomic Section, National Institute of Arthritis and Musculoskeletal and Skin Diseases, National Institutes of Health, Bethesda [14]

ALEXANDER KRATZ, MD, PhD, MPH
Assistant Professor of Clinical Pathology, Columbia University College of Physicians and Surgeons; Associate Director, Core Laboratory, Columbia University Medical Center, New York-Presbyterian Hospital; Director, Allen Pavilion Laboratory, New York [Appendix]

CAROL A. LANGFORD, MD, MHS
Associate Professor of Medicine; Director, Center for Vasculitis Care and Research, Department of Rheumatic and Immunologic Diseases, Cleveland Clinic, Cleveland [10, 12, 21, 22, 23]

PETER E. LIPSKY, MD
Chief, Autoimmunity Branch, National Institute of Arthritis, Musculoskeletal, and Skin Diseases, National Institutes of Health, Department of Health and Human Services, Bethesda [3, 5, 17]

ELYSE E. LOWER, MD
Professor of Medicine, University of Cincinnati, Cincinnati [13]

LAWRENCE C. MADOFF, MD
Associate Professor of Medicine, Harvard Medical School, Boston [20]

HARALAMPOS M. MOUTSOPOULOS, MD
Professor and Chair, Department of Pathophysiology, School of Medicine, National University of Athens, Greece [8, 11]

GERALD T. NEPOM, MD, PhD
Director, Benaroya Research Institute at Virginia Mason; Professor, University of Washington School of Medicine, Seattle [2]

MICHAEL A. PESCE, PhD
Clinical Professor of Pathology, Columbia University College of Physicians and Surgeons; Director of Specialty Laboratory, New York Presbyterian Hospital, Columbia University Medical Center, New York [Appendix]

JOSHUA SCHIFFER, MD
Department of Internal Medicine, The Johns Hopkins University School of Medicine, Baltimore [Review and Self-Assessment]

H. RALPH SCHUMACHER, MD
Professor of Medicine, University of Pennsylvania School of Medicine, Philadelphia [19]

DAVID C. SELDIN, MD, PhD
Professor of Medicine and Microbiology; Director, Amyloid Treatment and Research Program Section of Hematology-Oncology, Department of Medicine, Boston University School of Medicine and Boston Medical Center, Boston [15]

MARTHA SKINNER, MD
Professor of Medicine, Boston University School of Medicine; Director, Special Projects, Amyloid Treatment and Research Program, Boston [15]

---

†Deceased

KELLY A. SODERBERG, PhD, MPH
Director, Program Management, Duke Human Vaccine Institute,
Duke University School of Medicine, Durham [1]

ADAM SPIVAK, MD
Department of Internal Medicine, The Johns Hopkins University
School of Medicine, Baltimore [Review and Self-Assessment]

JOEL D. TAUROG, MD
Professor of Internal Medicine, William M. and Gatha Burnett
Professor for Arthritis Research, University of Texas Southwestern
Medical Center, Dallas [9]

JOHN VARGA, MD
Hughes Professor of Medicine, Northwestern University Feinberg
School of Medicine, Chicago [7]

CHARLES WIENER, MD
Professor of Medicine and Physiology;
Vice Chair, Department of Medicine;
Director, Osler Medical Training Program,
The Johns Hopkins University School of Medicine, Baltimore
[Review and Self-Assessment]

PREFACE

In 2006, the first *Harrison's Rheumatology* sectional was introduced with the goal of expanding the outreach of medical knowledge that began with the first edition of *Harrison's Principles of Internal Medicine*, which was published over 60 years ago. The sectional, which is comprised of the immunology and rheumatology chapters contained in *Harrison's Principles of Internal Medicine*, sought to provide readers with a current view of the science and practice of rheumatology. After its introduction, we were gratified to learn that this sectional was being utilized not only by young physicians gaining their first exposure to rheumatology, but also by a diversity of health care professionals seeking to remain updated on the latest advancements within this dynamic subspecialty of internal medicine. With this edition of the *Harrison's Rheumatology*, it remains our goal to provide the expertise of leaders in rheumatology and immunology to all students of medicine who wish to learn more about this important and constantly changing field.

The aspects of medical care encompassed by rheumatology greatly impact human health. Musculoskeletal symptoms are among the leading reasons that patients seek medical attention, and it is now estimated that one out of three people will be affected by arthritis. Joint and muscle pain not only affect quality of life and produce disability, they may also be heralding symptoms of serious inflammatory, infectious, or neoplastic diseases. Because of their frequency and the morbidity associated with the disease itself, as well as the therapeutic modalities employed, rheumatic diseases impact all physicians.

Although the connective tissues form the foundation of rheumatology, this specialty encompasses a wide spectrum of medical disorders which exemplify the diversity and complexity of internal medicine. Rheumatic diseases can range from processes characterized by monarticular arthropathy to multisystem illnesses that carry a significant risk of morbidity or mortality. The effective practice of rheumatology therefore requires broad-based diagnostic skills, a strong fundamental understanding of internal medicine, the ability to recognize life-threatening disease, and the knowledge of how to utilize and monitor a wide range of treatments in which benefit must be balanced against risk. Understanding these challenges provides an opportunity to improve the lives of patients, and it is these factors that make the practice of rheumatology an immensely rewarding area of internal medicine.

Another facet of rheumatology that has captivated the interest of both clinicians and biomedical researchers is its relationship to immunology and autoimmunity. From early studies in rheumatology, clinical and histologic evidence of inflammation supported the view that the immune system mediated many forms of joint and tissue injury. Laboratory-based investigations have not only provided firm evidence for the immunologic basis of these diseases, but they have identified specific mechanisms involved in the pathogenesis of individual clinical entities. Recognition of the pathways involved in disease and the potential to target specific immune effector functions have revolutionized the treatment of many rheumatic diseases. Such investigations will continue to shed insights regarding the pathogenesis of a wide range of rheumatic diseases, and will bring forth novel therapies that offer even greater potential to lessen pain, reduce joint and organ damage, and improve overall clinical outcome.

This sectional was originally developed in recognition of the importance of rheumatology to the practice of internal medicine as well as the rapid pace of scientific growth in this specialty. This assessment has been borne out by the numerous advancements in rheumatology that have been made even within the short period of time since the last sectional was published. The need for this sectional is a tribute to the hard work of many dedicated individuals at both the bench and the bedside whose contributions have greatly benefited our patients. It is the continued hope of the editors that this sectional will not only increase knowledge of the rheumatic diseases, but also serve to heighten appreciation for this fascinating specialty.

Anthony S. Fauci, MD
Carol A. Langford, MD, MHS

NOTICE

Medicine is an ever-changing science. As new research and clinical experience broaden our knowledge, changes in treatment and drug therapy are required. The authors and the publisher of this work have checked with sources believed to be reliable in their efforts to provide information that is complete and generally in accord with the standards accepted at the time of publication. However, in view of the possibility of human error or changes in medical sciences, neither the authors nor the publisher nor any other party who has been involved in the preparation or publication of this work warrants that the information contained herein is in every respect accurate or complete, and they disclaim all responsibility for any errors or omissions or for the results obtained from use of the information contained in this work. Readers are encouraged to confirm the information contained herein with other sources. For example, and in particular, readers are advised to check the product information sheet included in the package of each drug they plan to administer to be certain that the information contained in this work is accurate and that changes have not been made in the recommended dose or in the contraindications for administration. This recommendation is of particular importance in connection with new or infrequently used drugs.

Review and self-assessment questions and answers were taken from Wiener C, Fauci AS, Braunwald E, Kasper DL, Hauser SL, Longo DL, Jameson JL, Loscalzo J (editors) Bloomfield G, Brown CD, Schiffer J, Spivak A (contributing editors). *Harrison's Principles of Internal Medicine Self-Assessment and Board Review,* 17th ed. New York, McGraw-Hill, 2008, ISBN 978-0-07-149619-3.

 The global icons call greater attention to key epidemiologic and clinical differences in the practice of medicine throughout the world.

 The genetic icons identify a clinical issue with an explicit genetic relationship.

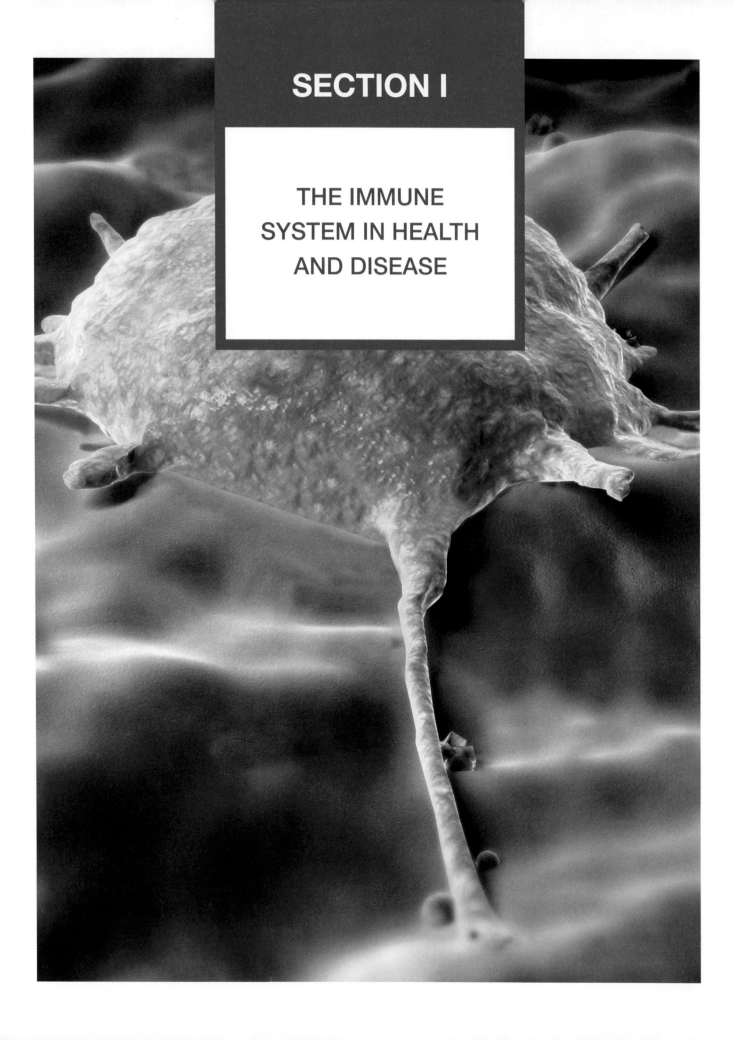

SECTION I

THE IMMUNE SYSTEM IN HEALTH AND DISEASE

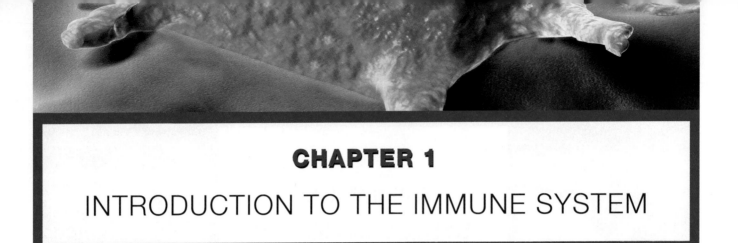

CHAPTER 1

INTRODUCTION TO THE IMMUNE SYSTEM

Barton F. Haynes ■ Kelly A. Soderberg ■ Anthony S. Fauci

DEFINITIONS

• *Adaptive immune system*—recently evolved system of immune responses mediated by T and B lymphocytes. Immune responses by these cells are based on specific antigen recognition by clonotypic receptors that are products of genes that rearrange during development and throughout the life of the organism. Additional cells of the adaptive immune system include various types of antigen–presenting cells.

• *Antibody*—B cell–produced molecules encoded by genes that rearrange during B cell development consisting of immunoglobulin heavy and light chains that together form the central component of the B cell receptor for antigen. Antibody can exist as B cell surface antigen-recognition molecules or as secreted molecules in plasma and other body fluids (Table 1-11).

• *Antigens*—foreign or self-molecules that are recognized by the adaptive and innate immune systems resulting in immune cell triggering, T cell activation, and/or B cell antibody production.

• *Antimicrobial peptides*—small peptides <100 amino acids in length that are produced by cells of the innate immune system and have anti-infectious agent activity (Table 1-2).

• *Apoptosis*—the process of *programmed cell death* where by signaling through various "death receptors" on the surface of cells [e.g., tumor necrosis factor (TNF) receptors, CD95] leads to a signaling cascade that involves activation of the caspase family of molecules and leads to DNA cleavage and cell death. Apoptosis, which does not lead to induction of inordinate inflammation, is to be contrasted with *cell necrosis*, which does lead to induction of inflammatory responses.

• *B lymphocytes*—bone marrow–derived or bursal-equivalent lymphocytes that express surface immunoglobulin (the B cell receptor for antigen) and secrete specific antibody after interaction with antigen (Figs. 1-2, 1-6).

• *B cell receptor for antigen*—complex of surface molecules that rearrange during postnatal B cell development, made up of surface immunoglobulin (Ig) and associated Ig αβ chain molecules that recognize nominal antigen via Ig heavy and light chain variable regions, and signal the B cell to terminally differentiate to make antigen-specific antibody (Fig. 1-8).

• *CD classification of human leukocyte differentiation antigens*—the development of monoclonal antibody technology led to the discovery of a large number of new leukocyte surface molecules. In 1982, the First International Workshop on Leukocyte Differentiation Antigens was held to establish a nomenclature for cell-surface molecules of human leukocytes. From this and subsequent leukocyte differentiation workshops has come the *cluster of differentiation (CD) classification* of leukocyte antigens (Table 1-1).

• *Chemokines*—soluble molecules that direct and determine immune cell movement and circulation pathways.

2

- *Complement*—cascading series of plasma enzymes and effector proteins whose function is to lyse pathogens and/or target them to be phagocytized by neutrophils and monocyte/macrophage lineage cells of the reticuloendothelial system (Fig. 1-5).
- *Co-stimulatory molecules*—molecules of antigen-presenting cells (such as B7-1 and B7-2 or CD40) that lead to T cell activation when bound by ligands on activated T cells (such as CD28 or CD40 ligand) (Fig. 1-7).
- *Cytokines*—soluble proteins that interact with specific cellular receptors that are involved in the regulation of the growth and activation of immune cells and mediate normal and pathologic inflammatory and immune responses (Tables 1-6, 1-8, 1-9).
- *Dendritic cells*—myeloid and/or lymphoid lineage antigen-presenting cells of the adaptive immune system. Immature dendritic cells, or dendritic cell precursors, are key components of the innate immune system by responding to infections with production of high levels of cytokines. Dendritic cells are key initiators both of innate immune responses via cytokine production and of adaptive immune responses via presentation of antigen to T lymphocytes (Figs. 1-2 and 1-3, Table 1-5).
- *Innate immune system*—ancient immune recognition system of host cells bearing germ line–encoded pattern recognition receptors (PRRs) that recognize pathogens and trigger a variety of mechanisms of pathogen elimination. Cells of the innate immune system include natural killer (NK) cell lymphocytes, monocytes/macrophages, dendritic cells, neutrophils, basophils, eosinophils, tissue mast cells, and epithelial cells (Tables 1-2, 1-3, 1-4, 1-5, 1-10).
- *Large granular lymphocytes*—lymphocytes of the innate immune system with azurophilic cytotoxic granules that have NK cell activity capable of killing foreign and host cells with few or no self–major histocompatibility complex (MHC) class I molecules (Fig. 1-4).
- *Natural killer cells*—large granular lymphocytes that kill target cells expressing few or no human leukocyte antigen (HLA) class I molecules, such as malignantly transformed cells and virally infected cells. NK cells express receptors that inhibit killer cell function when self–MHC class I is present (Fig. 1-4).
- *Pathogen-associated molecular patterns* (PAMPs)—Invariant molecular structures expressed by large groups of microorganisms that are recognized by host cellular pattern recognition receptors in the mediation of innate immunity (Fig. 1-1).
- *Pattern recognition receptors* (PRRs)—germ line–encoded receptors expressed by cells of the innate immune system that recognize pathogen-associated molecular patterns (Table 1-3).
- *T cells*—thymus-derived lymphocytes that mediate adaptive cellular immune responses including T helper, T regulatory, and cytotoxic T lymphocyte effector cell functions (Figs. 1-2, 1-3, 1-6).
- *T cell receptor for antigen*—complex of surface molecules that rearrange during postnatal T cell development made up of clonotypic T cell receptor (TCR) α and β chains that are associated with the CD3 complex composed of invariant γ, δ, ε, ζ, and η chains. TCR-α and -β chains recognize peptide fragments of protein antigen physically bound in antigen-presenting cell MHC class I or II molecules, leading to signaling via the CD3 complex to mediate effector functions (Fig. 1-7).
- *Tolerance*—B and T cell nonresponsiveness to antigens that results from encounter with foreign or self-antigens by B and T lymphocytes in the absence of expression of antigen-presenting cell co-stimulatory molecules. Tolerance to antigens may be induced and maintained by multiple mechanisms either centrally (in the thymus for T cells or bone marrow for B cells) or peripherally at sites throughout the peripheral immune system.

INTRODUCTION

The human immune system has evolved over millions of years from both invertebrate and vertebrate organisms to develop sophisticated defense mechanisms to protect the host from microbes and their virulence factors. The normal immune system has three key properties: a highly diverse repertoire of antigen receptors that enables recognition of a nearly infinite range of pathogens; immune memory, to mount rapid recall immune responses; and immunologic tolerance, to avoid immune damage to normal self-tissues. From invertebrates, humans have inherited the innate immune system, an ancient defense system that uses germ line–encoded proteins to recognize pathogens. Cells of the innate immune system, such as macrophages, dendritic cells, and natural killer (NK) lymphocytes, recognize pathogen-associated molecular patterns (PAMPs) that are highly conserved among many microbes and use a diverse set of pattern recognition receptor molecules (PRRs). Important components of the recognition of microbes by the innate immune system include (1) recognition by germ line–encoded host molecules, (2) recognition of key microbe virulence factors but not recognition of self-molecules, and (3) nonrecognition of benign foreign molecules or microbes. Upon contact with pathogens, macrophages and NK cells may kill pathogens directly or, in concert with dendritic cells, may activate a series of events that both slow the infection and recruit the more recently evolved arm of the human immune system, the adaptive immune system.

Adaptive immunity is found only in vertebrates and is based on the generation of antigen receptors on T and B lymphocytes by gene rearrangements, such that individual T or B cells express unique antigen receptors on their surface capable of specifically re cognizing diverse antigens of the myriad infectious agents in the environment. Coupled with finely tuned specific recognition mechanisms that maintain tolerance (nonreactivity) to self-antigens, T and B lymphocytes bring both *specificity* and *immune memory* to vertebrate host defenses.

This chapter describes the cellular components, key molecules (Table 1-1), and mechanisms that make up the

TABLE 1-1

HUMAN LEUKOCYTE SURFACE ANTIGENS—THE CD CLASSIFICATION OF LEUKOCYTE DIFFERENTIATION ANTIGENS

SURFACE ANTIGEN (OTHER NAMES)	FAMILY	MOLECULAR MASS, kDa	DISTRIBUTION	LIGAND(S)	FUNCTION
CD1a (T6, HTA-1)	Ig	49	CD, cortical thymocytes, Langerhans type of dendritic cells	TCRγδ T cells	CD1 molecules present lipid antigens of intracellular bacteria such as *M. leprae* and *M. tuberculosis* to TCRγδ T cells.
CD1b	Ig	45	CD, cortical thymocytes, Langerhans type of dendritic cells	TCRγδ T cells	
CD1c	Ig	43	DC, cortical thymocytes, subset of B cells, Langerhans type of dendritic cells	TCRγδ T cells	
CD1d	Ig	?	Cortical thymocytes, intestinal epithelium, Langerhans type of dendritic cells	TCRγδ T cells	
CD2 (T12, LFA-2)	Ig	50	T, NK	CD58, CD48, CD59, CD15	Alternative T cell activation, T cell anergy, T cell cytokine production, T- or NK-mediated cytolysis, T cell apoptosis, cell adhesion
CD3 (T3, Leu-4)	Ig	γ:25–28, δ:21–28, ε:20–25, η:21–22, ζ:16	T	Associates with the TCR	T cell activation and function; ζ is the signal transduction components of the CD3 complex
CD4 (T4, Leu-3)	Ig	55	T, myeloid	MHC-II, HIV, gp120, IL-16, SABP	T cell selection, T cell activation, signal transduction with p56*lck*, primary receptor for HIV
CD7 (3A1, Leu-9)	Ig	40	T, NK	K-12 (CD7L)	T and NK cell signal transduction and regulation of IFN-γ, TNF-α production
CD8 (T8, Leu-2)	Ig	34	T	MHC-I	T cell selection, T cell activation, signal transduction with p56*lck*
CD14 (LPS-receptor)	LRG	53–55	M, G (weak), not by myeloid progenitors	Endotoxin (lipopolysaccharide), lipoteichoic acid, PI	TLR4 mediates with LPS and other PAMP activation of innate immunity
CD19 (B4)	Ig	95	B (except plasma cells), FDC	Not known	Associates with CD21 and CD81 to form a complex involved in signal transduction in B cell development, activation, and differentiation
CD20 (B1)	Un-assigned	33–37	B (except plasma cells)	Not known	Cell signaling, may be important for B cell activation and proliferation
CD21 (B2, CR2, EBV-R, C3dR)	RCA	145	Mature B, FDC, subset of thymocytes	C3d, C3dg, iC3b, CD23, EBV	Associates with CD19 and CD81 to form a complex involved in signal transduction in B cell development, activation, and differentiation; Epstein-Barr virus receptor

(Continued)

TABLE 1-5

9

CHAPTER 1

Introduction to the Immune System

CELLS OF THE INNATE IMMUNE SYSTEM AND THEIR MAJOR ROLES IN TRIGGERING ADAPTIVE IMMUNITY

CELL TYPE	MAJOR ROLE IN INNATE IMMUNITY	MAJOR ROLE IN ADAPTIVE IMMUNITY
Macrophages	Phagocytose and kill bacteria; produce antimicrobial peptides; bind (LPS); produce inflammatory cytokines	Produce IL-1 and TNF-α to upregulate lymphocyte adhesion molecules and chemokines to attract antigen-specific lymphocyte. Produce IL-12 to recruit T_H1 helper T cell responses; upregulate co-stimulatory and MHC molecules to facilitate T and B lymphocyte recognition and activation. Macrophages and dendritic cells, after LPS signaling, upregulate co-stimulatory molecules B7-1 (CD80) and B7-2 (CD86) that are required for activation of antigen-specific anti-pathogen T cells. There are also Toll-like proteins on B cells and dendritic cells that, after LPS ligation, induce CD80 and CD86 on these cells for T cell antigen presentation
Plasmacytoid f dendritic cells (DCs) of lymphoid lineage	Produce large amounts of interferon-α (IFN-α), which has antitumor and antiviral activity, and are found in T cell zones of lymphoid organs; they circulate in blood	IFN-α is a potent activator of macrophage and mature DCs to phagocytose invading pathogens and present pathogen antigens to T and B cells
Myeloid dendritic cells are of two types; interstitial and Langerhans-derived	Interstitial DCs are strong producers of IL-12 and IL-10 and are located in T cell zones of lymphoid organs, circulate in blood, and are present in the interstices of the lung, heart, and kidney; Langerhans DCs are strong producers of IL-12; are located in T cell zones of lymph nodes, skin epithelia, and the thymic medulla; and circulate in blood	Interstitial DCs are potent activator of macrophage and mature DCs to phagocytose invading pathogens and present pathogen antigens to T and B cells
Natural killer (NK) cells	Kill foreign and host cells that have low levels of MHC+ self-peptides. Express NK receptors that inhibit NK function in the presence of high expression of self-MHC	Produce TNF-α and IFN-γ that recruit T_H1 helper T cell responses
NK-T cells	Lymphocytes with both T cell and NK surface markers that recognize lipid antigens of intracellular bacteria such as *M. tuberculosis* by CD1 molecules and kill host cells infected with intracellular bacteria	Produce IL-4 to recruit T_H2 helper T cell responses, IgG1 and IgE production
Neutrophils	Phagocytose and kill bacteria, produce antimicrobial peptides	Produce nitric oxide synthase and nitric oxide that inhibit apoptosis in lymphocytes and can prolong adaptive immune responses
Eosinophils	Kill invading parasites	Produce IL-5 that recruits Ig-specific antibody responses
Mast cells and basophils	Release TNF-α, IL-6, IFN-γ in response to a variety of bacterial PAMPs	Produce IL-4 that recruits T_H2 helper T cell responses and recruit IgG1- and IgE-specific antibody responses
Epithelial cells	Produce anti-microbial peptides; tissue specific epithelia produce mediator of local innate immunity, e.g., lung epithelial cells produce surfactant proteins (proteins within the collectin family) that bind and promote clearance of lung invading microbes	Produces TGF-β that triggers IgA-specific antibody responses.

Note: LPS, lipopolysaccharide; PAMP, pathogen-associated molecular patterns; TNF-α, tumor necrosis factor-alpha; IL-4, IL-5, IL-6, IL-10, and IL-12, interleukin 4, 5, 6, 10, and 12, respectively.

Source: Adapted with permission from R Medzhitov, CA Janeway: Innate immunity: Impact on the adaptive immune response. Curr Opinion Immunol 9:4-9, 1997.

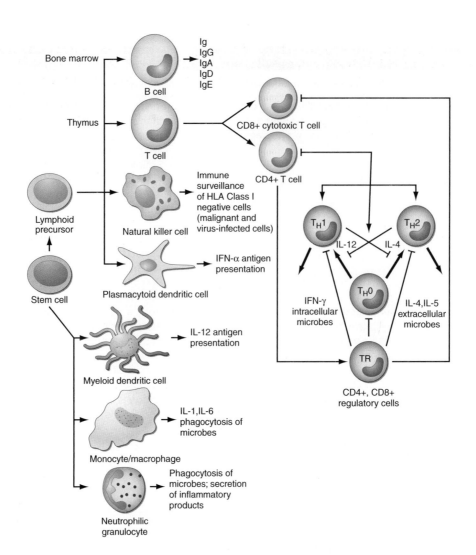

FIGURE 1-2

Schematic model of intercellular interactions of adaptive immune system cells. In this figure the arrows denote that cells develop from precursor cells or produce cytokines or antibodies; lines ending with bars indicate suppressive intercellular interactions. Stem cells differentiate into either T cells, antigen-presenting dendritic cells, natural killer cells, macrophages, granulocytes, or B cells. Foreign antigen is processed by dendritic cells, and peptide fragments of foreign antigen are presented to CD4+ and/or CD8+ T cells. CD8+ T cell activation leads to induction of cytotoxic T lymphocyte (CTL) or killer T cell generation, as well as induction of cytokine-producing CD8+ cytotoxic T cells. For antibody production against the same antigen, active antigen is bound to sIg within the B cell receptor complex and drives B cell maturation into plasma cells that secrete Ig. T_H1 or T_H2 CD4+ T cells producing interleukin (IL) 4, IL-5, or interferon (IFN)γ regulate the Ig class switching and determine the type of antibody produced. CD4+, CD25+ T regulatory cells produce IL-10 and downregulate T and B cell responses once the microbe has been eliminated. GM-CSF, granulocyte-macrophage colony stimulating factor; TNF, tumor necrosis factor.

(Kupffer cells), bone (osteoclasts), central nervous system (microglia cells), and synovium (type A lining cells).

In general, monocytes-macrophages are on the first line of defense associated with innate immunity and ingest and destroy microorganisms through the release of toxic products such as hydrogen peroxide (H_2O_2) and nitric oxide (NO). Inflammatory mediators produced by macrophages attract additional effector cells such as neutrophils to the site of infection. Macrophage mediators include prostaglandins; leukotrienes; platelet activating factor; cytokines such as interleukin (IL) 1, tumor necrosis factor (TNF) α, IL-6, and IL-12; and chemokines (**Tables 1-6** to **1-9**).

Although monocytes-macrophages were originally thought to be the major antigen-presenting cells (APCs) of the immune system, it is now clear that cell types called dendritic cells are the most potent and effective APCs in the body (see below). Monocytes-macrophages mediate innate immune effector functions such as destruction of antibody-coated bacteria, tumor cells, or even normal hematopoietic cells in certain types of autoimmune cytopenias. Monocytes-macrophages ingest

TABLE 1-6

CYTOKINES AND CYTOKINE RECEPTORS

CYTOKINE	RECEPTOR	CELL SOURCE	CELL TARGET	BIOLOGIC ACTIVITY
IL-1α,β	Type I IL-1r, Type II IL-1r	Monocytes/macrophages, B cells, fibroblasts, most epithelial cells including thymic epithelium, endothelial cells	All cells	Upregulated adhesion molecule expression, neutrophil and macrophage emigration, mimics shock, fever, upregulated hepatic acute phase protein production, facilitates hematopoiesis
IL-2	IL-2r α,β, common γ	T cells	T cells, B cells NK cells, monocytes/ macrophages	T cell activation and proliferation, B cell growth, NK cell proliferation and activation, enhanced monocyte/ macrophage cytolytic activity
IL-3	IL-3r, common β	T cells, NK cells, mast cells	Monocytes/ macrophages, mast cells, eosinophils, bone marrow progenitors	Stimulation of hematopoietic progenitors
IL-4	IL-4r α, common γ	T cells, mast cells, basophils	T cells, B cells, NK cells, monocytes/ macrophages, neutrophils, eosinophils, endothelial cells, fibroblasts	Stimulates T$_H$2 helper T cell differentiation and proliferation. Stimulates B cell Ig class switch to IgG1 and IgE anti-inflammatory action on T cells, monocytes
IL-5	IL-5r α, common γ	T cells, mast cells and eosinophils	Eosinophils, basophils, murine B cells	Regulates eosinophil migration and activation
IL-6	IL-6r, gp130	Monocytes/macrophages, B cells, fibroblasts, most epithelium including thymic epithelium, endothelial cells	T cells, B cells, epithelial cells, hepatocytes, monocytes/ macrophages	Induction of acute phase protein production, T and B cell differentiation and growth, myeloma cell growth, osteoclast growth and activation
IL-7	IL-7r α, common γ	Bone marrow, thymic epithelial cells	T cells, B cells, bone marrow cells	Differentiation of B, T and NK cell precursors, activation of T and NK cells
IL-8	CXCR1, CXCR2	Monocytes/macrophages, T cells, neutrophils, fibroblasts, endothelial cells, epithelial cells	Neutrophils, T cells, monocytes/ macrophages, endothelial cells, basophils	Induces neutrophil, monocyte and T cell migration, induces neutrophil adherence to endothelial cells, histamine release from basophils, stimulates angiogenesis. Suppresses proliferations of hepatic precursors
IL-9	IL-9r α, common γ	T cells	Bone marrow progenitors, B cells, T cells, mast cells	Induces mast cell proliferation and function, synergizes with IL-4 in IgG and IgE production, T cell growth, activation and differentiation
IL-10	IL-10r	Monocytes/macrophages, T cells, B cells, keratinocytes, mast cells	Monocytes/ macrophages, T cells, B cells, NK cells, mast cells	Inhibits macrophage proinflammatory cytokine production, downregulates cytokine class II antigen and B7-1 and B7-2 expression, inhibits differentiation of T$_H$1, helper T cells, inhibits NK cell function, stimulates mast cell proliferation and function, B cell activation and differentiation
IL-11	IL-11, gp130	Bone marrow stromal cells	Megakaryocytes, B cells, hepatocytes	Induces megakaryocyte colony formation and maturation, enhances antibody responses, stimulates acute-phase protein production
IL-12 (35 kD and 40 kD subunits)	IL-12r	Activated macrophages, dendritic cells, neutrophils	T cells, NK cells	Induces T$_H$1 helper T cell formation and lymphokine-activated killer cell formation. Increases CD8+ CTL cytolytic activity; $\downarrow$IL-17, $\uparrow\gamma$-IFN

TABLE 1-6 (CONTINUED)

CYTOKINES AND CYTOKINE RECEPTORS

CYTOKINE	RECEPTOR	CELL SOURCE	CELL TARGET	BIOLOGIC ACTIVITY
IL-13	IL-13/IL-4	T cells (T$_H$2)	Monocytes/ macrophages, B cells, endothelial cells, keratinocytes	Upregulation of VCAM-1 and C-C chemokine expression on endothelial cells, B cell activation and differentiation, inhibits macrophage proinflammatory cytokine production
IL-14	Unknown	T cells	Normal and malignant B cells	Induces B cell proliferation
IL-15	IL-15r α, common γ, IL2r β	Monocytes/macrophages, epithelial cells, fibroblasts	T cells, NK cells	T cell activation and proliferation. Promotes angiogenesis, and NK cells
IL-16	CD4	Mast cells, eosinophils, CD8+ T cells, respiratory epithelium	CD4+ T cells, monocytes/ macrophages, eosinophils	Chemoattraction of CD4+ T cells, monocytes, and eosinophils. Inhibits HIV replication. Inhibits T cell activation through CD3/T cell receptor
IL-17	IL17r	CD4+ T cells	Fibroblasts, endothelium, epithelium	Enhanced cytokine secretion
IL-18	IL-18r (IL-1R related protein)	Keratinocytes, macrophages	T cells, B cells, NK cells	Upregulated IFNγ production, enhanced NK cell cytotoxicity
IL-21	IL-δγ chain/ IL-21R	CD4 T cells	NK cells	Downregulates NK cell activating molecules, NKG2D/DAP10
IL-23	IL-12Rb1/ IL23R	Macrophages, other cell types	T cells	Opposite effects of IL-12 ↓(IL-17, ↑γ-IFN)
IFNα	Type I interferon receptor	All cells	All cells	Anti-viral activity. Stimulates T cell, macrophage, and NK cell activity. Direct anti-tumor effects. Upregulates MHC class I antigen expression. Used therapeutically in viral and autoimmune conditions
IFNβ	Type I interferon receptor	All cells	All cells	Anti-viral activity. Stimulates T cell, macrophage, and NK cell activity. Direct anti-tumor effects. Upregulates MHC class I antigen expression. Used therapeutically in viral and autoimmune conditions
IFNγ	Type II interferon receptor	T cells, NK cells	All cells	Regulates macrophage and NK cell activations. Stimulates immunoglobulin secretion by B cells. Induction of class II histocompatibility antigens. T$_H$1 T cell differentiation
TNFα	TNFrI, TNFrII	Monocytes/macrophages, mast cells, basophils, eosinophils, NK cells, B cells, T cells, keratinocytes, fibroblasts, thymic epithelial cells	All cells except erythrocytes	Fever, anorexia, shock, capillary leak syndrome, enhanced leukocyte cytotoxicity, enhanced NK cell function, acute phase protein synthesis, pro-inflammatory cytokine induction
TNFβ	TNFrI, TNFrII	T cells, B cells	All cells except erythrocytes	Cell cytotoxicity, lymph node and spleen development
LTβ	LTβR	T cells	All cells except erythrocytes	Cell cytotoxicity, normal lymph node development
G-CSF	G-CSFr; gp130	Monocytes/macrophages, fibroblasts, endothelial cells, thymic epithelial cells, stromal cells	Myeloid cells, endothelial cells	Regulates myelopoiesis. Enhances survival and function of neutrophils. Clinical use in reversing neutropenia after cytotoxic chemotherapy

(Continued)

TABLE 1-6 (CONTINUED)

13

CHAPTER 1

Introduction to the Immune System

CYTOKINES AND CYTOKINE RECEPTORS

CYTOKINE	RECEPTOR	CELL SOURCE	CELL TARGET	BIOLOGIC ACTIVITY
GM-CSF	GM-CSFr, common β	T cells, monocytes/ macrophages, fibroblasts, endothelial cells, thymic epithelial cells	Monocytes/ macrophages, neutrophils, eosinophils, fibroblasts, endothelial cells	Regulates myelopoiesis. Enhances macrophage bactericidal and tumoricidal activity. Mediator of dendritic cell maturation and function. Upregulates NK cell function. Clinical use in reversing neutropenia after cytotoxic chemotherapy
M-CSF	M-CSFr (c-fms pro-toooncogene)	Fibroblasts, endothelial cells, monocytes/ macrophages, T cells, B cells, epithelial cells including thymic epithelium	Monocytes/ macrophages	Regulates monocyte/macrophage production and function
LIF	LIFr; gp130	Activated T cells, bone marrow stromal cells, thymic epithelium	Megakaryocytes, monocytes, hepatocytes, possibly lymphocyte subpopulations	Induces hepatic acute phase protein production. Stimulates macrophage differentiation. Promotes growth of myeloma cells and hematopoietic progenitors. Stimulates thromboiesis
OSM	OSMr; LIFr; gp130	Activated monocytes/ macrophages and T cells, bone marrow stromal cells, some breast carcinoma cell lines, myeloma cells	Neurons, hepato-cytes, monocytes/ macrophages, adipocytes, alveolar epithelial cells, embryonic stem cells, melanocytes, endothelial cells, fibroblasts, myeloma cells	Induces hepatic acute phase protein production. Stimulates macrophage differentiation. Promotes growth of myeloma cells and hematopoietic progenitors. Stimulates thromboiesis. Stimulates growth of Kaposi's sarcoma cells
SCF	SCFr (c-kit protoonco-gene)	Bone marrow stromal cells and fibroblasts	Embryonic stem cells, myeloid and lymphoid precursors, mast cells	Stimulates hematopoietic progenitor cell growth, mast cell growth, promotes embryonic stem cell migration
TGFβ (3 iso-forms)	Type I, II, III TGFβ receptor	Most cell types	Most cell types	Downregulates T cell, macrophage and granulocyte responses. Stimulates synthesis of matrix proteins. Stimulates angiogenesis
Lympho-tactin/ SCM-1	Unknown	NK cells, mast cells, double negative thymocytes, activated CD8+ T cells	T cells, NK cells	Chemoattractant for lymphocytes. Only known chemokine of C class
MCP-1	CCR2	Fibroblasts, smooth muscle cells, activated PBMCs	Monocytes/ macrophages, NK cells, memory T cells, basophils	Chemoattractant for monocytes, activated memory T cells, and NK cells. Induces granule release from CD8+ T cells and NK cells. Potent histamine releasing factor for basophiles. Suppresses proliferation of hematopoietic precursors. Regulates monocyte protease production
MCP-2	CCR1, CCR2	Fibroblasts, activated PBMCs	Monocytes/ macrophages, T cells, eosinophils, basophils, NK cells	Chemoattractant for monocytes, memory and naïve T cells, eosinophils, ?NK cells. Activates basophils and eosinophils. Regulates monocyte protease production

CYTOKINES AND CYTOKINE RECEPTORS

CYTOKINE	RECEPTOR	CELL SOURCE	CELL TARGET	BIOLOGIC ACTIVITY
MCP-3	CCR1, CCR2	Fibroblasts, activated PBMCs	Monocytes/macrophages, T cells, eosinophils, basophils, NK cells, dendritic cells	Chemoattractant for monocytes, memory and naïve T cells, dendritic cells, eosinophils, ?NK cells. Activates basophils and eosinophils. Regulates monocyte protease production
MCP-4	CCR2, CCR3	Lung, colon, small intestinal epithelial cells, activated endothelial cells	Monocytes/macrophages, T cells eosinophils, basophils	Chemoattractant for monocytes, T cells, eosinophils and basophils
Eotaxin	CCR3	Pulmonary epithelial cells, heart	Eosinophils, basophils	Potent chemoattractant for eosinophils and basophils. Induces allergic airways disease. Acts in concert with IL-5 to activate eosinophils. Antibodies to eotaxin inhibit airway inflammation
TARC	CCR4	Thymus, dendritic cells, activated T cells	T cells, NK cells	Chemoattractant for T and NK cells
MDC	CCR4	Monocytes/macrophages, dendritic cells, thymus	Activated T cells	Chemoattractant for activated T cells. Inhibits infection with T cell tropic HIV
MIP-1α	CCR1, CCR5	Monocytes/macrophages, T cells	Monocytes/macrophages, T cells, dendritic cells, NK cells, eosinophils, basophils	Chemoattractant for monocytes, T cells, dendritic cells, NK cells, and weak chemoattractant for eosinophils and basophils. Activates NK cell function. Suppresses proliferation of hematopoietic precursors. Necessary for myocarditis associated with coxsackie virus infection. Inhibits infection with monocytotropic HIV
MIP-1β	CCR5	Monocytes/macrophages, T cells	Monocytes/macrophages, T cells, NK cells, dendritic cells	Chemoattractant for monocytes, T cells, and NK cells. Activates NK cell function. Inhibits infection with monocytotropic HIV
RANTES	CCR1, CCR2, CCR5	Monocytes/macrophages, T cells, fibroblasts, eosinophils	Monocytes/macrophages, T cells, NK cells, dendritic cells, eosinophils, basophils	Chemoattractant for monocytes/macrophages, CD4+ CD45Ro+T cells, CD8+ T cells, NK cells, eosinophils, and basophils. Induces histamine release from basophils. Inhibits infections with monocytotropic HIV
LARC/MIP-3α/Exodus-1	CCR6	Dendritic cells, fetal liver cells, activated T cells	T cells, B cells	Chemoattractant for lymphocytes
ELC/MIP-3β	CCR7	Thymus, lymph node, appendix	Activated T cells and B cells	Chemoattractant for B and T cells. Receptor upregulated on EBV infected B cells and HSV infected T cells
I-309/TCA-3	CCR8	Activated T cells	Monocytes/macrophages, T cells	Chemoattractant for monocytes. Prevents glucocorticoid-induced apoptosis in some T cell lines
SLC/TCA-4/Exodus-2	Unknown	Thymic epithelial cells, lymph node, appendix and spleen	T cells	Chemoattractant for T lymphocytes. Inhibits hematopoiesis
DC-CK1/PARC	Unknown	Dendritic cells in secondary lymphoid tissues	Naïve T cells	May have a role in induction of immune responses
TECK	Unknown	Dendritic cells, thymus, liver, small intestine	T cells, monocytes/macrophages, dendritic cells	Thymic dendritic cell-derived cytokine, possibly involved in T cell development

(Continued)

TABLE 1-6 (CONTINUED)

CYTOKINES AND CYTOKINE RECEPTORS

CYTOKINE	RECEPTOR	CELL SOURCE	CELL TARGET	BIOLOGIC ACTIVITY
GROα/ MGSA	CXCR2	Activated granulocytes, monocyte/macrophages, and epithelial cells	Neutrophils, epithelial cells, ?endothelial cells	Neutrophil chemoattractant and activator. Mitogenic for some melanoma cell lines. Suppresses proliferation of hematopoietic precursors. Angiogenic activity
GROβ/ MIP-2α	CXCR2	Activated granulocytes and monocyte/ macrophages	Neutrophils and ?endothelial cells	Neutrophil chemoattractant and activator. Angiogenic activity
NAP-2	CXCR2	Platelets	Neutrophils, basophils	Derived from platelet basic protein. Neutrophil chemoattractant and activator
IP-10	CXCR3	Monocytes/macrophages, T cells, fibroblasts, endothelial cells, epithelial cells	Activated T cells, tumor infiltrating lymphocytes, ?endothelial cells, ?NK cells	IFNγ-inducible protein that is a chemoattractant for T cells. Suppresses proliferation of hematopoietic precursors
MIG	CXCR3	Monocytes/macrophages, T cells, fibroblasts	Activated T cells, tumor infiltrating lymphocytes	IFNγ-inducible protein that is a chemoattractant for T cells. Suppresses proliferation of hematopoietic precursors
SDF-1	CXCR4	Fibroblasts	T cells, dendritic cells, ?basophils, ?endothelial cells	Low potency, high efficacy T cell chemoattractant. Required for B-lymphocyte development. Prevents infection of CD4+, CXCR4+ cells by T cell tropic HIV
Fractalkine	CX3CR1	Activated endothelial cells	NK cells, T cells, monocytes/ macrophages	Cell surface chemokine/mucin hybrid molecule that functions as a chemoattractant, leukocyte activator and cell adhesion molecule
PF-4	Unknown	Platelets, megakaryocytes	Fibroblasts, endothelial cells	Chemoattractant for fibroblasts. Suppresses proliferation of hematopoietic precursors. Inhibits endothelial cell proliferation and angiogenesis

Note: IL, interleukin; NK, natural killer; T$_H$1 and T$_H$2 helper T cell subsets; Ig, immunoglobulin; CXCR, CXC-type chemokine receptor; B7-1, CD80, B7-2, CD86; PBMC, peripheral blood mononuclear cells; VCAM, vascular cell adhesion molecule; IFN, interferon; MHC, major histocompatibility complex; TNF, tumor necrosis factor; G-CSF, granulocyte colony- stimulating factor; GM-CSF, granulocyte-macrophage CSF; M-CSF, macrophage CSF; HIV, human immunodeficiency virus; LIF, leukemia inhibitory factor; OSM, oncostatin M; SCF, stem cell factor; TGF, transforming growth factor; MCP, monocyte chemotactic protein; CCR, CC-type chemokine receptor; TARC, thymus and activation-regulated chemokine; MDC, macrophage-derived chemokine; MIP, macrophage inflammatory protein; RANTES, regulated on activation, normally T-cell expressed and secreted; LARC, liver and activation-regulated chemokine; EBV, Epstein-Barr virus; ELC, EB11 ligand chemokine (MIP-1β); HSV, herpes simplex virus; TCA, T-cell activation protein; DC-CK, dendritic cell chemokine; PARC, pulmonary and activation-regulated chemokine; SLC, secondary lymphoid tissue chemokine; TECK, thymus expressed chemokine; GRP, growth-related peptide; MGSA, melanoma growth-stimulating activity; NAP, neutrophil-activating protein; IP-10, IFN-γ-inducible protein-10; MIG, monoteine induced by IFN-γ; SDF, stromal cell-derived factor; PF, platelet factor.
Source: Used with permission from Sundy JS, Patel DD, and Haynes BF: Appendix B, in *Inflammation, Basic Principles and Clinical Correlates*, 3rd ed, J Gallin and R Snyderman (eds). Philadelphia, Lippincott Williams and Wilkins, 1999.

bacteria or are infected by viruses, and in doing so, they frequently undergo apoptosis. Macrophages that are "stressed" by intracellular infectious agents are recognized by dendritic cells as infected and apoptotic cells and are phagocytosed by dendritic cells. In this manner, dendritic cells "cross-present" infectious agent antigens of macrophages to T cells. Activated macrophages can also mediate antigen-nonspecific lytic activity and eliminate cell types such as tumor cells in the absence of antibody. This activity is largely mediated by cytokines (i.e., TNF-α

and IL-1). Monocytes-macrophages express lineage-specific molecules (e.g., the cell-surface LPS receptor, CD14) as well as surface receptors for a number of molecules, including the Fc region of IgG, activated complement components, and various cytokines (Table 1-6).

Dendritic Cells

Human dendritic cells (DCs) are heterogenous and contain two subsets, myeloid DCs and plasmacytoid DCs.

TABLE 1-7

CC, CXC$_1$, CX$_3$, C$_1$, AND XC FAMILIES OF CHEMOKINES AND CHEMOKINE RECEPTORS[a]

CHEMOKINE RECEPTOR	CHEMOKINE LIGANDS	CELL TYPES	DISEASE CONNECTION
CCR1	CCL3 (MIP-1α), CCL5 (RANTES), CCL7 (MCP-3), CCL14 (HCC1)	T cells, monocytes, eosinophils, basophils	Rheumatoid arthritis, multiple sclerosis
CCR2	CCL2 (MCP-1), CCL8 (MCP-2), CCL7 (MCP-3), CCL13 (MCP-4), CCL16 (HCC4)	Monocytes, dendritic cells (immature), memory T cells	Atherosclerosis, rheumatoid arthritis, multiple sclerosis, resistance to intracellular pathogens, Type 2 diabetes mellitus
CCR3	CCL11 (eotaxin), CCL13 (eotaxin-2), CCL7 (MCP-3), CCL5 (RANTES), CCL8 (MCP-2), CCL13 (MCP-4)	Eosinophils, basophils, mast cells, T$_H$2, platelets	Allergic asthma and rhinitis
CCR4	CCL17 (TARC), CCL22 (MDC)	T cells (T$_H$2) dendritic cells (mature), basophils, macrophages, platelets	Parasitic infection, graft rejection, T-cell homing to skin
CCR5	CCL3 (MIP-1α), CCL4 (MIP-1β), CCL5 (RANTES), CCL11 (eotaxin), CCL14 (HCC1), CCL16 (HCC4)	T cells, monocytes	HIV-1 coreceptor (T-tropic strains), transplant rejection
CCR6	CCL20 (MIP-3β, LARC)	T cells (T regulatory and memory), B cells, dendritic cells	Mucosal humoral immunity, allergic asthma, intestinal T-cell homing
CCR7	CCL19 (ELC), CCL21 (SLC)	T cells, dendritic cells (mature)	Transport of T cells and dendritic cells to lymph nodes, antigen presentation, and cellular immunity
CCR8	CCL1 (1309)	T cells (T$_H$2), monocytes, dendritic cells	Dendritic-cell migration to lymph node, type 2 cellular immunity, granuloma formation
CCR9	CCL25 (TECK)	T cells, IgA+ plasma cells	Homing of T cells and IgA+ plasma cells to the intestine, inflammatory bowel disease
CCR10	CCL27 (CTACK, CCL28 (MEC)	T cells	T-cell homing to intestine and skin
CXCR1	CXCL8 (interleukin-8), CXCL6 (GCP2)	Neutrophils, monocytes	Inflammatory lung disease, COPD
CXCR2	CXCL8, CXCL1 (GROα), CXCL2 (GROβ), CXCL3 (GROγ), CXCL5 (ENA-78), CXCL6	Neutrophils, monocytes, microvascular endothelial cells	Inflammatory lung disease, COPD, angiogenic for tumor growth
CXCR3-A	CXCL9 (MIG), CXCL10 (IP-10), CXCL11 (I-TAC)	Type 1 helper cells, mast cells, mesangial cells	Inflammatory skin disease, multiple sclerosis, transplant rejection
CXCR3-B	CXCL4 (PF4), CXCL9 (MIG), CXCL10 (IP-10), CXCL11 (I-TAC)	Microvascular endothelial cells, neoplastic cells	Angiostatic for tumor growth
CXCR4	CXCL12 (SDF-1)	Widely expressed	HIV-1 coreceptor (T-cell–tropic), tumor metastases, hematopoiesis
CXCR5	CXCL13 (BCA-1)	B cells, follicular helper T cells	Formation of B cell follicles
CXCR6	CXCL16 (SR-PSOX)	CD8+ T cells, natural killer cells, and memory CD4+ T cells	Inflammatory liver disease, atherosclerosis (CXCL16)
CX$_3$CR1	CX3CL1 (fractalkine)	Macrophages, endothelial cells, smooth-muscle cells	Atherosclerosis
XCR1	XCL1 (lymphotactin), XCL2	T cells, natural killer cells	Rheumatoid arthritis, IgA nephropathy, tumor response

[a]MIP denotes macrophage inflammatory protein, MCP monocyte chemoattractant protein, HCC hemofiltrate chemokine, T$_H$2 type 2 helper T cells, TARC thymus and activation-regulated chemokine, MDC macrophage-derived chemokine, LARC liver and activation-regulated chemokine, ELC Epstein-Barr I1-ligand chemokine, SLC secondary lymphoid-tissue chemokine, TECK thymus-expressed chemokine, CTACK cutaneous T-cell–attracting chemokine, and MEC mammary-enriched chemokine. GCP denotes granulocyte chemotactic protein, COPD chronic obstructive pulmonary disease, GRO growth-regulated oncogene, ENA epithelial-cell–derived neutrophil-activating peptide, MIG monokine induced by interferon-γ, IP-10 interferon inducible 10, I-TAC interferon-inducible T-cell alpha chemoattractant, PF platelet factor, SDF stromal-cell–derived factor, HIV human immunodeficiency virus, BCA-1 B cell chemoattractant 1, and SR-PSOX scavenger receptor for phosphatidylserinecontaining oxidized lipids
Source: From Charo and Ransohoff, 2006; with permission.

by binding of C3 directly to pathogens and "altered self" such as tumor cells. In the renal glomerular inflammatory disease *IgA nephropathy*, IgA activates the alternative complement pathway and causes glomerular damage and decreased renal function. Activation of the classic complement pathway via C1, C4, and C2 and activation of the alternative pathway via factor D, C3, and factor B both lead to cleavage and activation of C3. C3 activation fragments, when bound to target surfaces such as bacteria and other foreign antigens, are critical for opsonization (coating by antibody and complement) in preparation for phagocytosis. The MBL pathway substitutes MBL-associated serine proteases (MASPs) 1 and 2 for C1q, C1r, and C1s to activate C4. The MBL activation pathway is activated by mannose on the surface of bacteria and viruses.

The three pathways of complement activation all converge on the final common terminal pathway. C3 cleavage by each pathway results in activation of C5, C6, C7, C8, and C9, resulting in the membrane attack complex that physically inserts into the membranes of target cells or bacteria and lyses them.

Thus, complement activation is a critical component of innate immunity for responding to microbial infection. The functional consequences of complement activation by the three initiating pathways and the terminal pathway are shown in Fig. 1-5. In general the cleavage products of complement components facilitate microbe or damaged cell clearance (C1q, C4, C3), promote activation and enhancement of inflammation (anaphylatoxins, C3a, C5a), and promote microbe or opsonized cell lysis (membrane attack complex).

CYTOKINES

Cytokines are soluble proteins produced by a wide variety of hematopoietic and nonhematopoietic cell types (Tables 1-6 to 1-9). They are critical for both normal innate and adaptive immune responses, and their expression may be perturbed in most immune, inflammatory, and infectious disease states.

Cytokines are involved in the regulation of the growth, development, and activation of immune system cells and in the mediation of the inflammatory response. In general, cytokines are characterized by considerable redundancy; different cytokines have similar functions. In addition, many cytokines are pleiotropic in that they are capable of acting on many different cell types. This pleiotropism results from the expression on multiple cell types of receptors for the same cytokine (see below), leading to the formation of "cytokine networks." The action of cytokines may be (1) autocrine when the target cell is the same cell that secretes the cytokine, (2) paracrine when the target cell is nearby, and (3) endocrine when the cytokine is secreted into the circulation and acts distal to the source.

Cytokines have been named based on presumed targets or based on presumed functions. Those cytokines that are thought to primarily target leukocytes have been named interleukins (IL-1, -2, -3, etc.). Many cytokines that were originally described as having a certain function have retained those names (granulocyte colony-stimulating factor or G-CSF, etc.). Cytokines belong in general to three major structural families: the hemopoietin family; the TNF, IL-1, platelet-derived growth factor (PDGF), and transforming growth factor (TGF) β families; and the CXC and c-c chemokine families (Table 1-8). Chemokines are cytokines that regulate cell movement and trafficking; they act through G protein–coupled receptors and have a distinctive three-dimensional structure. IL-8 is the only chemokine that early on was named an interleukin (Table 1-6).

In general, cytokines exert their effects by influencing gene activation that results in cellular activation, growth, differentiation, functional cell-surface molecule expression, and cellular effector function. In this regard, cytokines can have dramatic effects on the regulation of immune responses and the pathogenesis of a variety of diseases. Indeed, T cells have been categorized on the basis of the pattern of cytokines that they secrete, which results in either humoral immune response (T_H2) or cell-mediated immune response (T_H1) (Fig. 1-3).

Cytokine receptors can be grouped into five general families based on similarities in their extracellular amino acid sequences and conserved structural domains. The *immunoglobulin (Ig) superfamily* represents a large number of cell-surface and secreted proteins. The IL-1 receptors (type 1, type 2) are examples of cytokine receptors with extracellular Ig domains.

The hallmark of the *hematopoietic growth factor (type 1) receptor* family is that the extracellular regions of each receptor contain two conserved motifs. One motif, located at the N terminus, is rich in cysteine residues. The other motif is located at the C terminus proximal to the transmembrane region and comprises five amino acid residues, tryptophan-serine-X-tryptophan-serine (WSXWS). This family can be grouped on the basis of the number of receptor subunits they have and on the utilization of shared subunits. A number of cytokine receptors, i.e., IL-6, IL-11, IL-12, and leukemia inhibitory factor, are paired with gp130. There is also a common 150-kDa subunit shared by IL-3, IL-5, and granulocyte-macrophage colony-stimulating factor (GM-CSF) receptors. The gamma chain (γ_c) of the IL-2 receptor is common to the IL-2, IL-4, IL-7, IL-9, and IL-15 receptors. Thus, the specific cytokine receptor is responsible for ligand-specific binding, while the subunits such as gp130, the 150-kDa subunit, and γ_c are important in signal transduction. The γ_c gene is on the X chromosome, and mutations in the γ_c protein result in the *X-linked form of severe combined immune deficiency syndrome (X-SCID)*.

The members of the *interferon (type II) receptor* family include the receptors for IFN-γ and -β, which share a similar 210-amino-acid binding domain with conserved cysteine pairs at both the amino and carboxy termini. The members of the *TNF (type III) receptor family* share a common binding domain composed of repeated cysteine-rich regions. Members of this family include the p55 and p75 receptors for TNF (TNFR1 and TNFR2, respectively); CD40 antigen, which is an important B cell–surface marker involved in immunoglobulin isotype switching; fas/Apo-1, whose triggering induces apoptosis; CD27 and CD30, which are found on activated T cells and B cells; and nerve growth factor receptor.

The common motif for the *seven transmembrane helix family* was originally found in receptors linked to GTP-binding proteins. This family includes receptors for chemokines (Table 1-7), β-adrenergic receptors, and retinal rhodopsin. It is important to note that two members of the chemokine receptor family, CXC chemokine receptor type 4 (CXCR4) and β chemokine receptor type 5 (CCR5), have been found to serve as the two major coreceptors for binding and entry of HIV into CD4-expressing host cells.

Significant advances have been made in defining the signaling pathways through which cytokines exert their effects intracellularly. The Janus family of protein tyrosine kinases (JAK) is a critical element involved in signaling via the hematopoietin receptors. Four JAK kinases, JAK1, JAK2, JAK3, and Tyk2, preferentially bind different cytokine receptor subunits. Cytokine binding to its receptor brings the cytokine receptor subunits into apposition and allows a pair of JAKs to transphosphorylate and activate one another. The JAKs then phosphorylate the receptor on the tyrosine residues and allow signaling molecules to bind to the receptor, where these molecules become phosphorylated. Signaling molecules bind the receptor because they have domains (SH2, or src homology 2 domains) that can bind phosphorylated tyrosine residues. There are a number of these important signaling molecules that bind the receptor, such as the adapter molecule SHC, which can couple the receptor to the activation of the mitogen-activated protein kinase pathway. In addition, an important class of substrate of the JAKs is the signal transducers and activators of transcription (STAT) family of transcription factors. STATs have SH2 domains that enable them to bind to phosphorylated receptors, where they are then phosphorylated by the JAKs. It appears that different STATs have specificity for different receptor subunits. The STATs then dissociate from the receptor and translocate to the nucleus, bind to DNA motifs that they recognize, and regulate gene expression. The STATs preferentially bind DNA motifs that are slightly different from one another and thereby control transcription of specific genes. The importance of this pathway is particularly relevant to lymphoid development. Mutations of JAK3 itself also

result in a disorder identical to X-SCID; however, since JAK3 is found on chromosome 19 and not on the X chromosome, JAK3 deficiency occurs in boys and girls.

THE ADAPTIVE IMMUNE SYSTEM

Adaptive immunity is characterized by antigen-specific responses to a foreign antigen or pathogen. A key feature of adaptive immunity is that following the initial contact with antigen (*immunologic priming*), subsequent antigen exposure leads to more rapid and vigorous immune responses (*immunologic memory*). The adaptive immune system consists of dual limbs of cellular and humoral immunity. The principal effectors of cellular immunity are T lymphocytes, while the principal effectors of humoral immunity are B lymphocytes. Both B and T lymphocytes derive from a common stem cell (**Fig. 1-6**).

The proportion and distribution of immunocompetent cells in various tissues reflect cell traffic, homing patterns, and functional capabilities. Bone marrow is the major site of maturation of B cells, monocytes-macrophages, dendritic cells, and granulocytes and contains pluripotent stem cells that, under the influence of various colony-stimulating factors, are capable of giving rise to all hematopoietic cell types. T cell precursors also arise from hematopoietic stem cells and home to the thymus for maturation. Mature T lymphocytes, B lymphocytes, monocytes, and dendritic cells enter the circulation and home to peripheral lymphoid organs (lymph nodes, spleen) and mucosal surface-associated lymphoid tissue (gut, genitourinary, and respiratory tracts) as well as the skin and mucous membranes and await activation by foreign antigen.

T Cells

The pool of effector T cells is established in the thymus early in life and is maintained throughout life both by new T cell production in the thymus and by antigen-driven expansion of virgin peripheral T cells into "memory" T cells that reside in peripheral lymphoid organs. The thymus exports ~2% of the total number of thymocytes per day throughout life, with the total number of daily thymic emigrants decreasing by ~3% per year during the first four decades of life.

Mature T lymphocytes constitute 70–80% of normal peripheral blood lymphocytes (only 2% of the total-body lymphocytes are contained in peripheral blood), 90% of thoracic duct lymphocytes, 30–40% of lymph node cells, and 20–30% of spleen lymphoid cells. In lymph nodes, T cells occupy deep paracortical areas around B cell germinal centers, and in the spleen, they are located in periarteriolar areas of white pulp. T cells are the primary effectors of cell-mediated immunity, with subsets of T cells maturing into CD8+ cytotoxic T cells capable of lysis of virus-infected or foreign cells

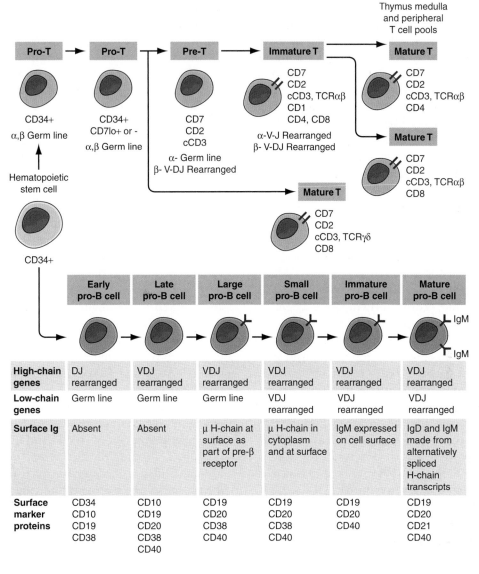

FIGURE 1-6

Development stages of T and B cells. Elements of the developing T and B cell receptor for antigen are shown schematically. The classification into the various stages of B cell development is primarily defined by rearrangement of the immunoglobulin (Ig), heavy (H), and light (L) chain genes and by the absence or presence of specific surface markers.

[Adapted from CA Janeway et al, (eds): Immunobiology. The Immune Systemic Health and Disease, 4th ed, New York, Garland, 1999, with permission.] The classification of stages of T cell development is primarily defined by cell surface marker protein expression (sCD3, surface CD3 expression; cCD3, cytoplasmic CD3 expression; TCR, T cell receptor).

(short-lived effector T cells). Two populations of long-lived memory T cells are triggered by infections: effector memory and central memory T cells. Effector memory T cells reside in nonlymphoid organs and respond rapidly to repeated pathogenic infections with cytokine production and cytotoxic functions to kill virus-infected cells. Central memory T cells home to lymphoid organs where they replenish long- and short-lived and effector memory T cells as needed.

In general, CD4+ T cells are also the primary regulatory cells of T and B lymphocyte and monocyte function by the production of cytokines and by direct cell contact (Fig. 1-2). In addition, T cells regulate erythroid

cell maturation in bone marrow, and through cell contact (CD40 ligand) have an important role in activation of B cells and induction of Ig isotype switching.

Human T cells express cell-surface proteins that mark stages of intrathymic T cell maturation or identify specific functional subpopulations of mature T cells. Many of these molecules mediate or participate in important T cell functions (Table 1-1, Fig. 1-6).

The earliest identifiable T cell precursors in bone marrow are CD34+ pro-T cells (i.e., cells in which TCR genes are neither rearranged nor expressed). In the thymus, CD34+ T cell precursors begin cytoplasmic (c) synthesis of components of the CD3 complex of

TCR-associated molecules (Fig. 1-6). Within T cell precursors, TCR for antigen gene rearrangement yields two T cell lineages, expressing either TCRαβ chains or TCRγδ chains. T cells expressing the TCRαβ chains constitute the majority of peripheral T cells in blood, lymph node, and spleen and terminally differentiate into either CD4+ or CD8+ cells. Cells expressing TCRγδ chains circulate as a minor population in blood; their functions, although not fully understood, have been postulated to be those of immune surveillance at epithelial surfaces and cellular defenses against mycobacterial organisms and other intracellular bacteria through recognition of bacterial lipids.

In the thymus, the recognition of self-peptides on thymic epithelial cells, thymic macrophages, and dendritic cells plays an important role in shaping the T cell repertoire to recognize foreign antigen (*positive selection*) and in eliminating highly autoreactive T cells (*negative selection*). As immature cortical thymocytes begin to express surface TCR for antigen, autoreactive thymocytes are destroyed (negative selection), thymocytes with TCRs capable of interacting with foreign antigen peptides in the context of self-MHC antigens are activated and develop to maturity (positive selection), and thymocytes with TCR that are incapable of binding to self-MHC antigens die of attrition (*no selection*). Mature thymocytes that are positively selected are either CD4+ helper T cells or MHC class II–restricted cytotoxic (killer) T cells, or they are CD8+ T cells destined to become MHC class I–restricted cytotoxic T cells. *MHC class I– or class II–restricted* means that T cells recognize antigen peptide fragments only when they are presented in the antigen-recognition site of a class I or class II MHC molecule, respectively (Chap. 2).

After thymocyte maturation and selection, CD4 and CD8 thymocytes leave the thymus and migrate to the peripheral immune system. The thymus continues to be a contributor to the peripheral immune system, well into adult life, both normally and when the peripheral T cell pool is damaged, such as occurs in AIDS and cancer chemotherapy.

Molecular Basis of T Cell Recognition of Antigen

The TCR for antigen is a complex of molecules consisting of an antigen-binding heterodimer of either αβ or γδ chains noncovalently linked with five CD3 subunits (γ, δ, ε, ζ, and η) (**Fig. 1-7**). The CD3 ζ chains are either disulfide-linked homodimers (CD3-ζ_2) or disulfide-linked heterodimers composed of one ζ chain and one η chain. TCRαβ or TCRγδ molecules must be associated with CD3 molecules to be inserted into the T cell surface membrane, TCRα being paired with TCRβ and TCRγ being paired with TCRδ. Molecules of the CD3 complex mediate transduction of T cell activation signals via TCRs, while TCRα and -β or -γ and -δ molecules combine to form the TCR antigen-binding site.

The α, β, γ, and δ TCR for antigen molecules have amino acid sequence homology and structural similarities to immunoglobulin heavy and light chains and are members of the *immunoglobulin gene superfamily* of molecules. The genes encoding TCR molecules are encoded as clusters of gene segments that rearrange during the course of T cell maturation. This creates an efficient and compact mechanism for housing the diversity requirements of antigen receptor molecules. The TCRα chain is on chromosome 14 and consists of a series of V (variable), J (joining), and C (constant) regions. The TCRβ chain is on chromosome 7 and consists of multiple V, D (diversity), J, and C TCRβ loci. The TCRγ chain is on chromosome 7, and the TCRδ chain is in the middle of the TCRα locus on chromosome 14. Thus, molecules of the TCR for antigen have constant (framework) and variable regions, and the gene segments encoding the α, β, γ, and δ chains of these molecules are recombined and selected in the thymus, culminating in synthesis of the completed molecule. In both T and B cell precursors (see below), DNA rearrangements of antigen receptor genes involve the same enzymes, recombinase activating gene (RAG)1 and RAG2, both DNA-dependent protein kinases.

TCR diversity is created by the different V, D, and J segments that are possible for each receptor chain by the many permutations of V, D, and J segment combinations, by "N-region diversification" due to the addition of nucleotides at the junction of rearranged gene segments, and by the pairing of individual chains to form a TCR dimer. As T cells mature in the thymus, the repertoire of antigen-reactive T cells is modified by selection processes that eliminate many autoreactive T cells, enhance the proliferation of cells that function appropriately with self-MHC molecules and antigen, and allow T cells with nonproductive TCR rearrangements to die.

TCRαβ cells do not recognize native protein or carbohydrate antigens. Instead, T cells recognize only short (~9–13 amino acids) peptide fragments derived from protein antigens taken up or produced in APCs. Foreign antigens may be taken up by endocytosis into acidified intracellular vesicles or by phagocytosis and degraded into small peptides that associate with MHC class II molecules (exogenous antigen-presentation pathway). Other foreign antigens arise endogenously in the cytosol (such as from replicating viruses) and are broken down into small peptides that associate with MHC class I molecules (endogenous antigen-presenting pathway). Thus, APCs proteolytically degrade foreign proteins and display peptide fragments embedded in the MHC class I or II antigen-recognition site on the MHC molecule surface, where foreign peptide fragments are available to bind to TCRαβ or TCRγδ chains of reactive T cells. CD4 molecules act as adhesives and, by direct binding to MHC class II (DR, DQ,

TABLE 1-11

29

PHYSICAL, CHEMICAL, AND BIOLOGIC PROPERTIES OF HUMAN IMMUNOGLOBULINS

PROPERTY	IgG	IgA	IgM	IgD	IgE
Usual molecular form	Monomer	Monomer, dimer	Pentamer, hexamer	Monomer	Monomer
Other chains	None	J chain, SC	J chain	None	None
Subclasses	G1, G2, G3, G4	A1, A2	None	None	None
Heavy chain allotypes	Gm (=30)	No A1, A2m (2)	None	None	None
Molecular mass, kDa	150	160, 400	950, 1150	175	190
Sedimentation constant, Sw20	6.6S	7S, 11S	19S	7S	8S
Carbohydrate content, %	3	7	10	9	13
Serum level in average adult, mg/mL	9.5–12.5	1.5–2.6	0.7–1.7	0.04	0.0003
Percentage of total serum Ig	75–85	7–15	5–10	0.3	0.019
Serum half-life, days	23	6	5	3	2.5
Synthesis rate, mg/kg per d	33	65	7	0.4	0.016
Antibody valence	2	2, 4	10, 12	2	2
Classical complement activation	+(G1, 2?, 3)	–	++	–	–
Alternate complement activation	+(G4)	+	–	+	–
Binding cells via Fc	Macrophages, neutrophils, large granular lymphocytes	Lymphocytes	Lymphocytes	None	Mast cells, basophils, B cells
Biologic properties	Placental transfer, secondary Ab for most antipathogen responses	Secretory immunoglobulin	Primary Ab responses	Marker for mature B cells	Allergy, antiparasite responses

Source: After L Carayannopoulos and JD Capra, in WE Paul (ed): *Fundamental Immunology*, 3d ed. New York, Raven, 1993; with permission.

idiotype portion of an antibody molecule are called *anti-idiotype antibodies*. The formation of such antibodies in vivo during a normal B cell antibody response may generate a negative (or "off") signal to B cells to terminate antibody production.

IgG constitutes ~75–85% of total serum immunoglobulin. The four IgG subclasses are numbered in order of their level in serum, IgG1 being found in greatest amounts and IgG4 the least. IgG subclasses have clinical relevance in their varying ability to bind macrophage and neutrophil Fc receptors and to activate complement (Table 1-11). Moreover, selective deficiencies of certain IgG subclasses give rise to clinical syndromes in which the patient is inordinately susceptible to bacterial infections. IgG antibodies are frequently the predominant antibody made after rechallenge of the host with antigen (secondary antibody response).

IgM antibodies normally circulate as a 950-kDa pentamer with 160-kDa bivalent monomers joined by a molecule called the *J chain*, a 15-kDa nonimmunoglobulin molecule that also effects polymerization of IgA molecules. IgM is the first immunoglobulin to appear in the immune response (primary antibody response) and is the initial type of antibody made by neonates. Membrane IgM in the monomeric form also functions as a major antigen receptor on the surface of mature B cells (Fig. 1–8). IgM is an important component of immune complexes in autoimmune diseases. For example, IgM antibodies against IgG molecules (rheumatoid factors) are present in high titers in *rheumatoid arthritis*, other collagen diseases, and some infectious diseases (*subacute bacterial endocarditis*).

IgA constitutes only 7–15% of total serum immunoglobulin but is the predominant class of immunoglobulin in secretions. IgA in secretions (tears, saliva, nasal secretions, gastrointestinal tract fluid, and human milk) is in the form of secretory IgA (sIgA), a polymer consisting of two IgA monomers, a joining molecule, again called the J chain, and a glycoprotein called the *secretory protein*. Of the two IgA subclasses, IgA1 is primarily found in serum, whereas IgA2 is more prevalent in secretions. IgA fixes complement via the alternative complement pathway and has potent antiviral activity in humans by prevention of virus binding to respiratory and gastrointestinal epithelial cells.

IgD is found in minute quantities in serum and, together with IgM, is a major receptor for antigen on the B cell surface. IgE, which is present in serum in very low concentrations, is the major class of immunoglobulin involved in arming mast cells and basophils by binding to these cells via the Fc region. Antigen cross-linking of IgE molecules on basophil and mast cell surfaces results in release of mediators of the immediate hypersensitivity response (Table 1-11).

CELLULAR INTERACTIONS IN REGULATION OF NORMAL IMMUNE RESPONSES

The net result of activation of the humoral (B cell) and cellular (T cell) arms of the adaptive immune system by foreign antigen is the elimination of antigen directly by specific effector T cells or in concert with specific antibody. Figure 1-2 is a simplified schematic diagram of the T and B cell responses indicating some of these cellular interactions.

The expression of adaptive immune cell function is the result of a complex series of immunoregulatory events that occur in phases. Both T and B lymphocytes mediate immune functions, and each of these cell types, when given appropriate signals, passes through stages, from activation and induction through proliferation, differentiation, and ultimately effector functions. The effector function expressed may be at the end point of a response, such as secretion of antibody by a differentiated plasma cell, or it might serve a regulatory function that modulates other functions, such as is seen with CD4+ and CD8+ T lymphocytes that modulate both differentiation of B cells and activation of CD8+ cytotoxic T cells.

CD4 helper T cells can be subdivided on the basis of cytokines produced (Fig. 1-2). Activated T_H1-type helper T cells secrete IL-2, IFN-γ, IL-3, TNF-α, GM-CSF, and TNF-β, while activated T_H2-type helper T cells secrete IL-3, -4, -5, -6, -10, and -13. T_H1 CD4+ T cells, through elaboration of IFN-γ, have a central role in mediating intracellular killing by a variety of pathogens. T_H1 CD4+ T cells also provide T cell help for generation of cytotoxic T cells and some types of opsonizing antibody, and they generally respond to antigens that lead to delayed hypersensitivity types of immune responses for many intracellular viruses and bacteria (such as HIV or *M. tuberculosis*). In contrast, T_H2 cells have a primary role in regulatory humoral immunity and isotype switching. T_H2 cells, through production of IL-4 and IL-10, have a regulatory role in limiting proinflammatory responses mediated by T_H1 cells (Fig. 1-2). In addition, T_H2 CD4+ T cells provide help to B cells for specific Ig production and respond to antigens that require high antibody levels for foreign antigen elimination (extracellular encapsulated bacteria such as *Streptococcus pneumoniae* and certain parasite infections). The type of T cell response generated in an immune response is determined by the microbe PAMPs presented to the dendritic cells, the TLRs on the dendritic cells that become activated, the types of dendritic cells that are activated, and the cytokines that are

produced (Table 1-4). Commonly, myeloid dendritic cells produce IL-12 and activate T_H1 T cell responses that result in IFN-γ and cytotoxic T cell induction, and plasmacytoid dendritic cells produce IFN-α and lead to T_H2 responses that result in IL-4 production and enhanced antibody responses.

As shown in Figs. 1-2 and 1-3, upon activation by dendritic cells, T cell subsets that produce IL-2, IL-3, IFN-γ, and/or IL-4, -5, -6, -10, and -13 are generated and exert positive and negative influences on effector T and B cells. For B cells, trophic effects are mediated by a variety of cytokines, particularly T cell–derived IL-3, -4, -5, and -6, that act at sequential stages of B cell maturation, resulting in B cell proliferation, differentiation, and ultimately antibody secretion. For cytotoxic T cells, trophic factors include inducer T cell secretion of IL-2, IFN-γ, and IL-12.

An important type of immunomodulatory T cell that controls immune responses is *CD4+ and CD8+ T regulatory cells*. These cells constitutively express the α chain of the IL-2 receptor (CD25), produce large amounts of IL-10, and can suppress both T and B cell responses. T regulatory cells are induced by immature dendritic cells and play key roles in maintaining tolerance to self-antigens in the periphery. Loss of T regulatory cells is the cause of organ-specific autoimmune disease in mice such as autoimmune thyroiditis, adrenalitis, and oophoritis (see "Immune Tolerance and Autoimmunity" later in the chapter). T regulatory cells also play key roles in controlling the magnitude and duration of immune responses to microbes. Normally, after the initial immune response to a microbe has eliminated the invader, T regulatory cells are activated to suppress the antimicrobe response and prevent host injury. Some microbes have adapted to induce T regulatory cell activation at the site of infection to promote parasite infection and survival. In *Leishmania* infection, the parasite locally induces T regulatory cell accumulation at skin infection sites that dampens anti-*Leishmania* T cell responses and prevents elimination of the parasite. It is thought that many chronic infections such as by *M. tuberculosis* are associated with abnormal T regulatory cell activation that prevents elimination of the microbe.

Although B cells recognize native antigen via B cell surface Ig receptors, B cells require T cell help to produce high-affinity antibody of multiple isotypes that are the most effective in eliminating foreign antigen. This T cell dependence likely functions in the regulation of B cell responses and in protection against excessive autoantibody production. T cell–B cell interactions that lead to high-affinity antibody production require (1) processing of native antigen by B cells and expression of peptide fragments on the B cell surface for presentation to T_H cells, (2) the ligation of B cells by both the TCR complex and the CD40 ligand, (3) induction of the process termed *antibody isotype switching* in antigen-specific

B cell clones, and (4) induction of the process of affinity maturation of antibody in the germinal centers of B cell follicles of lymph node and spleen.

Naïve B cells express cell-surface IgD and IgM, and initial contact of naïve B cells with antigen is via binding of native antigen to B cell–surface IgM. T cell cytokines, released following T_H2 cell contact with B cells or by a "bystander" effect, induce changes in Ig gene conformation that promote recombination of Ig genes. These events then result in the "switching" of expression of heavy chain exons in a triggered B cell, leading to the secretion of IgG, IgA, or, in some cases, IgE antibody with the same V region antigen specificity as the original IgM antibody, for response to a wide variety of extracellular bacteria, protozoa, and helminths. CD40 ligand expression by activated T cells is critical for induction of B cell antibody isotype switching and for B cell responsiveness to cytokines. Patients with mutations in T cell CD40 ligand have B cells that are unable to undergo isotype switching, resulting in lack of memory B cell generation and the immunodeficiency syndrome of *X-linked hyper-IgM syndrome*.

IMMUNE TOLERANCE AND AUTOIMMUNITY

Immune tolerance is defined as the absence of activation of pathogenic autoreactivity. *Autoimmune diseases* are syndromes caused by the activation of T or B cells or both, with no evidence of other causes such as infections or malignancies (Chap. 3). Once thought to be mutually exclusive, immune tolerance and autoimmunity are now both recognized to be present normally in health; when abnormal, they represent extremes from the normal state. For example, it is now known that low levels of autoreactivity of T and B cells with self-antigens in the periphery are critical to their survival. Similarly, low levels of autoreactivity and thymocyte recognition of self-antigens in the thymus are the mechanisms whereby (1) normal T cells are positively selected to survive and leave the thymus to respond to foreign microbes in the periphery, and (2) T cells highly reactive to self-antigens are negatively selected and die to prevent overly self-reactive T cells from getting into the periphery (central tolerance). However, not all self-antigens are expressed in the thymus to delete highly self-reactive T cells, and there are mechanisms for peripheral tolerance induction of T cells as well. Unlike the presentation of microbial antigens by mature dendritic cells, the presentation of self-antigens by immature dendritic cells neither activates nor matures the dendritic cells to express high levels of co-stimulatory molecules such as B7-1 (CD80) or B7-2 (CD86). When peripheral T cells are stimulated by dendritic cells expressing self-antigens in the context of HLA molecules, sufficient stimulation of T cells occurs to keep them alive, but otherwise they remain anergic, or nonresponsive, until they contact a dendritic cell with high levels of co-stimulatory molecules expressing microbial antigens. In the latter setting, normal T cells then become activated to respond to the microbe. If B cells have high-self-reactivity BCRs, they normally undergo receptor editing to express a less autoreactive receptor or are induced to die. Although many autoimmune diseases are characterized by abnormal or pathogenic autoantibody production (Table 1-12), most autoimmune diseases are caused by a combination of excess T and B cell reactivity.

Multiple factors contribute to the genesis of clinical autoimmune disease syndromes, including genetic susceptibility (Table 1-13), environmental immune stimulants such as drugs (e.g., procainamide and dilantin with drug-induced systemic lupus erythematosus), infectious agent triggers (such as Epstein-Barr virus and autoantibody production against red blood cells and platelets), and loss of T regulatory cells (leading to thyroiditis, adrenalitis, and oophoritis).

Immunity at Mucosal Surfaces

Mucosa covering the respiratory, digestive, and urogenital tracts; the eye conjunctiva; the inner ear; and the ducts of all exocrine glands contain cells of the innate and adaptive mucosal immune system that protect these surfaces against pathogens. In the healthy adult, mucosa-associated lymphoid tissue (MALT) contains 80% of all immune cells within the body and constitutes the largest mammalian lymphoid organ system.

MALT has three main functions: (1) to protect the mucous membranes from invasive pathogens; (2) to prevent uptake of foreign antigens from food, commensal organisms, and airborne pathogens and particulate matter; and (3) to prevent pathologic immune responses from foreign antigens if they do cross the mucosal barriers of the body.

MALT is a compartmentalized system of immune cells that functions independently from systemic immune organs. Whereas the systemic immune organs are essentially sterile under normal conditions and respond vigorously to pathogens, MALT immune cells are continuously bathed in foreign proteins and commensal bacteria, and they must select those pathogenic antigens that must be eliminated. MALT contains anatomically defined foci of immune cells in the intestine, tonsil, appendix, and peribronchial areas that are inductive sites for mucosal immune responses. From these sites immune T and B cells migrate to effector sites in mucosal parenchyma and exocrine glands where mucosal immune cells eliminate pathogen-infected cells. In addition to mucosal immune responses, all mucosal sites have strong mechanical and chemical barriers and cleansing functions to repel pathogens.

Key components of MALT include specialized epithelial cells called "membrane" or "M" cells that take up antigens

TABLE 1-12

RECOMBINANT OR PURIFIED AUTOANTIGENS RECOGNIZED BY AUTOANTIBODIES ASSOCIATED WITH HUMAN AUTOIMMUNE DISORDERS

AUTOANTIGEN	AUTOIMMUNE DISEASES	AUTOANTIGEN	AUTOIMMUNE DISEASES
Cell- or Organ-Specific Autoimmunity			
Acetylcholine receptor	Myasthenia gravis	Insulin receptor	Type B insulin resistance, acanthosis, systemic lupus erythematosus (SLE)
Actin	Chronic active hepatitis, primary bilary cirrhosis	Intrinsic factor type 1	Pernicious anemia
Adenine nucleotide translator (ANT)	Dilated cardiomyopathy, myocarditis	Leukocyte function-associated antigen (LFA-1)	Treatment-resistant Lyme arthritis
β-Adrenoreceptor	Dilated cardiomyopathy	Myelin-associated glycoprotein (MAG)	Polyneuropathy
Aromatic L-amino acid decarboxylase	Autoimmune polyendocrine syndrome type 1 (APS-1)		
Asialoglycoprotein receptor	Autoimmune hepatitis	Myelin-basic protein	Multiple sclerosis, demyelinating diseases
Bactericidal/permeability-increasing protein (Bpi)	Cystic fibrosis vasculitides	Myelin oligodendrocyte glycoprotein (MOG)	Multiple sclerosis
Calcium-sensing receptor	Acquired hypoparathyroidism	Myosin	Rheumatic fever
Cholesterol side-chain cleavage enzyme (CYPlla)	Autoimmune polyglandular syndrome-1	p-80-Collin	Atopic dermatitis
Collagen type IV-α3-chain	Goodpasture's syndrome	Pyruvate dehydrogenase complex-E2 (PDC-E2)	Primary biliary cirrhosis
Cytochrome P450 2D6 (CYP2D6)	Autoimmune hepatitis	Sodium iodide symporter (NIS)	Graves' disease, autoimmune hypothyroidism
Desmin	Crohn's disease, coronary artery disease	SOX-10	Vitiligo
		Thyroid and eye muscle shared protein	Thyroid-associated ophthalmopathy
Desmoglein 1	Pemphigus foliaceus	Thyroglobulin	Autoimmune thyroiditis
Desmoglein 3	Pemphigus vulgaris	Thyroid peroxidase	Autoimmune Hashimoto thyroiditis
F-actin	Autoimmune hepatitis	Throtropin receptor	Graves' disease
GM gangliosides	Guillain-Barré syndrome	Tissue transglutaminase	Celiac disease
Glutamate decarboxylase (GAD65)	Type 1 diabetes, stiff man syndrome	Transcription coactivator p75	Atopic dermatitis
Glutamate receptor (GLUR)	Rasmussen encephalitis	Tryptophan hydroxylase	Autoimmune polyglandular syndrome-1
H/K ATPase	Autoimmune gastritis		
17-α-Hydroxylase (CYP17)	Autoimmune polyglandular syndrome-1	Tyrosinase	Vitiligo, metastatic melanoma
21-Hydroxylase (CYP21)	Addison's disease	Tyrosine hydroxylase	Autoimmune polyglandular syndrome-1
IA-2 (ICA512)	Type 1 diabetes		
Insulin	Type 1 diabetes, insulin hypoglycemic syndrome (Hirata's disease)		
Systemic Autoimmunity			
ACTH	ACTH deficiency	Histone H2A-H2B-DNA	SLE
Aminoacyl-tRAN histidyl synthetase	Myositis, dermatomyositis	IgE receptor	Chronic idiopathic urticaria
		Keratin	RA
Aminoacyl-tRNA synthetase (several)	Polymyositis, dermatomyositis	Ku-DNA-protein kinase	SLE
		Ku-nucleoprotein	Connective tissue syndrome
Cardiolipin	SLE, anti-phospholipid syndrome	La phosphoprotein (La 55-B)	Sjögren's syndrome
Carbonic anhydrase II	SLE, Sjögren's syndrome, systemic sclerosis	Myeloperoxidase	Necrotizing and crescentic glomerulonephritis (NCGN), systemic vasculitis
Collagen (multiple types)	Rheumatoid arthritis (RA), SLE, progressive systemic sclerosis	Proteinase 3 (PR3)	Wegener granulomatosis, Churg-Strauss syndrome
Centromere-associated proteins	Systemic sclerosis		

TABLE 1-16

CURRENT STATUS OF DEVELOPMENT OF IMMUNOMODULATORY AGENTS

AGENTS	RATIONALE	STATUS
Cytokines and Cytokine Inhibitors to Inhibit Immune Responses and Inflammation		
Anti–TNF-α monoclonal antibody; humanized mouse chimeric MAb, infliximab, fully humanized MAb, adalimumab	Inhibit TNF-α	FDA approved for rheumatoid arthritis, Crohn's colitis (infliximab); FDA approved for rheumatoid arthritis (adalimumab)
Recombinant TNF-receptor-Ig fusion protein (etanercept)	Inhibit TNF-α	FDA approved for rheumatoid arthritis, juvenile rheumatoid arthritis, psoriasis
Recombinant IL-1 receptor antagonist (IL-1Ra) (anakinra)	Inhibit IL-1α and -β	FDA approved for rheumatoid arthritis
Monoclonal Antibodies or Toxins Against T or B Cells		
Anti-CD3 and T cell murine monoclonal antibody (OKT3)	Inhibit T cell function; induce T cell lymphopenia	FDA approved for treatment of cardiac and renal allograft rejection
Diphtheria toxin-IL2 fusion protein	Kills activated T cells	FDA approved for GVHD and transplant repertoire; understudy to kill T regulatory cell to embrace tumor vaccine efficacy
Humanized anti-CD3 monoclonal antibody (hOKT3 gamma-1)	Eliminates auto-reactive T cells	Human study underway in Type I diabetes, psoriasis
Humanized anti-CD25 (IL-2R) monoclonal antibody (daclizumab)	Eliminates activated T cells	FDA approved for graft versus host disease; studies underway in ulcerative colitis
Anti-CD40 ligand (CD154) monoclonal antibody	Inhibit CD40-CD40 ligand interaction; induces T cell tolerance	In primate trials for prevention of renal allograft rejection
Humanized anti-CD20 (anti-B cell) monoclonal antibody (rituximab)	Eliminates autoreactive B cells	Human study underway for treatment of ANCA+ vasculitis
Humanized anti-IgE monoclonal antibody (omalizumab)	Block allergy causing IgE	Human study underway for allergy (hay fever, allergic rhinitis)
Soluble T Cell Molecule		
Soluble CTLA-4 protein	Inhibit CD28-B7-1 and B7-2 interactions; induces tolerance to organ grafts; inhibit autoimmune T cell reactivity in autoimmune diseases	FDA approved for rheumatoid arthritis. In trials for preventing GVHD in bone marrow transplantation and for treatment of psoriasis, systemic lupus erythematosus, and certain forms of vasculitis.
Intravenous Immunoglobin		
IVIg	Reticuloendothelial cell blockage; complement inhibition; regulation of idiotype/anti-idiotype antibodies; modulation of cytokine production; modulation of lymphocyte production	FDA approved for Kawasaki's disease and immune thrombocytopenia purpura; treatment of GVHD, multiple sclerosis, myasthenia gravis, Guillain-Barré syndrome, and chronic inflammatory demyelinating polyneuropathy supported by clinical trials
Cytokines for Immune Reconstitution		
IL-2	Induce proliferation of peripheral memory CD4+ and CD8+ T cells	In trial for treatment of HIV infection
IL-7	Induce renewed thymopoiesis	Under consideration for treatment of disease associated with T cell deficiency
Hematopoietic Stem Cell Transplantation		
Hematopoietic stem transplantation for immune reconstitution	Remove pathologic autoreactive immune system and replace with less autoreactive immunity	In clinical trials for systemic lupus erythematosus, multiple sclerosis, and scleroderma

Note: FDA, Food and Drug Administration; GVHD, graft-versus-host disease; ANCA, anti-neutrophil cytoplasmic antibody.

results have also been found with the use of IL-1 ra in *autoinflammatory disease*. Similarly, anti–IL-6, IFN-β, and IL-11 act to inhibit pathogenic proinflammatory cytokines. Anti–IL-6 inhibits IL-6 activity, while IFN-β and IL-11 decrease IL-1 and TNF- production.

Of particular note has been the successful use of IFN-γ in the treatment of the phagocytic cell defect in *chronic granulomatous disease*. Intermittent infusions of IL-2 in HIV-infected individuals in the early or intermediate stages of disease have resulted in substantial and sustained increases in CD4+ T cells.

Monoclonal Antibodies to T and B Cells

The OKT3 MAb against human T cells has been used for several years as a T cell–specific immunosuppressive agent that can substitute for horse anti-thymocyte globulin (ATG) in the treatment of solid organ transplant rejection. OKT3 produces fewer allergic reactions than ATG but does induce human anti-mouse Ig antibody, thus limiting its use. Anti-CD4 MAb therapy has been used in trials to treat patients with rheumatoid arthritis. While inducing profound immunosuppression, anti-CD4 MAb treatment also induces susceptibility to severe infections. Treatment of patients with a MAb against the T cell molecule CD40 ligand (CD154) is under investigation to induce tolerance to organ transplants, with promising results reported in animal studies. Monoclonal antibodies to the CD25 (IL-2α) receptor are being used for treatment of graft-versus-host disease in bone marrow transplantation, and anti-CD20 MAb (rituximab) is being tested for Wegener's granulomatosis and microscopic polyangiitis that are associated with *antineutrophil cytoplasmic antibodies* (Chap. 10). Anti-IgE monoclonal antibody (omalizumab) is used in the treatment of asthma and is being tested for blocking antigen-specific IgE that causes *hay fever* and *allergic rhinitis*.

Tolerance Induction

Specific immunotherapy has moved into a new era with the introduction of soluble CTLA-4 protein, which is an approved treatment for rheumatoid arthritis (Chap. 5) and is being studied in a number of other clinical trials. Use of this molecule to block T cell activation via TCR/CD28 ligation during organ or bone marrow transplantation has showed promising results in animals and in human studies. Specifically, treatment of bone marrow with CTLA-4 protein reduces rejection of the graft in HLA-mismatched bone marrow transplantation. In addition, promising results with soluble CTLA-4 have been reported in the downmodulation of autoimmune T cell responses in the treatment of psoriasis; new trials of the drug are ongoing for treatment of systemic lupus erythematosus (Chap. 4), Wegener's granulomatosis, giant cell arteritis, and Takayasu's arteritis (Chap. 10).

Intravenous Immunoglobulin (IVIg)

IVIg has been used successfully to block reticuloendothelial cell function and immune complex clearance in various immune cytopenias such as immune thrombocytopenia. In addition, IVIg is useful for prevention of tissue damage in certain inflammatory syndromes such as Kawasaki disease (Chap. 10) and as Ig replacement therapy for certain types of immunoglobulin deficiencies. In addition, controlled clinical trials support the use of IVIg in selected patients with graft-versus-host disease, multiple sclerosis, myasthenia gravis, Guillain-Barré syndrome, and chronic demyelinating polyneuropathy (Table 1-16).

Stem Cell Transplantation

Hematopoietic stem cell transplantation (SCT) is now being comprehensively studied to treat several autoimmune diseases, including systemic lupus erythematosus, multiple sclerosis, and scleroderma. The goal of immune reconstitution in autoimmune disease syndromes is to replace a dysfunctional immune system with a normally reactive immune cell repertoire. Preliminary results in patients with scleroderma and lupus have showed encouraging results. Controlled clinical trials in these three diseases are now being launched in the United States and Europe to compare the toxicity and efficacy of conventional immunosuppression therapy with that of myeloablative autologous SCT.

Thus, a number of recent insights into immune system function have spawned a new field of interventional immunotherapy and have enhanced the prospect for development of specific and nontoxic therapies for immune and inflammatory diseases.

FURTHER READINGS

ANDREAKOS ETH et al: Role of cytokines, in *Rheumatoid Arthritis*, EW St. Clair et al (eds). Philadelphia, Lippincott Williams & Wilkins, 2004, pp 134–149

BACKHED F et al: Host-bacterial mutualism in the human intestine. Science 307:1915, 2005

BLANDER JM et al: Toll-dependent selection of microbial antigens for presentation by dendritic cells. Nature 440:808, 2006

COLONNA M et al: Dendritic cells at the host-pathogen interface. Nat Immunol 7:117, 2006

DAVIDSON A, DIAMOND B: Autoimmune diseases. N Engl J Med 345:340, 2001

DIAMOND B et al: The immune tolerance network and rheumatic disease: Immune tolerance comes to the clinic. Arthritis Rheum 44:1730, 2001

DI SANTO JP: Natural killer cells: diversity in search of a niche. Nat Immunol 9:473, 2008

DRAYTON DL et al: Lymphoid organ development: From ontogeny to neogenesis. Nat Immunol 7:344, 2006

HAYNES BF et al: The role of the thymus in immune reconstitution in aging bone marrow transplantation and AIDS. Annu Rev Immunol 18:529, 2000

HOLMGREN J et al: Mucosal immunity and vaccines. Nat Med 11(4 Suppl):S45, 2005

JANEWAY CA et al (eds): Immunobiology. The Immune System in Health and Disease, 5th ed. New York, Garland, 1999

KORETZKY GA et al: SLP76 and SLP65: Complex regulation of signalling in lymphocytes and beyond. Nat Rev Immunol 6:67, 2006

LERNMARK A: Autoimmune diseases: Are markers ready for prediction? J Clin Invest 108:1091, 2001

LUSTER AD et al: Immune cell migration in inflammation: Present and future therapeutic targets. Nat Immunol 6:1182, 2005

MACDONALD TT et al: Immunity, inflammation, and allergy in the gut. Science 307:1920, 2005

MORETTA A et al: Major histocompatibility complex class I–specific receptors on human natural killer and T lymphocytes. Immunol Rev 155:105, 1997

———— et al: What is a natural killer cell? Nat Immunol 3:6, 2002

MORETTA L et al: Human natural killer cells: Molecular mechanisms controlling NK cell activation and tumor cell lysis. Immunol Lett 100:7, 2005

MORLEY BJ, WALPORT MJ: The Complement Facts Books. London, Academic Press, 2000, Chap. 2

MULLAUER L et al: Mutations in apoptosis genes: A pathogenetic factor for human disease. Mutat Res 488:211, 2001

PAUST S et al: Regulatory T cells and autoimmune disease. Immunolog Rev 204:195, 2005

RIVERA J et al: Molecular regulation of mast cell activation. J Allergy Clin Immunol 6:1214, 2006

ROCHMAN Y et al: New insights into the regulation of T cells by gamma(c) family cytokines. Nat Rev Immunol 9:480, 2009

ROMAGNANI S: CD4 effector cells, in Inflammation: Basic Principles and Clinical Correlates, 3d ed, J Gallin, R Snyderman (eds). Philadelphia, Lippincott Williams & Wilkins, 1999, pp 177–184

SAKAGUCHI S: Regulatory T cells: Mediating compromises between host and parasite. Nat Immunol 4:10, 2003

SARTOR RB: Therapeutic manipulation of the enteric microflora in inflammatory bowel diseases: Antibiotics, probiotics, and prebiotics. Gastroenterology 6:1620, 2004

SCHRADER JW: Interleukin is as interleukin does. Trends Immunol 23:573, 2002

SHEVACH EM: Regulatory T cells in autoimmunity. Annu Rev Immunol 18:423, 2000

SHINKAI K et al: Helper T cells regulate type-2 innate immunity in vivo. Nature 420:825, 2002

TESMER LA et al: Th17 cells in human disease. Immunol Rev 223:87, 2008

VAN DUIN D et al: Triggering TLR signaling in vaccination. Trends Immunol 27:49, 2006

YOKOYAMA WM: Contact hypersensitivity: Not just T cells! Nat Immunol 7:437, 2006

ZHOU X et al: Plasticity of CD4(+) FoxP3(+) T cells. Curr Opin Immunol 21:281, 2009

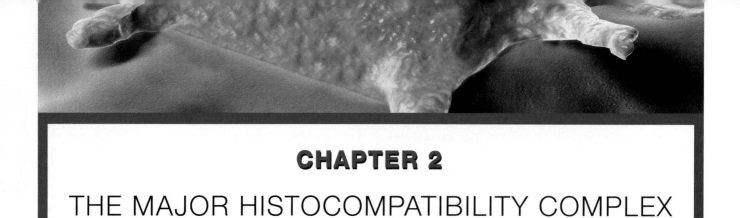

CHAPTER 2
THE MAJOR HISTOCOMPATIBILITY COMPLEX

Gerald T. Nepom

THE HLA COMPLEX AND ITS PRODUCTS

The human major histocompatibility complex (MHC), commonly called the human leukocyte antigen (HLA) complex, is a 4-megabase (Mb) region on chromosome 6 (6p21.3) that is densely packed with expressed genes. The best known of these genes are the HLA class I and class II genes, whose products are critical for immunologic specificity and transplantation histocompatibility, and they play a major role in susceptibility to a number of autoimmune diseases. Many other genes in the HLA region are also essential to the innate and antigen-specific functioning of the immune system. The HLA region shows extensive conservation with the MHC of other mammals in terms of genomic organization, gene sequence, and protein structure and function. Much of our understanding of the MHC has come from investigation of the MHC in mice, which is termed the *H-2 complex*, and to a lesser degree from other species as well. Nonetheless, in this chapter discussion is confined to information applicable to the MHC in humans.

The *HLA class I genes* are located in a 2-Mb stretch of DNA at the telomeric end of the HLA region (**Fig. 2-1**). The classic (MHC class Ia) HLA-A, -B, and -C loci, the products of which are integral participants in the immune response to intracellular infections, tumors, and allografts, are expressed in all nucleated cells and are highly polymorphic in the population. *Polymorphism* refers to a high degree of allelic variation within a genetic locus that leads to extensive variation between different individuals expressing different alleles. Over 450 alleles at HLA-A, 780 at HLA-B, and 230 at HLA-C have been identified in different human populations, making this the most highly polymorphic segment known within the human genome. Each of the alleles at these loci encodes a *heavy chain* (also called an α *chain*) that associates noncovalently with the nonpolymorphic light chain β_2-*microglobulin*, encoded on chromosome 15.

The nomenclature of HLA genes and their products reflects the grafting of newer DNA sequence information on an older system based on serology. Among class I genes, alleles of the HLA-A, -B, and -C loci were originally identified in the 1950s, 1960s, and 1970s by alloantisera, derived primarily from multiparous women, who in the course of normal pregnancy produce antibodies against paternal antigens expressed on fetal cells. The serologic allotypes were designated by consecutive numbers, e.g., HLA-A1, HLA-B8. Currently, under World Health Organization (WHO) nomenclature, class I alleles are given a single designation that indicates locus, serologic specificity, and sequence-based subtype. For example, HLA-A*0201 indicates subtype 1 of the serologically defined allele HLA-A2. Subtypes that differ from each other at the nucleotide but not the amino acid sequence level are designated by an extra numeral, e.g., HLA-B*07021 and

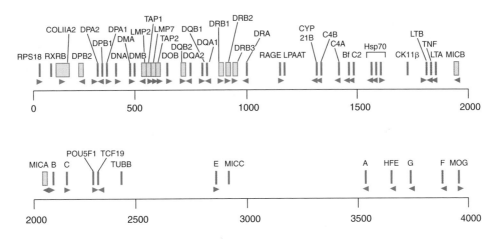

FIGURE 2-1

Physical map of the HLA region, showing the class I and class II loci, other immunologically important loci, and a sampling of other genes mapped to this region. Gene orientation is indicated by arrowheads. Scale is in kilobase (kb).

The approximate genetic distance from DP to A is 3.2 cM. This includes 0.8 cM between A and B (including 0.2 cM between C and B), 0.4–0.8 cM between B and DR-DQ, and 1.6–2.0 cM between DR-DQ and DP.

HLA-B*07022 are two variants of the HLA-B702 subtype of HLA-B*07. The nomenclature of class II genes, discussed below, is made more complicated by the fact that both chains of a class II molecule are encoded by closely linked HLA-encoded loci, both of which may be polymorphic, and by the presence of differing numbers of isotypic DRB loci in different individuals. It has become clear that accurate HLA genotyping requires DNA sequence analysis, and the identification of alleles at the DNA sequence level has contributed greatly to the understanding of the role of HLA molecules as peptide-binding ligands, to the analysis of associations of HLA

alleles with certain diseases, to the study of the population genetics of HLA, and to a clearer understanding of the contribution of HLA differences to allograft rejection and graft-vs-host disease. Current databases of HLA class I and class II sequences can be accessed by Internet (e.g., from the IMGT/HLA Database, *http://www.ebi.ac.uk/ imgt/hla*), and frequent updates of HLA gene lists are published in several journals.

The biologic significance of this MHC genetic diversity, resulting in extreme variation in the human population, is evident from the perspective of the structure of MHC molecules. As shown in **Fig. 2-2**, the MHC class I

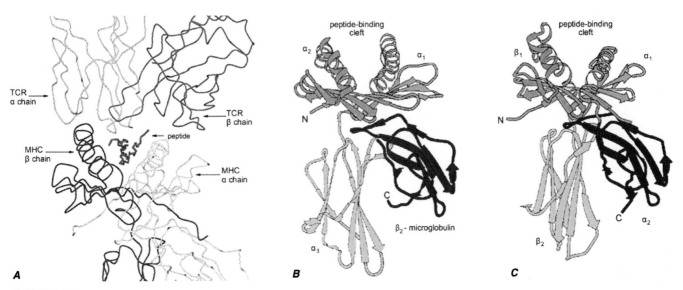

FIGURE 2-2

A. The trimolecular complex of TCR (*top*), MHC molecule (*bottom*), and a bound peptide form the structural determinants of specific antigen recognition. Other panels (**B** and **C**) show the domain structure of MHC class I (B) and class II (C) molecules. The α_1 and α_2 domains of class I and the α_1 and β_1 domains of class II form a β-sheet platform that forms the floor of the

peptide-binding groove, and α helices that form the sides of the groove. The α_3 (**A**) and β_2 domains (**B**) project from the cell surface and form the contact sites for CD8 and CD4, respectively. *(Adapted from EL Reinhertz et al: Science 286:1913, 1999; and C Janeway et al: Immunobiology Bookshelf, 2d ed, Garland Publishing, New York, 1997; with permission.)*

and class II genes encode MHC molecules that bind small peptides, and together this complex (pMHC; peptide-MHC) forms the ligand for recognition by T lymphocytes, through the antigen-specific T cell receptor. There is a direct link between the genetic variation and this structural interaction: The allelic changes in genetic sequence result in diversification of the peptide-binding capabilities of each MHC molecule and in differences for specific TCR binding. Thus, different pMHC complexes bind different antigens and are targets for recognition by different T cells.

The class I MHC and class II MHC structures, shown in Figs. 2-2B and 2-2C, are structurally closely related, although there are a few key differences. While both bind peptides and present them to T cells, the binding pockets have different shapes, which influences the types of immune responses that result (discussed below). In addition, there are structural contact sites for T cell molecules known as CD8 and CD4, expressed on the class I or class II membrane-proximal domains, respectively. This ensures that when peptide antigens are presented by class I molecules, the responding T cells are predominantly of the CD8 class, and similarly, that T cells responding to class II pMHC complexes are predominantly CD4.

The nonclassic, or class Ib, MHC molecules, HLA-E, -F, and -G, are much less polymorphic than MHC Ia and appear to have distinct functions. The HLA-E molecule, which has a peptide repertoire restricted to signal peptides cleaved from classic MHC class I molecules, is the major self-recognition target for the natural killer (NK) cell inhibitory receptors NKG2A or NKG2C paired with CD94 (see below and Chap. 1); four HLA-E alleles are known. HLA-G is expressed selectively in extravillous trophoblasts, the fetal cell population directly in contact with maternal tissues. It binds a wide array of peptides, is expressed in six different alternatively spliced forms, and provides inhibitory signals to both NK cells and T cells, presumably in the service of maintaining maternofetal tolerance. The function of HLA-F remains largely unknown.

Additional class I–like genes have been identified, some HLA-linked and some encoded on other chromosomes, that show only distant homology to the class Ia and Ib molecules but share the three-dimensional class I structure. Those on chromosome 6p21 include MIC-A and MIC-B, which are encoded centromeric to HLA-B, and HLA-HFE, located 3 to 4 cM (centi-Morgan) telomeric of HLA-F. MIC-A and MIC-B do not bind peptide but are expressed on gut and other epithelium in a stress-inducible manner and serve as activation signals for certain $\gamma\delta$ T cells, NK cells, CD8 T cells, and activated macrophages, acting through the activating NKG2D receptors. Sixty-one MIC-A and twenty-five MIC-B alleles are known, and additional diversification comes from variable alanine repeat sequences in the transmembrane domain. HLA-HFE encodes the gene defective in hereditary hemochromatosis. Among the non-HLA, class I–like genes, CD1 refers to a family of molecules that present glycolipids or other nonpeptide ligands to certain T cells, including T cells with NK activity; FcRn binds IgG within lysosomes and protects it from catabolism (Chap. 1); and Zn-α_2-glycoprotein 1 binds a nonpeptide ligand and promotes catabolism of triglycerides in adipose tissue. Like the HLA-A, -B, -C, -E, -F, and -G heavy chains, each of which forms a heterodimer with β_2-microglobulin (Fig. 2-2), the class I–like molecules, HLA-HFE, FcRn, and CD1 also bind to β_2-microglobulin, but MIC-A, MIC-B, and Zn-α_2-glycoprotein 1 do not.

The *HLA class II region* is also illustrated in Fig. 2-1. Multiple class II genes are arrayed within the centromeric 1 Mb of the HLA region, forming distinct haplotypes. A *haplotype* refers to an array of alleles at polymorphic loci along a chromosomal segment. Multiple class II genes are present on a single haplotype, clustered into three major subregions: HLA-DR, -DQ, and -DP. Each of these subregions contains at least one functional alpha (A) locus and one functional beta (B) locus. Together these encode proteins that form the α and β polypeptide chains of a mature class II HLA molecule. Thus, the DRA and DRB genes encode an HLA-DR molecule; products of the DQA1 and DQB1 genes form an HLA-DQ molecule; and the DPA1 and DPB1 genes encode an HLA-DP molecule. There are several DRB genes (DRB1, DRB2, DRB3, etc.), so that two expressed DR molecules are encoded on most haplotypes by combining the α-chain product of the DRA gene with separate β chains. More than 438 alleles have been identified at the HLA-DRB1 locus, with most of the variation occurring within limited segments encoding residues that interact with antigens. Detailed analysis of sequences and population distribution of these alleles strongly suggests that this diversity is actively selected by environmental pressures associated with pathogen diversity.

The class II region was originally termed the *D-region*. The allelic gene products were first detected by their ability to stimulate lymphocyte proliferation by *mixed lymphocyte reaction* and were named Dw1, Dw2, etc. Subsequently, serology was used to identify gene products on peripheral blood B cells, and the antigens were termed *DR* (D-related). After additional class II loci were identified, these came to be known as DQ and DP. In the DQ region, both DQA1 and DQB1 are polymorphic, with 34 DQA1 alleles and 71 DQB1 alleles. The current nomenclature is largely analogous to that discussed above for class I, using the convention "locus*allele." Thus, for example, subtypes of the serologically defined specificity DR4, encoded by the DRB1 locus, are termed DRB1*0401, -0402, etc. In addition to allelic polymorphism, products of different DQA1 alleles can, with some limitations, pair with products of different DQB1 alleles through both *cis* and *trans* pairing to create combinatorial complexity and expand the number of expressed class II molecules. Because of the enormous allelic diversity in the general population, most individuals are heterozygous at all of the class I and class II loci. Thus, most individuals express six classic class I molecules (two each of HLA-A, -B, and -C) and around eight class II molecules—two DP, two DR (more in the case of haplotypes with additional functional DRB genes), and up to four DQ (two *cis* and two *trans*).

OTHER GENES IN THE MHC

In addition to the class I and class II genes themselves, there are numerous genes interspersed among the HLA loci that have interesting and important immunologic functions. Our current concept of the function of MHC genes now encompasses many of these additional genes, some of which are also highly polymorphic. Indeed, direct comparison of the complete DNA sequences for two of the entire 4-Mb MHC regions from different haplotypes show >18,000 variations, encoding an extremely high potential for biologic diversity. Specific examples include the TAP and LMP genes, as discussed in more detail below, which encode molecules that participate in intermediate steps in the HLA class I biosynthetic pathway. Another set of HLA genes, DMA and DMB, perform an analogous function for the class II pathway. These genes encode an intracellular molecule that facilitates the proper complexing of HLA class II molecules with antigen (see below). The *HLA class III region* is a name given to a cluster of genes between the class I and class II complexes, which includes genes for the two closely related cytokines tumor necrosis factor (TNF)-α and lymphotoxin (TNF-β); the complement components C2, C4, and Bf; heat shock protein (HSP)70; and the enzyme 21-hydroxylase.

The class I genes HLA-A, -B, and -C are expressed in all nucleated cells, although generally to a higher degree on leukocytes than on nonleukocytes. In contrast, the class II genes show a more restricted distribution: HLA-DR and HLA-DP genes are constitutively expressed on most cells of the myeloid cell lineage, whereas all three class II gene families (HLA-DR, -DQ, and -DP) are inducible by certain stimuli provided by inflammatory cytokines such as interferon γ. Within the lymphoid lineage, expression of these class II genes is constitutive on B cells and inducible on human T cells. Most endothelial and epithelial cells in the body, including the vascular endothelium and the intestinal epithelium, are also inducible for class II gene expression. Thus, while these somatic tissues normally express only class I and not class II genes, during times of local inflammation they are recruited by cytokine stimuli to express class II genes as well, thereby becoming active participants in ongoing immune responses. Class II expression is controlled largely at the transcriptional level through a conserved set of promoter elements that interact with a protein known as *CIITA*. Cytokine-mediated induction of CIITA is a principal method by which tissue-specific expression of HLA gene expression is controlled. Other HLA genes involved in the immune response, such as TAP and LMP, are also susceptible to upregulation by signals such as interferon γ. Sequence data for the entire HLA region can be accessed on the Internet (e.g., *http://www.sanger.ac.uk/HGP/Chr6/MHC*). Many new genes have been discovered, the functions of which remain to be determined, as well as numerous microsatellite regions and other genetic elements. The gene density of the class II region is high, with approximately one protein encoded every 30 kb, and that of the class I and class III regions is even higher, with approximately one protein encoded every 15 kb.

LINKAGE DISEQUILIBRIUM

In addition to extensive polymorphism at the class I and class II loci, another characteristic feature of the HLA complex is *linkage disequilibrium*. This is formally defined as a deviation from Hardy-Weinberg equilibrium for alleles at linked loci. This is reflected in the very low recombination rates between certain loci within the HLA complex. For example, recombination between DR and DQ loci is almost never observed in family studies, and characteristic haplotypes with particular arrays of DR and DQ alleles are found in every population. Similarly, the complement components C2, C4, and Bf are almost invariably inherited together, and the alleles at these loci are found in characteristic haplotypes. In contrast, there is a recombinational hotspot between DQ and DP, which are separated by 1–2 cM of genetic distance, despite their close physical proximity. Certain extended haplotypes encompassing the interval from DQ into the class I region are commonly found, the most notable being the haplotype DR3-B8-A1, which is found, in whole or in part, in 10–30% of northern European Caucasians. It has been hypothesized that selective pressures may maintain linkage disequilibrium in HLA, but this remains to be determined. As discussed below under HLA and immunologic disease, one consequence of the phenomenon of linkage disequilibrium has been the resulting difficulty in assigning HLA-disease associations to a single allele at a single locus.

MHC STRUCTURE AND FUNCTION

Class I and class II molecules display a distinctive structural architecture, which contains specialized functional domains responsible for the unique genetic and immunologic properties of the HLA complex. The principal known function of both class I and class II HLA molecules is to bind antigenic peptides in order to present antigen to an appropriate T cell. The ability of a particular peptide to satisfactorily bind to an individual HLA molecule is a direct function of the molecular fit between the amino acid residues on the peptide with respect to the amino acid residues of the HLA molecule. The bound peptide forms a tertiary structure called the *MHC-peptide complex*, which communicates with T lymphocytes through binding to the T cell receptor (TCR) molecule. The first site of TCR-MHC-peptide interaction in the life of a T cell occurs in the thymus, where self-peptides are presented to developing thymocytes by MHC molecules expressed on thymic epithelium and hematopoietically derived antigen-presenting cells, which are primarily responsible for positive and negative selection, respectively (Chap. 1). Thus, the population of MHC–T cell complexes expressed in the thymus shapes the TCR repertoire. Mature T cells encounter MHC molecules in the periphery both in the maintenance of tolerance (Chap. 3) and in the initiation of immune responses. The MHC-peptide-TCR interaction is the central event in the initiation of most antigen-specific immune responses, since it is the structural determinant of the specificity. For potentially immunogenetic peptides, the ability of a given peptide to be generated and bound by an HLA molecule is a primary feature of whether or not an immune response to that peptide can be generated, and the repertoire of peptides that a particular individual's HLA molecules can bind exerts a major influence over the specificity of that individual's immune response.

When a TCR molecule binds to an HLA-peptide complex, it forms intermolecular contacts with both the antigenic peptide and with the HLA molecule itself. The outcome of this recognition event depends on the density and duration of the binding interaction, accounting for a dual specificity requirement for activation of the T cell. That is, the TCR must be specific both for the antigenic peptide and for the HLA molecule. The polymorphic nature of the presenting molecules, and the influence that this exerts on the peptide repertoire of each molecule, results in the phenomenon of *MHC restriction* of the T cell specificity for a given peptide. The binding of CD8 or CD4 molecules to the class I or class II molecule, respectively, also contributes to the interaction between the T cell and the HLA-peptide complex, by providing for the selective activation of the appropriate T cell.

CLASS I STRUCTURE

(Fig. 2-2B) As noted above, MHC class I molecules provide a cell-surface display of peptides derived from intracellular proteins, and they also provide the signal for self-recognition by NK cells. Surface-expressed class I molecules consist of an MHC-encoded 44-kD glycoprotein

heavy chain, a non-MHC-encoded 12-kD light chain β_2-microglobulin, and an antigenic peptide, typically 8–11 amino acids in length and derived from intracellularly produced protein. The heavy chain displays a prominent peptide-binding groove. In HLA-A and -B molecules, the groove is ~3 nm in length by 1.2 nm in maximum width (30 Å × 12 Å), whereas it is apparently somewhat wider in HLA-C. Antigenic peptides are noncovalently bound in an extended conformation within the peptide-binding groove, with both N- and C-terminal ends anchored in pockets within the groove (A and F pockets, respectively) and, in many cases, with a prominent kink, or arch, approximately one-third of the way from the N-terminus that elevates the peptide main chain off the floor of the groove.

A remarkable property of peptide binding by MHC molecules is the ability to form highly stable complexes with a wide array of peptide sequences. This is accomplished by a combination of peptide sequence–independent and peptide sequence–dependent bonding. The former consists of hydrogen bond and van der Waals interactions between conserved residues in the peptide-binding groove and charged or polar atoms along the peptide backbone. The latter is dependent upon the six side pockets that are formed by the irregular surface produced by protrusion of amino acid side chains from within the binding groove. The side chains lining the pockets interact with some of the peptide side chains. The sequence polymorphism among different class I alleles and isotypes predominantly affects the residues that line these pockets, and the interactions of these residues with peptide residues constitute the sequence-dependent bonding that confers a particular sequence "motif" on the range of peptides that can bind any given MHC molecule.

CLASS I BIOSYNTHESIS

(Fig. 2-3A) The biosynthesis of the classic MHC class I molecules reflects their role in presenting endogenous peptides. The heavy chain is cotranslationally inserted into the membrane of the endoplasmic reticulum (ER), where it becomes glycosylated and associates sequentially with the chaperone proteins calnexin and ERp57. It then forms a complex with β_2-microglobulin, and this complex associates with the chaperone calreticulin and the MHC-encoded molecule tapasin, which physically links the class I complex to TAP, the MHC-encoded transporter associated with antigen processing. Meanwhile, peptides generated within the cytosol from intracellular proteins by the multisubunit, multicatalytic proteasome complex are actively transported into the ER by TAP, where they are trimmed by a peptidase known as *ERAAP* (ER aminopeptidase associated with antigen processing). At this point, peptides with appropriate sequence complementarity bind specific class I molecules to form complete,

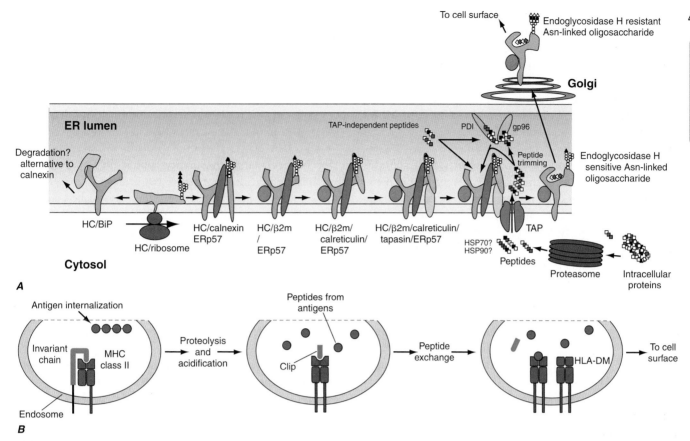

FIGURE 2-3

Biosynthesis of class I (*A*) and class II (*B*) molecules.
A. Nascent heavy chain (HC) becomes associated with β_2-microglobulin (β_2m) and peptide through interactions with a series of chaperones. Peptides generated by the proteasome are transported into the endoplasmic reticulum (ER) by TAP. Peptides undergo N-terminal trimming in the ER and become associated with chaperones, including gp96 and PDI. Once peptide binds to HC-β_2m, the HC-β_2m-peptide trimeric complex exits the ER and is transported by the secretory pathway to the cell surface. In the Golgi, the N-linked oligosaccharide undergoes maturation, with addition of sialic acid residues. Molecules are not necessarily drawn to scale. ***B.*** Pathway of HLA class II molecule assembly and antigen processing. After transport through the Golgi and post-Golgi compartment, the class II–invariant chain complex moves to an acidic endosome, where the invariant chain is proteolytically cleaved into fragments and displaced by antigenic peptides, facilitated by interactions with the DMA-DMB chaperone protein. This class II molecule–peptide complex is then transported to the cell surface.

folded heavy chain–β_2-microglobulin–peptide trimer complexes. These are transported rapidly from the ER, through the *cis*- and *trans*-Golgi where the N-linked oligosaccharide is further processed, and thence to the cell surface.

Most of the peptides transported by TAP are produced in the cytosol by proteolytic cleavage of intracellular proteins by the multisubunit, multicatalytic proteasome, and inhibitors of the proteasome dramatically reduce expression of class I–presented antigenic peptides. A thiol-dependent oxidoreductase ERp57, which mediates disulfide bond rearrangements, also appears to play an important role in folding the class I–peptide complex into a stable multicomponent molecule. The MHC-encoded proteasome subunits LMP2 and LMP7 may influence the spectrum of peptides produced but are not essential for proteasome function.

CLASS I FUNCTION

Peptide Antigen Presentation

On any given cell, a class I molecule occurs in 100,000–200,000 copies and binds several hundred to several thousand distinct peptide species. The vast majority of these peptides are self-peptides to which the host immune system is tolerant by one or more of the mechanisms that maintain tolerance, e.g., clonal deletion in the thymus or clonal anergy or clonal ignorance in the periphery (Chaps. 1 and 3). However, class I molecules bearing foreign peptides expressed in a permissive immunologic context activate CD8 T cells, which, if naïve, will then differentiate into cytolytic T lymphocytes (CTLs). These T cells and their progeny, through their $\alpha\beta$ TCRs, are then capable of Fas/CD95- and/or perforin-mediated cytotoxicity and/or cytokine secretion (Chap. 1) upon further encounter with the class I–peptide combination that originally activated it, and also with other combinations of class I molecule plus peptide that present a similar immunochemical stimulus to the TCR. As alluded to above, this phenomenon by which T cells recognize foreign antigens in the context of specific MHC alleles is termed *MHC restriction*, and the specific MHC molecule is termed the *restriction element*. The most common source of foreign peptides presented by class I molecules is viral infection, in the course of which peptides from viral proteins enter the class I pathway. The generation of a strong CTL response that destroys virally infected cells represents an important antigen-specific defense against many viral infections (Chap. 1). In the case of some viral infections—hepatitis B, for example—CTL-induced target cell apoptosis is thought to be a more important mechanism of tissue damage than any direct cytopathic effect of the virus itself. The importance of the class I pathway in the defense against viral infection is underscored by the identification of a number of viral products that interfere with the normal class I biosynthetic pathway and thus block the immunogenetic expression of viral antigens.

Other examples of intracellularly generated peptides that can be presented by class I molecules in an immunogenic manner include peptides derived from nonviral intracellular infectious agents (e.g., *Listeria*, *Plasmodium*), tumor antigens, minor histocompatibility antigens, and certain autoantigens. There are also situations in which cell surface–expressed class I molecules are thought to acquire and present exogenously derived peptides.

HLA Class I Receptors and NK Cell Recognition

(Chap. 1) NK cells, which play an important role in innate immune responses, are activated to cytotoxicity and cytokine secretion by contact with cells that lack MHC class I expression, and NK cell activation is inhibited by cells that express MHC class I. In humans, the recognition of class I molecules by NK cells is carried out by three classes of receptor families, the killer cell–inhibitory cell receptor (KIR) family, the leukocyte Ig-like receptor (LIR) family, and the CD94/NKG2 family. The KIR family, also called CD158, is encoded on chromosome 19q13.4. KIR gene nomenclature is based on the number of domains (2D or 3D) and the presence of long (L) or short (S) cytoplasmic domains. The KIR2DL1 and S1 molecules primarily recognize alleles of HLA-C, which possess a lysine at position 80 (HLA-Cw2,-4, -5, and -6), while the KIR2DL2/S2 and KIR2DL3/S3 families primarily recognize alleles of HLA-C with asparagine at this position (HLA-Cw1,-3, -7, and -8). The KIR3DL1 and S1 molecules predominantly recognize HLA-B alleles that fall into the HLA-Bw4 class determined by residues 77–83 in the α_1 domain

of the heavy chain, while the KIR3DL2 molecule is an inhibitory receptor for HLA-A*03. One of the KIR products, KIR2DL4, is known to be an activating receptor for HLA-G. The most common KIR haplotype in Caucasians contains one activating KIR and six inhibitory KIR genes, although there is a great deal of diversity in the population, with >100 different combinations. It appears that most individuals have at least one inhibitory KIR for a self-HLA class I molecule, providing a structural basis for NK cell target specificity, which helps prevent NK cells from attacking normal cells.

The LIR gene family (CD85, also called ILT) is encoded centromeric of the KIR locus on 19q13.4, and it encodes a variety of inhibitory immunoglobulin-like receptors expressed on many lymphocyte and other hematopoietic lineages. Interaction of LIR-1 (ILT2) with NK or T cells inhibits activation and cytotoxicity, mediated by many different HLA class I molecules, including HLA-G. HLA-F also appears to interact with LIR molecules, although the functional context for this is not understood.

The third family of NK receptors for HLA is encoded in the NK complex on chromosome 12p12.3-13.1 and consists of CD94 and five NKG2 genes, A/B, C, E/H, D, and F. These molecules are C-type (calcium-binding) lectins, and most function as disulfide-bonded heterodimers between CD94 and one of the NKG2 glycoproteins. The principle ligand of CD94/NKG2A receptors is the HLA-E molecule, complexed to a peptide derived from the signal sequence of classic HLA class I molecules and HLA-G. Thus, analogous to the way in which KIR receptors recognize HLA-C, the NKG2 receptor monitors self–class I expression, albeit indirectly through peptide recognition in the context of HLA-E. NKG2C, -E, and -H appear to have similar specificities but act as activating receptors. NKG2D is expressed as a homodimer and functions as an activating receptor expressed on NK cells, γδ TCR T cells, and activated CD8 T cells. When complexed with an adaptor called DAP10, NKG2D recognizes MIC-A and MIC-B molecules and activates the cytolytic response. NKG2D also binds a class of molecules known as *ULBP*, structurally related to class I molecules but not encoded in the MHC. The function of NK cells in immune responses is discussed in Chap. 1.

CLASS II STRUCTURE

(Fig. 2-2C) A specialized functional architecture similar to that of the class I molecules can be seen in the example of a class II molecule depicted in Fig. 2-2C, with an antigen-binding cleft arrayed above a supporting scaffold that extends the cleft toward the external cellular environment. However, in contrast to the HLA class I molecular structure, β_2-microglobulin is not associated with class II molecules. Rather, the class II molecule is a heterodimer, composed of a 29-kD α chain and a 34-kD β chain. The amino-terminal domains of each chain form the antigen-binding elements which, like the class I molecule, cradle a bound peptide in a groove bounded by extended α-helical loops, one encoded by the A (α chain) gene and one by the B (β chain) gene. Like the class I groove, the class II antigen-binding groove is punctuated by pockets that contact the side chains of amino acid residues of the bound peptide, but unlike the class I groove, it is open at both ends. Therefore, peptides bound by class II molecules vary greatly in length, since both the N- and C-terminal ends of the peptides can extend through the open ends of this groove. Approximately 11 amino acids within the bound peptide form intimate contacts with the class II molecule itself, with backbone hydrogen bonds and specific side chain interactions combining to provide, respectively, stability and specificity to the binding (**Fig. 2-4**).

The genetic polymorphisms that distinguish different class II genes correspond to changes in the amino acid composition of the class II molecule, and these variable sites are clustered predominantly around the pocket structures within the antigen-binding groove. As with class I, this is a critically important feature of the class II

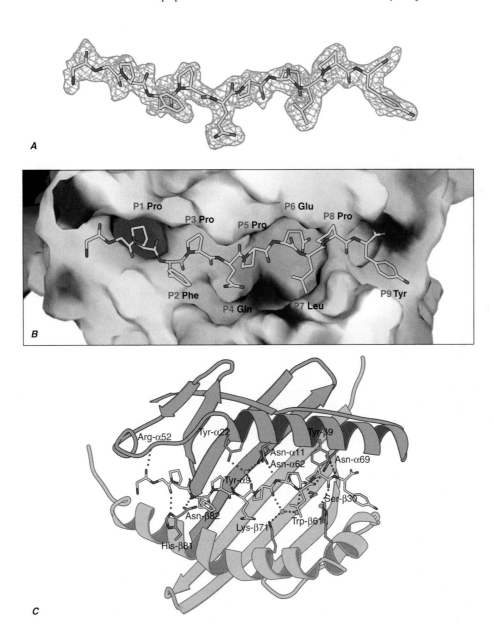

FIGURE 2-4

Specific intermolecular interactions determine peptide binding to MHC class II molecules. A short peptide sequence derived from alpha-gliadin (**A**) is accommodated within the MHC class II binding groove by specific interactions between peptide side chains (the P1–P9 residues illustrated in **B**) and corresponding pockets in the MHC class II structure. The latter are determined by the genetic polymorphisms of the MHC gene, in this case encoding an HLA-DQ2 molecule. **C.** This shows the extensive hydrogen bond and salt bridge network that tightly constrains the pMHC complex and presents the complex of antigen and restriction element for CD4 T cell recognition. (*From Kim et al.*)

molecule, which explains how genetically different individuals have functionally different HLA molecules.

BIOSYNTHESIS AND FUNCTION OF CLASS II MOLECULES

(Fig. 2-3B) The intracellular assembly of class II molecules occurs within a specialized compartmentalized pathway that differs dramatically from the class I pathway described above. As illustrated in Fig. 2-3B, the class II molecule assembles in the ER in association with a chaperone molecule, known as the *invariant chain*. The invariant chain performs at least two roles. First, it binds to the class II molecule and blocks the peptide-binding groove, thus preventing antigenic peptides from binding. This role of the invariant chain appears to account for one of the important differences between class I and class II MHC pathways, since it can explain why class I molecules present endogenous peptides from proteins newly synthesized in the ER but class II molecules generally do not. Second, the invariant chain contains molecular localization signals that direct the class II molecule to traffic into post-Golgi compartments known as *endosomes*, which develop into specialized acidic compartments where proteases cleave the invariant chain, and antigenic peptides can now occupy the class II groove. The specificity and tissue distribution of these proteases appear to be an important way in which the immune system regulates access to the peptide-binding groove and T cells become exposed to specific self-antigens. Differences in protease expression in the thymus and in the periphery may in part determine which specific peptide sequences comprise the peripheral repertoire for T cell recognition. It is at this stage in the intracellular pathway, after cleavage of the invariant chain, that the MHC-encoded DM molecule catalytically facilitates the exchange of peptides within the class II groove to help optimize the specificity and stability of the MHC-peptide complex.

Once this MHC-peptide complex is deposited in the outer cell membrane it becomes the target for T cell recognition via a specific TCR expressed on lymphocytes. Because the endosome environment contains internalized proteins retrieved from the extracellular environment, the class II–peptide complex often contains bound antigens that were originally derived from extracellular proteins. In this way, the class II peptide–loading pathway provides a mechanism for immune surveillance of the extracellular space. This appears to be an important feature that permits the class II molecule to bind foreign peptides, distinct from the endogenous pathway of class I–mediated presentation.

ROLE OF HLA IN TRANSPLANTATION

The development of modern clinical transplantation in the decades since the 1950s provided a major impetus for elucidation of the HLA system, as allograft survival is highest when donor and recipient are HLA-identical. Although many molecular events participate in transplantation rejection, allogeneic differences at class I and class II loci play a major role. Class I molecules can promote T cell responses in several different ways. In the cases of allografts in which the host and donor are mismatched at one or more class I loci, host T cells can be activated by classic *direct alloreactivity*, in which the antigen receptors on the host T cells react with the foreign class I molecule expressed on the allograft. In this situation, the response of any given TCR may be dominated by the allogeneic MHC molecule, the peptide bound to it, or some combination of the two. Another type of host antigraft T cell response involves the uptake and processing of donor MHC antigens by host antigen-presenting cells and the subsequent presentation of the resulting peptides by host MHC molecules. This mechanism is termed *indirect alloreactivity*.

In the case of class I molecules on allografts that are shared by the host and the donor, a host T cell response may still be triggered because of peptides that are presented by the class I molecules of the graft but not of the host. The most common basis for the existence of these endogenous antigen peptides, called *minor histocompatibility antigens*, is a genetic difference between donor and host at a non-MHC locus encoding the structural gene for the protein from which the peptide is derived. These loci are termed *minor histocompatibility loci*, and nonidentical individuals typically differ at many such loci. CD4 T cells react to analogous class II variation, both direct and indirect, and class II differences alone are sufficient to drive allograft rejection.

ASSOCIATION OF HLA ALLELES WITH SUSCEPTIBILITY TO DISEASE

It has long been postulated that infectious agents provide the driving force for the allelic diversification seen in the HLA system. An important corollary of this hypothesis is that resistance to specific pathogens may differ between individuals, based on HLA genotype. Observations of specific HLA genes associated with resistance to malaria or dengue fever, persistence of hepatitis B, and to disease progression in HIV infection are consistent with this model. For example, failure to clear persistent hepatitis B or C viral infection may reflect the inability of particular HLA molecules to present viral antigens effectively to T cells. Similarly, both protective and susceptible HLA allelic associations have been described for human papilloma virus–associated cervical neoplasia, implicating the MHC as an influence in mediating viral clearance in this form of cancer.

Pathogen diversity is probably also the major selective pressure favoring HLA heterozygosity. The extraordinary scope of HLA allelic diversity increases the likelihood that most new pathogens will be recognized by some HLA molecules, helping to assure immune fitness to the host. However, another consequence of diversification is that some alleles may become preferentially selective for recognition of self-antigens as well. Indeed, particular HLA alleles are strongly associated with certain disease states, particularly for some common autoimmune diseases (Chap. 3). By comparing allele frequencies in patients with any particular disease and in control populations, >100 such associations have been identified, some of which are listed in (Table 2-1). The strength of genetic association is reflected in the term *relative risk*,

TABLE 2-1

SIGNIFICANT HLA CLASS I AND CLASS II ASSOCIATIONS WITH DISEASE

	MARKER	GENE	STRENGTH OF ASSOCIATION
Spondyloarthropathies			
Ankylosing spondylitis	B27	B*2702, -04, -05	++++
Reiter's syndrome	B27		++++
Acute anterior uveitis	B27		+++
Reactive arthritis (*Yersinia, Salmonella, Shigella, Chlamydia*)	B27		+++
Psoriatic spondylitis	B27		+++
Collagen-Vascular Diseases			
Juvenile arthritis, pauciarticular	DR8		++
	DR5		++
Rheumatoid arthritis	DR4	DRB1*0401, -04, -05	+++
Sjögren's syndrome	DR3		++
Systemic lupus erythematosus			
Caucasian	DR3		+
Japanese	DR2		++
Autoimmune Gut and Skin			
Gluten-sensitive enteropathy (celiac disease)	DQ2	DQA1*0501	+++
		DQB1*0201	
Chronic active hepatitis	DR3		++
Dermatitis herpetiformis	DR3		+++
Psoriasis vulgaris	Cw6		++
Pemphigus vulgaris	DR4	DRB1*0402	+++
	DQ1	DQB1*0503	
Bullous pemphigoid variant	DQ7	DQB1*0301	+
Autoimmune Endocrine			
Type 1 diabetes mellitus	DR4	DQB1*0302	+++
	DQ8	DRB1*0401, -04	
	DR3		++
	DR2	DQB1*0602	—ᵃ
Hyperthyroidism (Graves')	B8		+
	DR3		+
Hyperthyroidism (Japanese)	B35		+
Adrenal insufficiency	DR3		++
Autoimmune Neurologic			
Myasthenia gravis	B8		+
	DR3		+
Multiple sclerosis	DR2	DRB1*1501	++
		DRB5*0101	
Other			
Behçet's disease	B51		++
Congenital adrenal hyperplasia	B47	21·OH (Cyp21B)	+++
Narcolepsy	DR2	DQB1*0602	++++
Goodpasture's syndrome (anti-GBM)	DR2		++

ᵃStrong negative association; i.e., genetic association with protection from diabetes.

an arthritogenic peptide; it may favor the expansion of a type of self-reactive T lymphocyte; or it may itself form part of the pMHC ligand recognized by TCR that initiates synovial tissue recognition.

MOLECULAR MECHANISMS FOR HLA-DISEASE ASSOCIATIONS

As noted above, HLA molecules play a key role in the selection and establishment of the antigen-specific T cell repertoire and a major role in the subsequent activation of those T cells during the initiation of an immune response. Precise genetic polymorphisms characteristic of individual alleles dictate the specificity of these interactions and thereby instruct and guide antigen-specific immune events. These same genetically determined pathways are therefore implicated in disease pathogenesis when specific HLA genes are responsible for autoimmune disease susceptibility.

The fate of developing T cells within the thymus is determined by the affinity of interaction between T cell receptor and HLA molecules bearing self-peptides, and thus the particular HLA types of each individual control the precise specificity of the T cell repertoire (Chap. 1). The primary basis for HLA-associated disease susceptibility may well lie within this thymic maturation pathway. The positive selection of potentially autoreactive T cells, based on the presence of specific HLA susceptibility genes, may establish the threshold for disease risk in a particular individual.

At the time of onset of a subsequent immune response, the primary role of the HLA molecule is to bind peptide and present it to antigen-specific T cells. The HLA complex can therefore be viewed as encoding genetic determinants of precise immunologic activation events. Antigenic peptides that bind particular HLA molecules are capable of stimulating T cell immune responses; peptides that do not bind are not presented to T cells and are not immunogenic. This genetic control of the immune response is mediated by the polymorphic sites within the HLA antigen–binding groove that interact with the bound peptides. In autoimmune and immune-mediated diseases, it is likely that specific tissue antigens that are targets for pathogenic lymphocytes are complexed with the HLA molecules encoded by specific susceptibility alleles. In autoimmune diseases with an infectious etiology, it is likely that immune responses to peptides derived from the initiating pathogen are bound and presented by particular HLA molecules to activate T lymphocytes that play a triggering or contributory role in disease pathogenesis. The concept that early events in disease initiation are triggered by specific HLA-peptide complexes offers some prospects for therapeutic intervention, since it may be possible to design compounds that interfere with the formation or function of specific HLA-peptide–T cell receptor interactions.

When considering mechanisms of HLA associations with immune response and disease, it is good to remember that just as HLA genetics are complex, so are the mechanisms likely to be heterogeneous. Immune-mediated disease is a multistep process in which one of the HLA-associated functions is to establish a repertoire of potentially reactive T cells, while another HLA-associated function is to provide the essential peptide-binding specificity for T cell recognition. For diseases with multiple HLA genetic associations, it is possible that both of these interactions occur and synergize to advance an accelerated pathway of disease.

FURTHER READINGS

Brewerton DA: Discovery: HLA and disease. Curr Opin Rheumatol 15:369, 2003

Colbert RA: The immunobiology of HLA-B27: Variations on a theme. Curr Mol Med 4:21, 2004

Hertl M et al: T cell control in autoimmune bullous skin disorders. J Clin Invest 116:1159, 2006

Jones EY et al: MHC class II proteins and disease: A structural perspective. Nat Rev Immunol 6:271, 2006

Kim C et al: Structural basis for HLA-DQ2-mediated presentation of gluten epitopes in celiac disease. Proc Natl Acad Sci USA 101:4175, 2004

Martin M, Carrington M: Immunogenetics of viral infections. Curr Opin Immunol 17:510, 2005

Nepom GT: Major histocompatibility complex-directed susceptibility to rheumatoid arthritis. Adv Immunol 68:315, 1998

———, Kwok WW: Molecular basis for HLA-DQ associations with IDDM. Diabetes 47:1177, 1998

Shiina T et al: An update of the HLA genomic region, locus information and disease associations: 2004. Tissue Antigens 64:631, 2004

Taurog JD: The mystery of HLA B27: If it isn't one thing, it's another. Arthritis Rheum 56:2478, 2007

Trowsdale J: HLA genomics in the third millennium. Curr Opin Immunol 17:498, 2005

Wellcome Trust Case Control Consortium et al: Association scan of 14,500 nonsynonymous SNPs in four diseases identifies autoimmunity variants. Nat Genet 39:1329, 2007

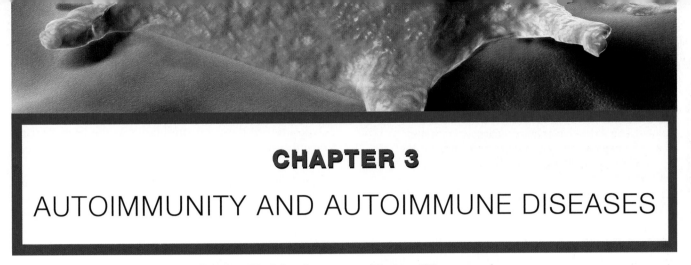

CHAPTER 3

AUTOIMMUNITY AND AUTOIMMUNE DISEASES

Peter E. Lipsky ■ **Betty Diamond**

One of the classically accepted features of the immune system is the capacity to distinguish self from nonself. Although animals are able to recognize and generate reactions to a vast array of foreign materials, most do not mount immune responses to self-antigens under ordinary circumstances and thus are tolerant to self. Whereas recognition of self plays an important role in shaping both the T cell and B cell repertoires of immune receptors and an essential role in the recognition of nominal antigen by T cells, the development of potentially harmful immune responses to self-antigens is, in general, precluded. Autoimmunity therefore represents the end result of the breakdown of one or more of the basic mechanisms regulating immune tolerance.

The essential feature of an autoimmune disease is that tissue injury is caused by the immunologic reaction of the organism with its own tissues. Autoimmunity, on the other hand, refers merely to the presence of antibodies or T lymphocytes that react with self-antigens, and does not necessarily imply that the development of self-reactivity has pathogenic consequences.

Autoimmunity may be seen in normal individuals and in higher frequency in normal older people. In addition, autoreactivity may develop during various infectious conditions. The expression of autoimmunity may be self-limited, as occurs with many infectious processes, or persistent. When autoimmunity is induced by an inciting event, such as infection or tissue damage from trauma or infarction, there may or may not be ensuing pathology. Even in the presence of organ pathology, it may be difficult to determine whether the damage is mediated by autoreactivity. Thus, the presence of self-reactivity may be either the cause or a consequence of an ongoing pathologic process.

MECHANISMS OF AUTOIMMUNITY

Since Ehrlich first postulated the existence of mechanisms to prevent the generation of self-reactivity in 1900, ideas concerning the nature of this inhibition have developed in parallel with the progressive increase in understanding of the immune system. Burnet's clonal selection theory included the idea that interaction of lymphoid cells with their specific antigens during fetal or early postnatal life would lead to elimination of such "forbidden clones." This idea became untenable, however, when it was shown by a number of investigators that autoimmune diseases could be induced by simple immunization procedures, that autoantigen-binding cells could be demonstrated easily in the circulation of normal individuals, and that self-limited autoimmune phenomena frequently developed during infections. These observations indicated that clones of cells capable of responding to autoantigens were present in the repertoire of antigen-reactive cells in normal adults and suggested that mechanisms in addition to clonal deletion were responsible for preventing their activation.

TABLE 3-1

MECHANISMS PREVENTING AUTOIMMUNITY
I. Sequestration of self-antigen
II. Generation and maintenance of tolerance
A. Central deletion of autoreactive lymphocytes
B. Peripheral anergy of autoreactive lymphocytes
C. Receptor replacement by autoreactive lymphocytes
III. Regulatory mechanisms

Currently, three general processes are thought to be involved in the maintenance of selective unresponsiveness to autoantigens (**Table 3-1**): (1) sequestration of self-antigens, rendering them inaccessible to the immune system; (2) specific unresponsiveness (tolerance or anergy) of relevant T or B cells; and (3) limitation of potential reactivity by regulatory mechanisms.

Derangements of these normal processes may predispose to the development of autoimmunity (**Table 3-2**). In general, these abnormal responses relate to stimulation by exogenous agents, usually bacterial or viral, or endogenous abnormalities in the cells of the immune system. Microbial superantigens, such as staphylococcal protein A and staphylococcal enterotoxins, are substances that can stimulate a broad range of T and B cells based upon specific interactions with selected families of immune receptors, irrespective of their antigen specificity. If autoantigen-reactive T and/or B cells express these receptors, autoimmunity might develop. Alternatively, molecular mimicry or cross-reactivity between a microbial product and a self-antigen might lead to activation of autoreactive lymphocytes. One of the best

TABLE 3-2

MECHANISMS OF AUTOIMMUNITY
I. Exogenous
A. Molecular mimicry
B. Superantigenic stimulation
C. Microbial adjuvanticity
II. Endogenous
A. Altered antigen presentation
1. Loss of immunologic privilege
2. Presentation of novel or crytic epitopes (epitope spreading)
3. Alteration of self-antigen
4. Enhanced function of antigen-presenting cells
a. Costimulatory molecule expression
b. Cytokine production
B. Increased T cell help
1. Cytokine production
2. Co-stimulatory molecules
C. Increased B cell function
D. Apoptotic defects
E. Cytokine imbalance
F. Altered immunoregulation

examples of autoreactivity and autoimmune disease resulting from molecular mimicry is rheumatic fever, in which antibodies to the M protein of streptococci cross-react with myosin, laminin, and other matrix proteins. Deposition of these autoantibodies in the heart initiates an inflammatory response. Molecular mimicry between microbial proteins and host tissues has been reported in Type 1 diabetes mellitus, rheumatoid arthritis, and multiple sclerosis. The capacity of nonspecific stimulation of the immune system to predispose to the development of autoimmunity has been explored in a number of models; one is provided by the effect of adjuvants on the production of autoimmunity. Autoantigens become much more immunogenic when administered with adjuvant. It is presumed that infectious agents may be able to overcome self-tolerance because they possess molecules, such as bacterial endotoxin, that have adjuvant-like effects on the immune system by stimulating cells through Toll-like receptors.

Endogenous derangements of the immune system may also contribute to the loss of immunologic tolerance to self-antigens and the development of autoimmunity (Table 3-2). Many autoantigens reside in immunologically privileged sites, such as the brain or the anterior chamber of the eye. These sites are characterized by the inability of engrafted tissue to elicit immune responses. Immunologic privilege results from a number of events, including the limited entry of proteins from those sites into lymphatics, the local production of immunosuppressive cytokines such as transforming growth factor β, and the local expression of molecules such as Fas ligand that can induce apoptosis of activated T cells. Lymphoid cells remain in a state of immunologic ignorance (neither activated nor anergized) to proteins expressed uniquely in immunologically privileged sites. If the privileged site is damaged by trauma or inflammation, or if T cells are activated elsewhere, proteins expressed at this site can become the targets of immunologic assault. Such an event may occur in multiple sclerosis and sympathetic ophthalmia, in which antigens uniquely expressed in the brain and eye, respectively, become the target of activated T cells.

Alterations in antigen presentation may also contribute to autoimmunity. This may occur by epitope spreading, in which protein determinants (*epitopes*) not routinely seen by lymphocytes (*cryptic epitopes*) are recognized as a result of immunologic reactivity to associated molecules. For example, animals immunized with one protein component of a multimolecular complex may be induced to produce antibodies to the other components of the complex. Finally, inflammation, drug exposure, or normal senescence may cause a primary chemical alteration in proteins, resulting in the generation of immune responses that cross-react with normal self-proteins. Alterations in the availability and presentation of autoantigens may be important components of immunoreactivity in certain models of organ-specific autoimmune diseases. In addition, these factors may be relevant in understanding the pathogenesis of various drug-induced autoimmune conditions. However, the diversity of autoreactivity manifest in non–organ-specific systemic autoimmune diseases suggests that these conditions might result from a more general activation of the immune system rather than from an alteration in individual self-antigens.

A number of experimental models have suggested that intense stimulation of T lymphocytes can produce non-specific signals that bypass the need for antigen-specific helper T cells and lead to polyclonal B cell activation with the formation of multiple autoantibodies. For example, antinuclear, antierythrocyte, and antilymphocyte antibodies are produced during the chronic graft-versus-host reaction. In addition, true autoimmune diseases, including autoimmune hemolytic anemia and immune complex–mediated glomerulonephritis, can also be induced in this manner. While it is clear that such diffuse activation of helper T cell activity can cause autoimmunity, nonspecific stimulation of B lymphocytes can also lead to the production of autoantibodies. Thus, the administration of polyclonal B cell activators, such as bacterial endotoxin, to normal mice leads to the production of a number of autoantibodies, including those directed to DNA and IgG (rheumatoid factor).

Aberrant selection of the B or T cell repertoire at the time of antigen receptor expression can also predispose to autoimmunity. For example, B cell immunodeficiency caused by an absence of the B cell receptor–associated kinase, Bruton's tyrosine kinase, leads to X-linked agammaglobulinemia. This syndrome is characterized by reduced B cell activation, but also by diminished negative selection of autoreactive B cells, resulting in increased autoreactivity within a deficient B cell repertoire. Likewise, negative selection of autoreactive T cells in the thymus requires expression of the autoimmune regulator (AIRE) gene that enables the expression of tissue-specific proteins in thymic medullary epithelial cells. Peptides from these proteins are expressed in the context of MHC molecules and mediate the elimination of autoreactive T cells. The absence of AIRE gene expression leads to a failure of negative selection of autoreactive cells, autoantibody production, and severe inflammatory destruction of multiple organs. Individuals deficient in AIRE gene expression develop autoimmune polyendocrinopathy-candidiasis-ectodermal dystrophy (APECED).

Primary alterations in the activity of T and/or B cells, cytokine imbalances, or defective immunoregulatory circuits may also contribute to the emergence of autoimmunity. For example, decreased apoptosis, as can be seen in animals with defects in Fas (CD95) or Fas ligand, or in patients with related abnormalities, can be associated with the development of autoimmunity. Similarly, diminished production of tumor necrosis factor (TNF) and interleukin (IL)-10 has been reported to be associated with the development of autoimmunity.

Autoimmunity may also result from an abnormality of immunoregulatory mechanisms. Observations made in both human autoimmune disease and animal models suggest that defects in the generation and expression of regulatory T cell activity may allow for the production of autoimmunity. It has recently been appreciated that the IPEX (immunodysregulation, polyendocrinopathy, enteropathy X-linked) syndrome results from the failure to express the FOXP3 gene, which encodes a molecule critical in the differentiation of regulatory T cells. Administration of normal regulatory T cells or factors derived from them can prevent the development of autoimmune disease in rodent models of autoimmunity.

It should be apparent that no single mechanism can explain all the varied manifestations of autoimmunity. Furthermore, genetic evaluation has shown that a number of abnormalities often need to converge to induce an autoimmune disease. Additional factors that appear to be important determinants in the induction of autoimmunity include age, sex (many autoimmune diseases are far more common in women), genetic background, exposure to infectious agents, and environmental contacts. How all of these disparate factors affect the capacity to develop self-reactivity is currently being intensively investigated.

GENETIC CONSIDERATIONS

Evidence in humans that there are susceptibility genes for autoimmunity comes from family studies and especially from studies of twins. Studies in Type 1 diabetes mellitus, rheumatoid arthritis, multiple sclerosis, and systemic lupus erythematosus (SLE) have shown that approximately 15–30% of pairs of monozygotic twins show disease concordance, compared with <5% of dizygotic twins. The occurrence of different autoimmune diseases within the same family has suggested that certain susceptibility genes may predispose to a variety of autoimmune diseases. Genetic mapping has begun to identify chromosomal regions that predispose to specific autoimmune diseases. One gene is a phosphatase expressed by a variety of hematopoietic cells that downregulates antigen receptor–mediated stimulation, PTPN22. A loss-of-function polymorphism of this gene is associated with both Type 1 diabetes mellitus and rheumatoid arthritis in some populations. In addition to this evidence from humans, certain inbred mouse strains reproducibly develop specific spontaneous or experimentally induced autoimmune diseases, whereas others do not. These findings have led to an extensive search for genes that determine susceptibility to autoimmune disease.

The most consistent association for susceptibility to autoimmune disease has been with particular alleles of the major histocompatibility complex (MHC). It has been suggested that the association of MHC genotype with autoimmune disease relates to differences in the ability of different allelic variations of MHC molecules to present autoantigenic peptides to autoreactive T cells. An alternative hypothesis involves the role of MHC alleles in shaping the T cell receptor repertoire during T cell ontogeny in the thymus. Additionally, specific MHC gene products may be themselves the source of peptides that can be recognized by T cells. Cross-reactivity between such MHC peptides and peptides derived from proteins produced by common microbes may trigger autoimmunity by molecular mimicry. However, MHC genotype alone does not determine the development of autoimmunity. Identical twins are far more likely to develop the same autoimmune disease than MHC-identical nontwin siblings, suggesting that genetic factors other than the MHC also affect disease susceptibility. Recent studies of the genetics of Type 1 diabetes mellitus, SLE, rheumatoid arthritis, and multiple sclerosis in humans and mice have shown that there are several independently segregating disease susceptibility loci in addition to the MHC.

There is evidence that several other genes are important in increasing susceptibility to autoimmune disease. In humans, inherited homozygous deficiency of the early proteins of the classic pathway of complement (C1, C4, or C2) is very strongly associated with the development of SLE. In mice and humans, abnormalities in the genes encoding proteins involved in the regulation of apoptosis, including Fas (CD95, tumor necrosis factor receptor superfamily 6) and Fas ligand (CD95 ligand; CD178, tumor necrosis factor ligand superfamily 6), are strongly associated with the development of autoimmunity. There is also evidence that inherited variation in the level of expression of certain cytokines, such as TNF or IL-10, may also increase susceptibility to autoimmune disease.

A further important factor in disease susceptibility is the hormonal status of the patient. Many autoimmune diseases show a strong sex bias, which appears in most cases to relate to the hormonal status of women.

IMMUNOPATHOGENIC MECHANISMS IN AUTOIMMUNE DISEASES

The mechanisms of tissue injury in autoimmune diseases can be divided into antibody-mediated and cell-mediated processes. Representative examples are listed in Table 3-3.

The pathogenicity of autoantibodies can be mediated through several mechanisms, including opsonization of soluble factors or cells, activation of an inflammatory cascade via the complement system, and interference with the physiologic function of soluble molecules or cells.

In autoimmune thrombocytopenic purpura, opsonization of platelets targets them for elimination by phagocytes. Likewise, in autoimmune hemolytic anemia, binding of immunoglobulin to red cell membranes leads to phagocytosis and lysis of the opsonized cell. Goodpasture's syndrome, a disease characterized by lung hemorrhage and severe glomerulonephritis, represents an example of antibody binding leading to local activation

TABLE 3-3

MECHANISMS OF TISSUE DAMAGE IN AUTOIMMUNE DISEASE			
EFFECTOR	**MECHANISM**	**TARGET**	**DISEASE**
Autoantibody	Blocking or inactivation	α (Chain of the nicotinic acetylcholine receptor	Myasthenia gravis
		Phospholipid–β₂-glycoprotein 1 complex	Antiphospholipid syndrome
		Insulin receptor	Insulin-resistant diabetes mellitus
		Intrinsic factor	Pernicious anemia
	Stimulation	TSH receptor (LATS)	Graves' disease
		Proteinase-3 (ANCA)	Wegener's granulomatosis
		Epidermal cadherin₁ Desmoglein 3	Pemphigus vulgaris
	Complement activation	α₃ Chain of collagen IV	Goodpasture's syndrome
	Immune-complex formation	Double-strand DNA Ig	Systemic lupus erythematosus Rheumatoid arthritis
	Opsonization	Platelet GpIIb:IIIa Rh antigens, I antigen	Autoimmune thrombocytopenic purpura Autoimmune hemolytic anemia
	Antibody-dependent cellular cytotoxicity	Thyroid peroxidase, thyroglobulin	Hashimoto's thyroiditis
T cells	Cytokine production	?	Rheumatoid arthritis, multiple sclerosis, Type 1 diabetes mellitus
	Cellular cytotoxicity	?	Type 1 diabetes mellitus

Note: ANCA, antineutrophil cytoplasmic antibody; LATS, long-acting thyroid stimulator; TSH, thyroid-stimulating hormone.

for T or B cell activation, by eliminating the effector T cells or B cells, or by using autoantigen itself to induce tolerance. One major advance in inhibiting effector mechanisms has been the introduction of cytokine blockade, targeting TNF or IL-1 receptor, which appears to limit organ damage in some diseases. Biologicals that interface with T cell activation (abatacept) or deplete B cells (rituximab) have also recently been approved for the treatment of rheumatoid arthritis. Therapies that prevent target organ damage or support target organ function remain an important therapeutic approach to autoimmune disease.

FURTHER READINGS

BANCHEREAU J, PASCUAL V, PALUCKA AK: Autoimmunity through cytokine-induced dendritic cell activation. Immunity 20:539, 2004

BECHLER EC et al: Gene expression profiling in human autoimmunity. Immunol Rev 210:120, 2006

CARLONT VE et al: PTPN22 genetic variation: Evidence for multiple variants associated with rheumatoid arthritis. Am J Hum Genet 77:567, 2005

CHEN M et al: Dendritic cell apoptosis in the maintenance of immune tolerance. Science 311(5764):1160, 2006

CHRISTENSEN SR et al: Toll-like receptor 9 controls anti-DNA autoantibody production in murine lupus. J Exp Med 202:321, 2005

FIJINAMI RS et al: Molecular mimicry, bystander activation, or viral persistence: Infections and autoimmune disease. Clin Microbiol Rev 19:80, 2006

FRANCO A, ALBANI S: Translating the concept of suppressor/regulatory T cells to clinical applications. Int Rev Immunol 25:27, 2006

GEULD SB et al: Silencing of autoreactive B cells by anergy: A fresh perspective. Curr Opin Immunol 18:292, 2006

HINKS A et al: Association between PTPN22 gene and rheumatoid arthritis and juvenile idiopathic arthritis in a UK population: Further support that PTPN22 is an autoimmunity gene. Arthritis Rheum 52:1694, 2005

HOYNE GF, GOODNOW CC: The use of genomewide ENU mutagenesis screens to unravel complex mammalian traits: Identifying genes that regulate organ-specific and systemic autoimmunity. Immunol Rev 210:27, 2006

JIANG W et al: Modifier loci condition autoimmunity provoked by AIRE deficiency. J Exp Med 202:805, 2005

KANG HK, DATTA SK: Regulatory T cells in lupus. Int Rev Immunol 25(1–2):5, 2006

KELLY KM et al: "Endogenous adjuvant" activity of the RNA components of lupus autoantigens Sm/RNP and Ro 60. Arthritis Rheum 54:1557, 2006

KIROU KA et al: Soluble mediators as therapeutic targets in systemic lupus erythematosus: Cytokines, immunoglobulin receptors, and the complement system. Rheum Dis Clin North Am 32:103, 2006

KOCHI Y et al: A functional variant in the FCRL3, encoding Fc receptor-like 3, is associated with rheumatoid arthritis and several autoimmunities. Nat Genet 37:478, 2005

LARSEN CE, ALPER CA: The genetics of HLA-associated disease. Curr Opin Immunol 16:660, 2004

LEE E, SINHA AA: T cell targeted immunotherapy for autoimmune disease. Autoimmunity 38:577, 2005

MAHONEY JA, ROSE A: Apoptosis and autoimmunity. Curr Opin Immunol 17:583, 2005

MARTIN F, CHAN AC: B cell immunobiology in disease: Evolving concepts from the clinic. Annu Rev Immunol 24:467, 2006

MCCLAIN MT et al: Early events in lupus humoral autoimmunity suggest initiation through molecular mimicry. Nat Med 11:85, 2005

NOTARANGELO LD et al: Immunodeficiencies with autoimmune consequences. Adv Immunol 89:321, 2006

OCHES HD et al: FOXP3 acts as a rheostat of the immune response. Immunol Rev 203:156, 2005

OKAZAKI T, WANG J: PD-1/PD-1 pathway and autoimmunity. Autoimmunity 38:353, 2005

OLIVEIRA JB, FLEISHER T: Autoimmune lymphoproliferative syndrome. Curr Opin Allergy Clin Immunol 4:497, 2004

PRESCOTT NJ et al: A general autoimmunity gene (PTPN22) is not associated with inflammatory bowel disease in a British population. Tissue Antigens 66:318, 2005

RICE JS et al: Molecular mimicry: Anti-DNA antibodies bind microbial and nonnucleic acid self-antigens. Curr Top Microbiol Immunol 296:137, 2005

SEELEN MA et al: Role of complement in innate and autoimmunity. J Nephrol 18:642, 2005

SHEPSHELOVICH D, SHOENFELD Y: Prediction and prevention of autoimmune diseases: Additional aspects of the mosaic of autoimmunity. Lupus 15:183, 2006

SHERIFF A et al: Apoptosis and systemic lupus erythematosus. Rheum Dis Clin North Am 30:505, 2004

SIGAL LH: Protecting against autoimmunity-tolerance: Mechanisms of negative selection in the thymus. J Clin Rheumatol 12:99, 2006

VILLASENOR J et al: Molecular insights into an autoimmune disease. Immunol Rev 204:156, 2005

YOUINOU P et al: B lymphocytes on the front line of autoimmunity. Autoimmun Rev 5:215, 2006

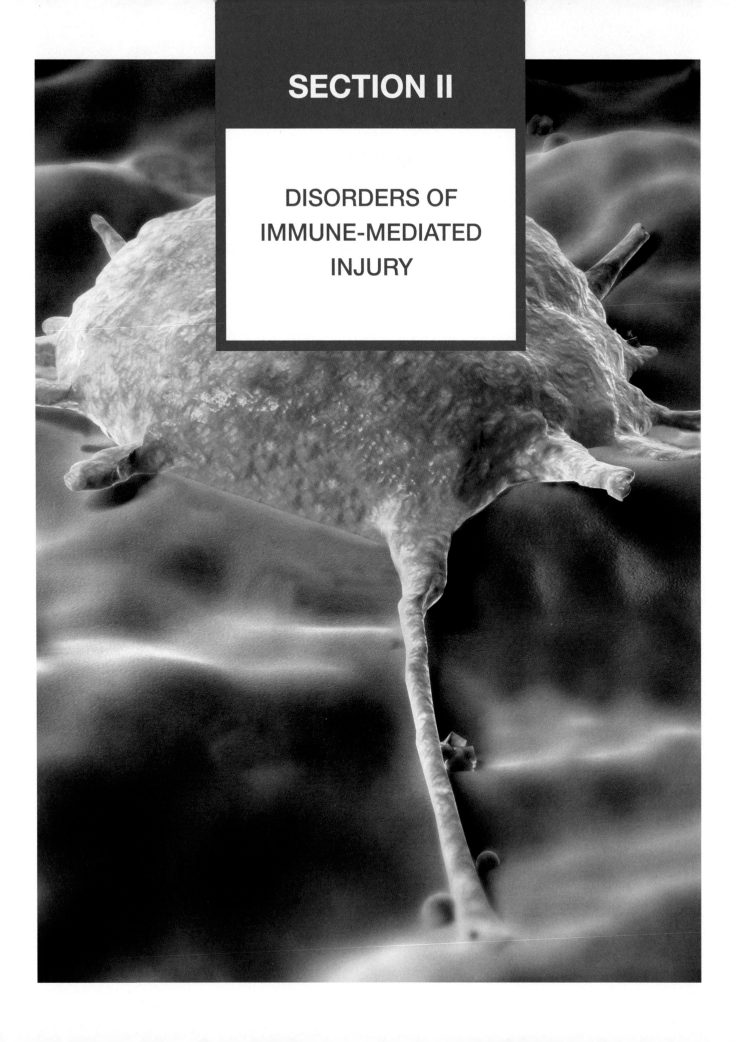

SECTION II

DISORDERS OF IMMUNE-MEDIATED INJURY

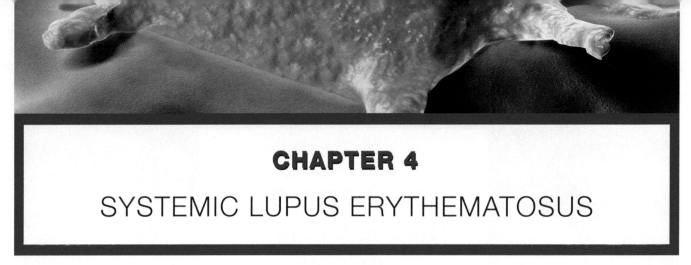

CHAPTER 4
SYSTEMIC LUPUS ERYTHEMATOSUS

Bevra Hannahs Hahn

DEFINITION AND PREVALENCE

Systemic lupus erythematosus (SLE) is an autoimmune disease in which organs and cells undergo damage mediated by tissue-binding autoantibodies and immune complexes. Ninety percent of patients are women of child-bearing years; people of both sexes, all ages, and all ethnic groups are susceptible. Prevalence of SLE in the United States is 15–50 per 100,000; the highest prevalence among ethnic groups studied is in African Americans.

PATHOGENESIS AND ETIOLOGY

The proposed pathogenic mechanisms of SLE are illustrated in **Fig. 4-1**. Interactions between susceptibility genes and environmental factors result in abnormal immune responses. Those responses include (1) activation of innate immunity (dendritic cells) by CpG DNA, DNA in immune complexes, and RNA in RNA/protein self-antigens; (2) lowered activation thresholds of adaptive immunity cells (antigen-specific T and B lymphocytes); (3) ineffective regulatory and inhibitory CD4+ and CD8+ T cells; and (4) reduced clearance of apoptotic cells and of immune complexes. Self-antigens (nucleosomal DNA/protein; RNA/protein in Sm, Ro, and La; phospholipids) are available for recognition by the immune system in surface blebs of apoptotic cells; thus antigens, autoantibodies, and immune complexes persist for prolonged periods of time, allowing inflammation and disease to develop. Immune activation of circulating and tissue-bound cells is accompanied by increased secretion of proinflammatory tumor necrosis factor (TNF) α and type 1 and 2 interferons (IFNs), and the B cell–driving cytokines B lymphocyte stimulator (BLyS) and interleukin (IL)-10. Upregulation of genes induced by interferons is a genetic "signature" of SLE. However, lupus T and natural killer (NK) cells fail to produce enough IL-2 and transforming growth factor (TGF) to induce regulatory CD4+ and inhibitory CD8+ T cells. The result of these abnormalities is sustained production of pathogenic autoantibodies (referred to in Fig. 4-1 and described in **Table 4-1**) and immune complexes, which bind to target tissues, with activation of complement and phagocytic cells that recognize Ig-coated circulating blood cells. Activation of complement and immune cells leads to release of chemotaxins, cytokines, chemokines, vasoactive peptides, and destructive enzymes. In the setting of chronic inflammation, accumulation of growth factors and products of chronic oxidation contribute to irreversible tissue damage in glomeruli, arteries, lungs, and other tissues.

SLE is a multigenic disease. In most genetically susceptible individuals, normal alleles of multiple normal genes each contribute a small amount to abnormal immune responses; if enough variations accumulate, disease results. Some predisposing genes confirmed in at least two independent cohorts are listed in Fig. 4-1. Homozygous

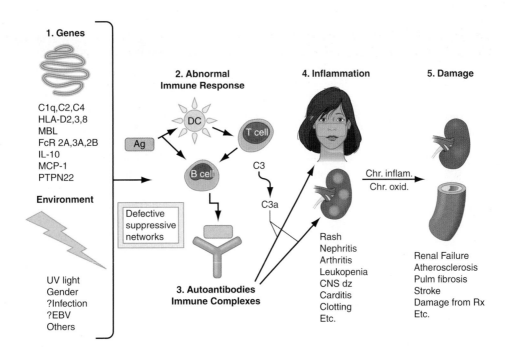

FIGURE 4-1

Pathogenesis of SLE. Genes confirmed in more than one independent cohort as increasing susceptibility to SLE or lupus nephritis are listed. Gene-environment interactions result in abnormal immune responses that generate pathogenic autoantibodies and immune complexes that deposit in tissue, activate complement, cause inflammation, and over time lead to irreversible organ damage. Ag, antigen; C1q, complement system; C3, complement component; CNS, central nervous system; DC, dendritic cell; EBV, Epstein-Barr virus; HLA, human leukocyte antigen; FcR, immunoglobulin Fc-binding receptor; IL, interleukin; MBL, mannose-binding ligand; MCP, monocyte chemotactic protein; PTPN, phosphotyrosine phosphatase; UV, ultraviolet.

deficiencies of early components of complement (C1q,r,s; C2; C4) confer strong predisposition to SLE, but such deficiencies are rare. Each of the other genes listed increases risk for SLE by only 1.5- to 3-fold. Some gene alleles probably contribute to disease susceptibility by influencing clearance of apoptotic cells (C1q, MBL) or immune complexes (FcR 2A and 3A), antigen presentation (HLA-DR2,3,8), B cell maturation (IL-10), T cell activation (PTPN22), or chemotaxis (MCP-1). None of these hypotheses is proven. In addition to influencing disease susceptibility in various ethnic groups, some genes influence clinical manifestations of disease (e.g., FcR 2A/3A, MBL, PDCD1 for nephritis; MCP-1 for arthritis and vasculitis). A region on chromosome 16 contains genes that predispose to SLE, rheumatoid arthritis, psoriasis, and Crohn's disease, suggesting the presence of "autoimmunity genes" that, when interacting with other genes, predispose to different autoimmune diseases. There are likely to be protective gene alleles as well. All these gene combinations influence immune responses to the external and internal environment; when such responses are too high and/or too prolonged, autoimmune disease results.

Female sex is permissive for SLE; females of many mammalian species make higher antibody responses than males. Women exposed to estrogen-containing oral contraceptives or hormone replacements have an increased risk of developing SLE (1.2- to 2-fold). Estradiol binds to receptors on T and B lymphocytes, increasing activation and survival of those cells, thus favoring prolonged immune responses.

Several environmental stimuli may influence SLE (Fig. 4-1). Exposure to ultraviolet light causes flares of SLE in approximately 70% of patients, possibly by increasing apoptosis in skin cells or by altering DNA and intracellular proteins to make them antigenic. It is likely that some infections induce a normal immune response that matures to contain some T and B cells that recognize self-antigens; such cells are not appropriately regulated, and autoantibody production occurs. Most SLE patients have autoantibodies for 3 years or more before the first symptoms of disease, suggesting that regulation controls the degree of autoimmunity for years before quantities and qualities of autoantibodies and pathogenic B and T cells actually cause clinical disease. Epstein-Barr virus (EBV) may be one infectious agent that can trigger SLE in susceptible individuals. Children and adults with SLE are more likely to be infected by EBV than age-, sex-, and ethnicity-matched controls—an observation confirmed in African-American adults in another population. EBV activates and infects B lymphocytes and survives in those cells for decades; it also contains amino acid sequences that mimic sequences on human spliceosomes (RNA/protein antigens often recognized by autoantibodies in people with SLE). Thus, interplay

TABLE 4-1

AUTOANTIBODIES IN SYSTEMIC LUPUS ERYTHEMATOSUS (SLE)

ANTIBODY	PREVALENCE, %	ANTIGEN RECOGNIZED	CLINICAL UTILITY
Antinuclear antibodies	98	Multiple nuclear	Best screening test; repeated negative tests make SLE unlikely
Anti-dsDNA	70	DNA (double-stranded)	High titers are SLE specific and in some patients correlate with disease activity, nephritis, vasculitis
Anti-Sm	25	Protein complexed to 6 species of nuclear U1 RNA	Specific for SLE; no definite clinical correlations; most patients also have anti-RNP; more common in African Americans and Asians than Caucasians
Anti-RNP	40	Protein complexed to U1 RNAγ	Not specific for SLE; high titers associated with syndromes that have overlap features of several rheumatic syndromes including SLE; more common in African Americans than Caucasians
Anti-Ro (SS-A)	30	Protein complexed to hY RNA, primarily 60 kDa and 52 kDa	Not specific for SLE; associated with sicca syndrome, subacute cutaneous lupus, and neonatal lupus with congenital heart block; associated with decreased risk for nephritis
Anti-La (SS-B)	10	47-kDa protein complexed to hY RNA	Usually associated with anti-Ro; associated with decreased risk for nephritis
Antihistone	70	Histones associated with DNA (in nucleosome, chromatin)	More frequent in drug-induced lupus than in SLE
Antiphospholipid	50	Phospholipids, β_2 glycoprotein 1 cofactor, prothrombin	Three tests available—ELISAs for cardiolipin and β_2G1, sensitive prothrombin time (DRVVT); predisposes to clotting, fetal loss, thrombocytopenia
Antierythrocyte	60	Erythrocyte membrane	Measured as direct Coombs' test; a small proportion develops overt hemolysis
Antiplatelet	30	Surface and altered cytoplasmic antigens in platelets	Associated with thrombocytopenia but sensitivity and specificity are not good; this is not a useful clinical test
Antineuronal (includes anti-glutamate receptor)	60	Neuronal and lymphocyte surface antigens	In some series a positive test in CSF correlates with active CNS lupus
Antiribosomal P	20	Protein in ribosomes	In some series a positive test in serum correlates with depression or psychosis due to CNS lupus

Note: CNS, central nervous system; CSF, cerebrospinal fluid; DRVVT, dilute Russell viper venom time; ELISA, enzyme-linked immunosorbent assay.

between genetic susceptibility, environment, sex, and abnormal immune responses results in autoimmunity (Chap. 3).

PATHOLOGY

In SLE, biopsies of affected skin show deposition of Ig at the dermal-epidermal junction (DEJ), injury to basal keratinocytes, and inflammation dominated by T lymphocytes in the DEJ and around blood vessels and dermal appendages. Clinically unaffected skin may also show Ig deposition at the DEJ.

In renal biopsies, the pattern and severity of injury are important in diagnosis and in selecting the best therapy. Most published clinical studies of lupus nephritis have used the World Health Organization (WHO) classification of lupus nephritis. However, the International Society of Nephrology (ISN) and the Renal Pathology Society (RPS) have published a new, similar classification (Table 4-2) that will probably replace the WHO standards. An advantage of the ISN/RPS classification is the addition of "a" for active and "c" for chronic changes, giving the physician information regarding the potential reversibility of disease. All the classification systems

TABLE 4-5 (CONTINUED) 75

MEDICATIONS FOR THE MANAGEMENT OF SLE

MEDICATION	DOSE RANGE	DRUG INTERACTIONS	SERIOUS OR COMMON ADVERSE EFFECTS
Azathioprine[b]	2–3 mg/kg per day PO; decrease frequency of dose if CrCl <50 mL/min	ACE inhibitors, allopurinol, bone marrow suppressants, interferons, mycophenolate mofetil, rituximab, warfarin, zidovudine	Infection, VZV infection, bone marrow suppression, leukopenia, anemia, thrombocytopenia, pancreatitis, hepatotoxicity, malignancy, alopecia, fever, flulike illness, GI symptoms

[a]Indicates medication is approved for use in SLE by the U.S. Food and Drug Administration.
[b]Indicates the medication has been used with glucocorticoids in the trials showing efficacy.
Note: A2R, angiotensin 2 receptor; ACE, angiotensin-converting enzyme; CHF, congestive heart failure; CrCl, creatinine clearance; FDA, U.S. Food and Drug Administration; GI, gastrointestinal; NSAIDs, nonsteroidal anti-inflammatory drugs; SPF, sun protection factor; VZV, varicella-zoster virus.

steroids along with appropriate supportive therapy for heart failure, arrhythmia, or embolic events. As discussed above, patients with SLE are at increased risk for myocardial infarction, usually due to accelerated atherosclerosis, which probably results from chronic inflammation and/or chronic oxidative damage to lipids and to organs.

Hematologic Manifestations

The most frequent hematologic manifestation of SLE is anemia, usually normochromic normocytic, reflecting chronic illness. Hemolysis can be rapid in onset and severe, requiring high-dose glucocorticoid therapy, which is effective in most patients. Leukopenia is also common and almost always consists of lymphopenia, not granulocytopenia; this rarely predisposes to infections and by itself usually does not require therapy. Thrombocytopenia may be a recurring problem. If platelet counts are >40,000/μL and abnormal bleeding is absent, therapy may not be required. High-dose glucocorticoid therapy (e.g., 1 mg/kg per day of prednisone or equivalent) is usually effective for the first few episodes of severe thrombocytopenia. Recurring or prolonged hemolytic anemia or thrombocytopenia, or disease requiring an unacceptably high dose of daily glucocorticoids, should be treated with an additional strategy (see "Treatment" later in the chapter).

Gastrointestinal Manifestations

Nausea, sometimes with vomiting, and diarrhea can be manifestations of an SLE flare, as can diffuse abdominal pain caused by autoimmune peritonitis and/or intestinal vasculitis. Increases in serum aspartate aminotransferase (AST) and alanine aminotransferase (ALT) are common when SLE is active. These manifestations usually improve promptly during systemic glucocorticoid therapy. Vasculitis involving the intestine may be life-threatening; perforations,

ischemia, bleeding, and sepsis are frequent complications. Aggressive immunosuppressive therapy with high-dose glucocorticoids is recommended for short-term control; evidence of recurrence is an indication for additional therapies.

Ocular Manifestations

Sicca syndrome (Sjögren's syndrome; Chap. 8) and nonspecific conjunctivitis are common in SLE and rarely threaten vision. In contrast, retinal vasculitis and optic neuritis are serious manifestations: blindness can develop over days to weeks. Aggressive immunosuppression is recommended, although there are no controlled trials to prove effectiveness. Complications of glucocorticoid therapy include cataracts (common) and glaucoma.

LABORATORY TESTS

Laboratory tests serve (1) to establish or rule out the diagnosis; (2) to follow the course of disease, particularly to suggest that a flare is occurring or organ damage is developing; and (3) to identify adverse effects of therapies.

Tests for Autoantibodies

(Tables 4-1 and 4-3) Diagnostically, the most important autoantibodies to detect are ANA since the test is positive in >95% of patients, usually at the onset of symptoms. A few patients develop ANA within 1 year of symptom onset; repeated testing may thus be useful. ANA-negative lupus exists but is very rare in adults and is usually associated with other autoantibodies (anti-Ro or anti-DNA). High-titer IgG antibodies to double-stranded DNA (dsDNA) (but not to single-stranded DNA) are specific for SLE. There is no international standardized test for ANA; variability between different service laboratories is high. Enzyme-linked immunosorbent assays (ELISA) and immunofluorescent reactions of sera with the dsDNA in the flagellate *Crithidia luciliae* have ~60% sensitivity for SLE; identification of high-avidity anti–dsDNA in the Farr assay is not as sensitive but may correlate better with risk for nephritis. Titers of anti–dsDNA vary over time. In some patients, increases in quantities of anti–dsDNA herald a flare, particularly of nephritis or vasculitis. Antibodies to Sm are also specific for SLE and assist in diagnosis; anti–Sm antibodies do not usually correlate with disease activity or clinical manifestations. aPL are not specific for SLE, but their presence fulfills one classification criterion and they identify patients at increased risk for venous or arterial clotting, thrombocytopenia, and fetal loss. There are two widely accepted tests that measure different antibodies (anticardiolipin and the lupus anticoagulant): (1) ELISA for anticardiolipin (internationally standardized with good reproducibility) and (2) a sensitive phospholipid-based activated prothrombin time such as the dilute Russell venom viper test. Some centers also recommend measurement of antibodies to β_2 glycoprotein 1, a serum protein cofactor that is the target of most antibodies to cardiolipin and some lupus anticoagulants. High titers of IgG anticardiolipin (>50 IU) indicate high risk for a clinical episode of clotting. Quantities of aPL may vary markedly over time; repeated testing is justified if clinical manifestations of the antiphospholipid antibody syndrome (APS) appear. To make a diagnosis of APS, with or without SLE, requires the presence of clotting and/or repeated fetal losses plus at least two positive tests for aPL, at least 12 weeks apart.

An additional autoantibody test with predictive value (not used for diagnosis) detects anti–Ro, which indicates increased risk for neonatal lupus, sicca syndrome, and SCLE. Women with child-bearing potential and SLE should be screened for aPL and anti–Ro.

Standard Tests for Diagnosis

Screening tests for complete blood count, platelet count, and urinalysis may detect abnormalities that contribute to the diagnosis and influence management decisions.

Tests for Following Disease Course

It is useful to follow tests that indicate the status of organ involvement known to be present during SLE flares. These might include hemoglobin levels, platelet counts, urinalysis, and serum levels of creatinine or albumin. There is great interest in identification of additional markers of disease activity. Candidates include levels of anti–DNA antibodies, several components of complement (C3 is most widely available), activated complement products (including those that bind to the C4d receptor on erythrocytes), IFN-inducible genes, soluble IL-2, and urinary adiponectin or monocyte chemotactic protein 1. None is uniformly agreed upon as a reliable indicator of flare or of response to therapeutic interventions. The physician should determine for each patient whether certain laboratory test changes predict flare. If so, altering therapy in response to these changes has been shown to prevent flares. In addition, given the increased prevalence of atherosclerosis in SLE, it is advisable to follow the recommendations of the National Cholesterol Education Program for testing and treatment, including scoring of SLE as an independent risk factor, similar to diabetes mellitus.

℞ Treatment: SYSTEMIC LUPUS ERYTHEMATOSUS

There is no cure for SLE, and complete sustained remissions are rare. Therefore, the physician should plan to control acute, severe flares and then develop maintenance strategies that suppress symptoms to an acceptable level and prevent organ damage. Usually patients will endure some adverse effects of medications. Therapeutic choices depend on (1) whether disease manifestations are life-threatening or likely to cause organ damage, justifying aggressive therapies; (2) whether manifestations are potentially reversible; and (3) the best approaches to preventing complications of disease and its treatments. Therapies, doses, and adverse effects are listed in Table 4-5.

CONSERVATIVE THERAPIES FOR MANAGEMENT OF NON–LIFE-THREATENING DISEASE Among patients with fatigue, pain, and autoantibodies of SLE, but without major organ involvement, management can be directed to suppression of symptoms. Analgesics and antimalarials are mainstays. NSAIDs are useful analgesics/anti-inflammatories, particularly for arthritis/ arthralgias. However, two major issues currently indicate caution in using NSAIDs. First, SLE patients compared with the general population are at increased risk for NSAID-induced aseptic meningitis, elevated serum transaminases, hypertension, and renal dysfunction. Second, all NSAIDs, particularly those that inhibit cyclooxygenase-2 specifically, may increase risk for myocardial infarction. Acetaminophen to control pain may be a good strategy, but NSAIDs may be more effective in some patients, and the relative hazards of NSAIDs compared with low-dose glucocorticoid therapy have not been established. Antimalarials (hydroxychloroquine, chloroquine, and quinacrine) often reduce dermatitis, arthritis, and fatigue. A randomized, placebo-controlled, prospective trial has shown that hydroxychloroquine reduces the number of disease flares; it may also reduce accrual of tissue damage over time. Because of potential retinal toxicity, patients receiving antimalarials should musculoskeletal symptoms until the appearance of synovitis becomes apparent. This prodrome may persist for weeks or months and defy diagnosis. Specific symptoms usually appear gradually as several joints, especially those of the hands, wrists, knees, and feet, become affected in a symmetric fashion. In ~10% of individuals, the onset is more acute, with a rapid development of polyarthritis, often accompanied by constitutional symptoms, including fever, lymphadenopathy, and splenomegaly. In approximately one-third of patients, symptoms may initially be confined to one or a few joints. Although the pattern of joint involvement may remain asymmetric in some patients, a symmetric pattern is more typical.

Signs and Symptoms of Articular Disease

Pain, swelling, and tenderness may initially be poorly localized to the joints. Pain in affected joints, aggravated by movement, is the most common manifestation of established RA. It corresponds in pattern to the joint involvement but does not always correlate with the degree of apparent inflammation. Generalized stiffness is frequent and is usually greatest after periods of inactivity. Morning stiffness of >1-h duration is an almost invariable feature of inflammatory arthritis. Notably, however, the presence of morning stiffness may not reliably distinguish between chronic inflammatory and noninflammatory arthritides, as it is also found frequently in the latter. The majority of patients will experience constitutional symptoms such as weakness, easy fatigability, anorexia, and weight loss. Although fever to 40°C occurs on occasion, temperature elevation of >38°C is unusual and suggests the presence of an intercurrent problem such as infection.

Clinically, synovial inflammation causes swelling, tenderness, and limitation of motion. Initially, impairment in physical function is caused by pain and inflammation, and disability owing to this is a frequent early feature of aggressive RA. Warmth is usually evident on examination, especially of large joints such as the knee, but erythema is infrequent. Pain originates predominantly from the joint capsule, which is abundantly supplied with pain fibers and is markedly sensitive to stretching or distention. Joint swelling results from accumulation of synovial fluid, hypertrophy of the synovium, and thickening of the joint capsule. Initially, motion is limited by pain. The inflamed joint is usually held in flexion to maximize joint volume and minimize distention of the capsule. Later, fibrous or bony ankylosis or soft tissue contractures lead to fixed deformities.

Although inflammation can affect any diarthrodial joint, RA most often causes symmetric arthritis with characteristic involvement of certain specific joints such as the proximal interphalangeal and metacarpophalangeal joints. The distal interphalangeal joints are rarely involved. Synovitis of the wrist joints is a nearly uniform feature of RA and may lead to limitation of motion,

deformity, and median nerve entrapment (carpal tunnel syndrome). Synovitis of the elbow joint often leads to flexion contractures that may develop early in the disease. The knee joint is commonly involved with synovial hypertrophy, chronic effusion, and frequently ligamentous laxity. Pain and swelling behind the knee may be caused by extension of inflamed synovium into the popliteal space (Baker's cyst). Arthritis in the forefoot, ankles, and subtalar joints can produce severe pain with ambulation as well as a number of deformities. Axial involvement is usually limited to the upper cervical spine. Involvement of the lumbar spine is not seen, and lower back pain cannot be ascribed to rheumatoid inflammation. On occasion, inflammation from the synovial joints and bursae of the upper cervical spine leads to atlantoaxial subluxation. This usually presents as pain in the occiput but on rare occasions may lead to compression of the spinal cord.

With persistent inflammation, a variety of characteristic joint changes develop. These can be attributed to a number of pathologic events, including laxity of supporting soft tissue structures; damage or weakening of ligaments, tendons, and the joint capsule; cartilage degradation; muscle imbalance; and unopposed physical forces associated with the use of affected joints. Characteristic changes of the hand include (1) radial deviation at the wrist with ulnar deviation of the digits, often with palmar subluxation of the proximal phalanges ("Z" deformity); (2) hyperextension of the proximal interphalangeal joints, with compensatory flexion of the distal interphalangeal joints (swan-neck deformity); (3) flexion contracture of the proximal interphalangeal joints and extension of the distal interphalangeal joints (boutonnière deformity); and (4) hyperextension of the first interphalangeal joint and flexion of the first metacarpophalangeal joint with a consequent loss of thumb mobility and pinch. Typical joint changes may also develop in the feet, including eversion at the hindfoot (subtalar joint), plantar subluxation of the metatarsal heads, widening of the forefoot, hallux valgus, and lateral deviation and dorsal subluxation of the toes. Later in the disease, disability is more related to structural damage to articular structures.

Extraarticular Manifestations

RA is a systemic disease with a variety of extraarticular manifestations. It is estimated that as many as 40% of patients may have extraarticular manifestations, and in ~15% these are severe. On occasion, extraarticular manifestations may be the major evidence of disease activity and source of morbidity and require management per se. As a rule, these manifestations occur in individuals with high titers of autoantibodies to the Fc component of immunoglobulin G (rheumatoid factors) or with antibodies to CCP. Although the frequency of patients with severe extraarticular manifestations appears to be declining, these patients have an increased mortality compared to other persons with RA or age-matched normal controls.

Rheumatoid nodules may develop in 20–30% of persons with RA. They are usually found on periarticular structures, extensor surfaces, or other areas subjected to mechanical pressure, but they can develop elsewhere, including the pleura and meninges. Common locations include the olecranon bursa, the proximal ulna, the Achilles tendon, and the occiput. Nodules vary in size and consistency and are rarely symptomatic, but on occasion they break down as a result of trauma or become infected. They are found almost invariably in individuals with circulating rheumatoid factor. Histologically, rheumatoid nodules consist of a central zone of necrotic material including collagen fibrils, noncollagenous filaments, and cellular debris; a midzone of palisading macrophages that express HLA-DR antigens; and an outer zone of granulation tissue. Examination of early nodules has suggested that the initial event may be a focal vasculitis. In some patients, treatment with methotrexate can increase the number of nodules dramatically.

Clinical weakness and atrophy of skeletal muscle are common. Muscle atrophy may be evident within weeks of the onset of RA and is usually most apparent in musculature approximating affected joints. Muscle biopsy may show type II fiber atrophy and muscle fiber necrosis with or without a mononuclear cell infiltrate.

Rheumatoid vasculitis (Chap. 10), which can affect nearly any organ system, is seen in patients with severe RA and high titers of circulating rheumatoid factor. Rheumatoid vasculitis is very uncommon in African Americans. In its most aggressive form, rheumatoid vasculitis can cause polyneuropathy and mononeuritis multiplex, cutaneous ulceration and dermal necrosis, digital gangrene, and visceral infarction. While such widespread vasculitis is very rare, more limited forms are not uncommon, especially in white patients with high titers of rheumatoid factor. Neurovascular disease presenting either as a mild distal sensory neuropathy or as mononeuritis multiplex may be the only sign of vasculitis. Cutaneous vasculitis usually presents as crops of small brown spots in the nail beds, nail folds, and digital pulp. Larger ischemic ulcers, especially in the lower extremity, may also develop. Myocardial infarction secondary to rheumatoid vasculitis has been reported, as has vasculitic involvement of lungs, bowel, liver, spleen, pancreas, lymph nodes, and testes. Renal vasculitis is rare.

Pleuropulmonary manifestations, which are more commonly observed in men, include pleural disease, interstitial fibrosis, pleuropulmonary nodules, pneumonitis, and arteritis. Evidence of pleuritis is found commonly at autopsy, but symptomatic disease during life is infrequent. Typically, the pleural fluid contains very low levels of glucose in the absence of infection. Pleural fluid complement is also low compared with the serum level

when these are related to the total protein concentration. Pulmonary fibrosis can produce impairment of the diffusing capacity of the lung. Pulmonary nodules may appear singly or in clusters. When they appear in individuals with pneumoconiosis, a diffuse nodular fibrotic process (Caplan's syndrome) may develop. On occasion, pulmonary nodules may cavitate and produce a pneumothorax or bronchopleural fistula. Rarely, pulmonary hypertension secondary to obliteration of the pulmonary vasculature occurs. In addition to pleuropulmonary disease, upper airway obstruction from cricoarytenoid arthritis or laryngeal nodules may develop.

Clinically apparent heart disease attributed to the rheumatoid process was thought previously to be rare, but evidence of asymptomatic pericarditis is found at autopsy in 50% of cases. Pericardial fluid has a low glucose level and is frequently associated with the occurrence of pleural effusion. Although pericarditis is usually asymptomatic, on rare occasions death has occurred from tamponade. Chronic constrictive pericarditis may also occur. More recently, an increased incidence of congestive heart failure and death from cardiovascular disease has been associated with RA. This relates to the level of disease activity and can be mitigated with appropriate anti-inflammatory therapy.

RA tends to spare the central nervous system directly, although vasculitis can cause peripheral neuropathy. *Neurologic manifestations* may also result from atlantoaxial or midcervical spine subluxations. Nerve entrapment secondary to proliferative synovitis or joint deformities may produce neuropathies of median, ulnar, radial (interosseous branch), or anterior tibial nerves.

The rheumatoid process involves the *eye* in <1% of patients. Affected individuals usually have long-standing disease and nodules. The two principal manifestations are episcleritis, which is usually mild and transient, and scleritis, which involves the deeper layers of the eye and is a more serious inflammatory condition. Histologically, the lesion is similar to a rheumatoid nodule and may result in thinning and perforation of the globe (scleromalacia perforans). From 15–20% of persons with RA may develop Sjögren's syndrome with attendant keratoconjunctivitis sicca.

Felty's syndrome consists of chronic RA, splenomegaly, neutropenia, and, on occasion, anemia and thrombocytopenia. It is most common in individuals with long-standing disease. These patients frequently have high titers of rheumatoid factor, subcutaneous nodules, and other manifestations of systemic rheumatoid disease. Felty's syndrome is very uncommon in African Americans. It may develop after joint inflammation has regressed. Circulating immune complexes are often present, and evidence of complement consumption may be seen. The leukopenia is a selective neutropenia with polymorphonuclear leukocyte counts of <1500 cells/μL and sometimes <1000 cell/μL. Bone marrow examination usually reveals moderate hypercellularity with a paucity of mature neutrophils. However, the bone marrow may be normal, hyperactive, or hypoactive; maturation arrest may be seen. Hypersplenism has been proposed as one of the causes of leukopenia, but splenomegaly is not invariably found and splenectomy does not always correct the abnormality. Excessive margination of granulocytes caused by antibodies to these cells, complement activation, or binding of immune complexes may contribute to granulocytopenia. Patients with Felty's syndrome have increased frequency of infections usually associated with neutropenia. The cause of the increased susceptibility to infection is related to the defective function of PMNLs as well as the decreased number of cells.

Osteoporosis secondary to rheumatoid involvement is common and may be aggravated by glucocorticoid therapy. Glucocorticoid treatment may cause significant loss of bone mass, especially early in the course of therapy, even when low doses are employed. Osteopenia in RA involves both juxtaarticular bone and long bones distant from involved joints. RA is associated with a modest decrease in mean bone mass and a moderate increase in the risk of fracture. Bone mass appears to be adversely affected by functional impairment and active inflammation, especially early in the course of the disease.

RA is associated with an increased incidence of lymphoma, especially large B cell lymphoma. Notably, this is particularly observed in those with persistent inflammatory disease.

RA in the Elderly

The incidence of RA continues to increase past age 60. It has been suggested that elderly-onset RA might have a poorer prognosis, as manifested by more persistent disease activity, more frequent radiographically evident deterioration, more frequent systemic involvement, and more rapid functional decline. Aggressive disease is largely restricted to those patients with high titers of rheumatoid factor. By contrast, elderly patients who develop RA without elevated titers of rheumatoid factor (seronegative disease) generally have less severe, often self-limited disease.

LABORATORY FINDINGS

No tests are specific for diagnosing RA. However, rheumatoid factors, which are autoantibodies reactive with the Fc portion of IgG, are found in more than two-thirds of adults with the disease and have classically been used to evaluate patients with RA. Widely utilized tests largely detect IgM rheumatoid factors. The presence of rheumatoid factor is not specific for RA, as rheumatoid factor is found in 5% of healthy persons. The frequency of rheumatoid factor in the general population increases with age, and 10–20% of individuals >65 years have a positive test. In addition, a number of conditions besides

RA are associated with the presence of rheumatoid factor. These include systemic lupus erythematosus, Sjögren's syndrome, chronic liver disease, sarcoidosis, interstitial pulmonary fibrosis, infectious mononucleosis, hepatitis B, tuberculosis, leprosy, syphilis, subacute bacterial endocarditis, visceral leishmaniasis, schistosomiasis, and malaria. In addition, rheumatoid factor may appear transiently in normal individuals after vaccination or transfusion and may also be found in relatives of individuals with RA.

The presence of rheumatoid factor does not establish the diagnosis of RA, as the predictive value of the presence of rheumatoid factor in determining a diagnosis of RA is poor. Thus less than one-third of unselected patients with a positive test for rheumatoid factor will be found to have RA. Therefore, the rheumatoid factor test is not useful as a screening procedure. However, the presence of rheumatoid factor can be of prognostic significance because patients with high titers tend to have more severe and progressive disease with extraarticular manifestations. Rheumatoid factor is uniformly found in patients with nodules or vasculitis. In summary, a test for the presence of rheumatoid factor can be employed to confirm a diagnosis in individuals with a suggestive clinical presentation and, if present in high titer, to designate patients at risk for severe systemic disease.

Antibodies to CCP (designated anti-CCP) can also be used to evaluate patients with RA. Although these antibodies are most commonly found in rheumatoid factor–positive patients, on occasion they can be detected in the absence of rheumatoid factor. In addition, the anti-CCP test has a similar sensitivity and a better specificity for RA than does rheumatoid factor, and, therefore, some have advocated its use to evaluate RA patients instead of rheumatoid factor. This is particularly the case in individuals with early RA, in whom assessment of anti-CCP may be the most useful to confirm the diagnosis and establish a likely prognosis. The presence of anti-CCP is most common in persons with aggressive disease, with a tendency for developing bone erosions. The development of anti-CCP is most frequent in individuals with an RA associated HLA-β1 allele and in those who smoke cigarettes, and may occur before the development of clinical manifestations of RA. However, as with rheumatoid factor, the presence of anti-CCP is not useful to predict the future development of RA because it can be found in ~1.5% of normal individuals, most of whom will not develop RA, and occasionally in persons with other rheumatic diseases. However, it is a useful test to confirm a diagnosis of RA and to estimate prognosis.

Normochromic, normocytic anemia is frequently present in active RA. It is thought to reflect ineffective erythropoiesis; large stores of iron are found in the bone marrow. In general, anemia and thrombocytosis correlate with disease activity. The white blood cell count is usually normal, but a mild leukocytosis may be present. Leukopenia may also exist without the full-blown picture of Felty's syndrome. Eosinophilia, when present, usually reflects severe systemic disease.

The erythrocyte sedimentation rate (ESR) is increased in nearly all patients with active RA. The levels of a variety of other acute-phase reactants including ceruloplasmin and C-reactive protein are also elevated, and generally such elevations correlate with disease activity and the likelihood of progressive joint damage.

Synovial fluid analysis confirms the presence of inflammatory arthritis, although none of the findings are specific. The fluid is usually turbid, with reduced viscosity, increased protein content, and a slightly decreased or normal glucose concentration. The white cell count varies between 5 and 50,000/μL; PMNLs predominate. A synovial fluid white blood cell count >2000/μL with >75% polymorphonuclear leukocytes is highly characteristic of inflammatory arthritis, although not diagnostic of RA. Total hemolytic complement, C3, and C4 are markedly diminished in synovial fluid relative to total protein concentration as a result of activation of the classic complement pathway by locally produced immune complexes.

RADIOGRAPHIC EVALUATION

Early in the disease, radiographic evaluations of the affected joints are usually not helpful in establishing a diagnosis. They reveal only that which is apparent from physical examination, namely, evidence of soft tissue swelling and joint effusion. As the disease progresses, abnormalities become more pronounced, but none of the radiographic findings is diagnostic of RA. The diagnosis, however, is supported by a characteristic pattern of abnormalities, including the tendency toward symmetric involvement. Juxtaarticular osteopenia may become apparent within weeks of onset. Loss of articular cartilage and bone erosions develop after months of sustained activity. The primary value of radiography is to determine the extent of cartilage destruction and bone erosion produced by the disease, particularly when one is attempting to estimate the aggressive nature of the disease, monitoring the impact of therapy with disease-modifying drugs, or determining the need for surgical intervention. Other means of imaging bones and joints, including ^{99m}Tc bisphosphonate bone scanning and MRI, may be capable of detecting early inflammatory changes that are not apparent from standard radiography but are rarely necessary in the routine evaluation of patients with RA.

CLINICAL COURSE AND PROGNOSIS

The course of RA is quite variable and difficult to predict in an individual patient. The current therapeutic approach of early aggressive intervention appears to have mitigated the clinical course of RA, resulting in less persistent inflammation, disability, joint damage, and mortality. Classically, most patients had experienced persistent

but fluctuating disease activity, accompanied by a variable degree of joint abnormalities and functional impairment. After 10–12 years, <20% of patients had no evidence of disability or joint abnormalities. Moreover, within 10 years, ~50% of patients had work disability. All of these outcomes are thought to be positively influenced by early aggressive intervention. A number of features are correlated with a greater likelihood of developing joint abnormalities or disabilities. These include the presence of >20 inflamed joints, a markedly elevated ESR, radiographic evidence of bone erosions, the presence of rheumatoid nodules, high titers of serum rheumatoid factor or anti-CCP antibodies, the presence of functional disability, persistent inflammation, advanced age at onset, the presence of comorbid conditions, low socioeconomic status or educational level, or the presence of HLA-DR,1*0401 or -DR,*0404. The presence of one or more of these implies the presence of more aggressive disease with a greater likelihood of developing progressive joint abnormalities and disability. Persistent elevation of the ESR, disability, and pain on longitudinal follow-up are good predictors of work disability, whereas persistent synovitis of >12 weeks is associated with an increased likelihood of developing bone erosions. Patients who lack these features have more indolent disease with a slower progression to joint abnormalities and disability. The pattern of disease onset does not appear to predict the development of disabilities. Approximately 15% of patients with RA will have a short-lived inflammatory process that remits without major disability. These individuals tend to lack the aforementioned features associated with more aggressive disease.

Several features of patients with RA appear to have prognostic significance. Remissions of disease activity are most likely to occur during the first year. White females tend to have more persistent synovitis and more progressively erosive disease than males. Persons who present with high titers of rheumatoid factor, anti-CCP antibodies, C-reactive protein, and haptoglobin also have a worse prognosis, as do individuals with subcutaneous nodules or radiographic evidence of erosions at the time of initial evaluation. Sustained disease activity of >1 year's duration portends a poor outcome, and persistent elevation of acute-phase reactants appears to correlate strongly with radiographic progression. Before the use of early aggressive therapy, a large proportion of inflamed joints manifested erosions within 2 years, whereas the subsequent course of erosions was highly variable; however, in general, radiographic damage appears to progress at a constant rate in patients with RA. Foot joints are affected more frequently than hand joints. Despite the decrease in the rate of progressive joint damage with time, functional disability, which develops early in the course of the disease, continues to worsen at the same rate, although the most rapid rate of functional loss occurs within the first 2 years of disease. Early in the course of RA, disability is more associated with pain and inflammation, whereas later in the course of the disease, damage to articular structures makes a greater contribution.

The median life expectancy of persons with RA is shortened by 3–7 years. Of the 2.5-fold increase in mortality rate, RA itself is a contributing feature in 15–30%. The increased mortality rate seems to be limited to patients with more severe articular disease and can be attributed largely to infection and gastrointestinal bleeding and an increased risk of cardiovascular disease. Recent evidence has emphasized the important role of cardiovascular disease in the increased mortality of RA patients, and this appears to diminish with effective anti-inflammatory therapy. Drug therapy may also play a role in the increased mortality rate seen in individuals with RA. Factors correlated with early death include disability, disease duration or severity, persistent inflammation, glucocorticoid use, age at onset, and low socioeconomic or educational status.

DIAGNOSIS

The diagnosis of RA can be delayed because of the nonspecific nature of initial symptoms. The diagnosis of RA is easily made in persons with typical established disease. The typical picture of bilateral symmetric inflammatory polyarthritis involving small and large joints in both the upper and lower extremities with sparing of the axial skeleton except the cervical spine suggests the diagnosis. Constitutional features indicative of the inflammatory nature of the disease, such as morning stiffness, support the diagnosis. Demonstration of subcutaneous nodules is a helpful diagnostic feature. Additionally, the presence of rheumatoid factor, anti-CCP antibodies, inflammatory synovial fluid with increased numbers of PMNLs, and radiographic findings of juxtaarticular bone demineralization and erosions of the affected joints substantiate the diagnosis.

The diagnosis is somewhat more difficult early in the course when only constitutional symptoms or intermittent arthralgias or arthritis in an asymmetric distribution may be present. A period of observation may be necessary before the diagnosis can be established. A definitive diagnosis of RA depends predominantly on characteristic clinical features and the exclusion of other inflammatory processes. The isolated finding of a positive test for rheumatoid factor, anti-CCP antibody, or an elevated ESR or C-reactive protein (CRP), especially in an older person with joint pains, should not itself be used as evidence of RA.

In 1987, the American College of Rheumatology developed revised criteria for the classification of RA (**Table 5-1**). These criteria demonstrate a sensitivity of 91–94% and a specificity of 89% when used to classify patients with RA compared with control subjects with rheumatic diseases other than RA. Although these criteria were developed as a means of disease classification for

---

TABLE 5-1

THE 1987 REVISED CRITERIA FOR THE CLASSIFICATION OF RA

1. Guidelines for classification
   a. Four of seven criteria are required to classify a patient as having rheumatoid arthritis (RA).
   b. Patients with two or more clinical diagnoses are not excluded.
2. Criteria[a]
   a. Morning stiffness: Stiffness in and around the joints lasting 1 h before maximal improvement.
   b. Arthritis of three or more joint areas: At least three joint areas, observed by a physician simultaneously, have soft tissue swelling or joint effusions, not just bony overgrowth. The 14 possible joint areas involved are right or left proximal interphalangeal, metacarpophalangeal, wrist, elbow, knee, ankle, and metatarsophalangeal joints.
   c. Arthritis of hand joints: Arthritis of wrist, metacarpophalangeal joint, or proximal interphalangeal joint.
   d. Symmetric arthritis: Simultaneous involvement of the same joint areas on both sides of the body.
   e. Rheumatoid nodules: Subcutaneous nodules over bony prominences, extensor surfaces, or juxtaarticular regions observed by a physician.
   f. Serum rheumatoid factor: Demonstration of abnormal amounts of serum rheumatoid factor by any method for which the result has been positive in less than 5% of normal control subjects.
   g. Radiographic changes: Typical changes of RA on posteroanterior hand and wrist radiographs that must include erosions or unequivocal bony decalcification localized in or most marked adjacent to the involved joints.

[a]Criteria a–d must be present for at least 6 weeks. Criteria b–e must be observed by a physician.
Source: From Arnett et al.

---

investigational purposes, they can be useful as guidelines for establishing the diagnosis. Failure to meet these criteria, however, especially during the early stages of the disease, does not exclude the diagnosis. Indeed, these criteria do not effectively differentiate patients with new-onset RA from those with a variety of other forms of early inflammatory arthritis. Moreover, in patients with early arthritis, the criteria do not discriminate effectively between patients who subsequently develop persistent, disabling, or erosive disease and those who do not.

℞ **Treatment:**
RHEUMATOID ARTHRITIS

GENERAL PRINCIPLES The goals of therapy for RA are (1) relief of pain, (2) reduction of inflammation, (3) protection of articular structures, (4) maintenance of function, and (5) control of systemic involvement. Since the etiology of RA is unknown, the pathogenesis is not completely delineated, and the mechanisms of action of some of the therapeutic agents employed are uncertain, therapy remains somewhat empirical. None of the therapeutic interventions is curative, and therefore all must be viewed as palliative, aimed at relieving the signs and symptoms of the disease. The various therapies employed are directed at nonspecific suppression of the inflammatory or immunologic process with the expectation of ameliorating symptoms and preventing progressive damage to articular structures.

Management of patients with RA involves an interdisciplinary approach, which attempts to deal with the various problems that these individuals encounter with functional as well as psychosocial interactions. A variety of physical therapy modalities may be useful in decreasing the symptoms of RA. Rest ameliorates symptoms and can be an important component of the total therapeutic program. In addition, splinting to reduce unwanted motion of inflamed joints may be useful. Exercise directed at maintaining muscle strength and joint mobility without exacerbating joint inflammation is also an important aspect of the therapeutic regimen. A variety of orthotic and assistive devices can be helpful in supporting and aligning deformed joints to reduce pain and improve function. Education of the patient and family is an important component of the therapeutic plan to help those involved become aware of the potential impact of the disease and make appropriate accommodations in lifestyle to maximize satisfaction and minimize stress on joints.

Medical management of RA involves five general approaches. The first is the use of nonsteroidal anti-inflammatory drugs (NSAIDs) and simple analgesics to control the symptoms and signs of the local inflammatory process. These agents are rapidly effective at mitigating signs and symptoms, but they appear to exert minimal effect on the progression of the disease. Recently, specific inhibitors of the isoform of cyclooxygenase (COX) that is upregulated at inflammatory sites (COX-2) have been developed. COX inhibitors (known as Coxibs), which selectively inhibit COX-2 and not COX-1, have been shown to be as effective as classic NSAIDs, which inhibit both isoforms of COX, but to cause significantly less gastroduodenal ulceration. However, these agents are associated with an increased risk of cardiovascular events, and therefore their use must be guided by a careful assessment of risk/benefit ratio. An important additional second line of therapy involves the use of low-dose oral glucocorticoids. Although low-dose glucocorticoids have been widely used to suppress signs and symptoms of inflammation, recent evidence indicates that they may also retard the development and progression of bone erosions. In addition, the use of low-dose glucocorticoids increases the anti-inflammatory

effects of agents such as methotrexate as well as the protective effect of these agents on bone damage. An initial course of low-dose glucocorticoids should be considered in patients either alone or when therapy with disease modifying anti-rheumatic drugs (DMARDs) is considered. Intraarticular glucocorticoids can often provide transient symptomatic relief when systemic medical therapy has failed to resolve inflammation. The third line of agents includes the DMARDs just mentioned. These agents appear to have the capacity to decrease elevated levels of acute-phase reactants in treated patients and, therefore, are thought to modify the inflammatory component of RA and thus its destructive capacity. These agents include methotrexate, sulfasalazine, hydroxychloroquine, gold salts, or D-penicillamine, although the latter two are now used infrequently. Combinations of DMARDs appear to be more effective than single agents in controlling the signs and symptoms of RA. A fourth group of agents are the biologics, which include TNF-neutralizing agents (infliximab, etanercept, and adalimumab), IL-1-neutralizing agents (anakinra), those that deplete B cells (rituximab), and those that interfere with T cell activation (abatacept). These agents have been shown to have a major impact on the signs and symptoms of RA and also to slow progressive damage to articular structures. A fifth group of agents are the immunosuppressive and cytotoxic drugs, including leflunomide, cyclosporine, azathioprine, and cyclophosphamide, that have been shown to ameliorate the disease process in some patients. Additional approaches have been employed in an attempt to control the signs and symptoms of RA. Substituting omega-3 fatty acids, such as eicosapentaenoic acid found in certain fish oils, for dietary omega-6 essential fatty acids found in meat has also been shown to provide symptomatic improvement in patients with RA. A variety of nontraditional approaches have also been claimed to be effective in treating RA, including diets, plant and animal extracts, vaccines, hormones, and topical preparations of various sorts. Many of these are costly, and none has been shown to be effective. However, belief in their efficacy ensures their continued use by some patients.

DRUGS

Disease-Modifying Anti-Rheumatic Drugs

Clinical experience has delineated a number of agents— the DMARDs—that appear to have the capacity to alter the course of RA. Despite having no chemical or pharmacologic similarities, in practice these agents share a number of characteristics. They exert minimal direct nonspecific anti-inflammatory or analgesic effects, and therefore NSAIDs must be continued during their administration, except in a few cases when true remissions are induced with them. The appearance of benefit from DMARD therapy is usually delayed for weeks or months. As many as two-thirds of patients develop some clinical improvement as a result of therapy with any of these agents, although the induction of true remissions is unusual. In addition to clinical improvement, there is frequently an improvement in serologic evidence of disease activity, and titers of rheumatoid factor and C-reactive protein and the ESR frequently decline. Moreover, DMARD therapy, especially early in the disease course, retards the development of bone erosions.

No characteristic features of patients have emerged that predict responsiveness to a DMARD. Moreover, the indications for the initiation of therapy with one of these agents are not well defined. Recently, evidence has emerged that the initiation of DMARD therapy early in the course of RA clearly has a major impact on the development of bone erosions and the progression to disability. It is now felt that DMARD therapy should be begun as soon as the diagnosis of RA is established, especially in those with any evidence of aggressive disease with a poor prognosis.

Which DMARD should be the drug of first choice remains controversial, and trials have failed to demonstrate a consistent advantage of one over the other. Despite this, methotrexate has emerged as the DMARD of choice especially in individuals with risk factors for development of bone erosions or persistent synovitis of >3 months' duration, because of its relatively rapid onset of action, its capacity to effect sustained improvement with ongoing therapy, and the higher level of patient retention on therapy. Methotrexate is usually employed on a weekly schedule of 7.5–25 mg given either orally in divided doses or, if necessary, SC or IM to avoid gastrointestinal toxicity. Recent trials have documented the efficacy of methotrexate and have indicated that its onset of action is more rapid than other DMARDs, and patients tend to remain on therapy with methotrexate longer than they remain on other DMARDs because of better clinical responses and less toxicity. Long-term trials have indicated that methotrexate does not induce remission but rather suppresses symptoms while it is being administered. Maximal improvement is observed after 6 months of therapy, with little additional improvement thereafter. Major toxicity includes gastrointestinal upset, oral ulceration, and liver function abnormalities that appear to be dose related and reversible and hepatic fibrosis that can be quite insidious, requiring liver biopsy for detection in its early stages. Drug-induced pneumonitis has also been reported. Liver biopsy is recommended for individuals with persistent or repetitive liver function abnormalities. Concurrent administration of folic acid or folinic acid may diminish the frequency of some side effects, although efficacy may be diminished somewhat. In this regard,

each of the DMARDs is associated with toxicity, and therefore careful patient monitoring is necessary. Toxicity of the various agents also becomes important in determining the drug of first choice. Of note, failure to respond or development of toxicity to one DMARD does not preclude responsiveness to another. Thus, a similar percentage of RA patients who have failed to respond to one DMARD will respond to another when it is given as the second disease-modifying drug.

GLUCOCORTICOID THERAPY Systemic glucocorticoid therapy can provide effective symptomatic therapy in patients with RA. Low-dose (<7.5 mg/d) prednisone is a useful additive therapy to control symptoms. Moreover, recent evidence suggests that low-dose glucocorticoid therapy may retard the progression of bone erosions and that an initial course of low-dose glucocorticoids may have a long-term protective effect against bone damage. Monthly pulses with high-dose glucocorticoids may be useful in some patients and may hasten the response when therapy with a DMARD is initiated. Finally, a course of low-dose oral glucocorticoids combined with DMARD therapy can be beneficial in controlling signs and symptoms rapidly and affording long-term retardation of bone erosion.

BIOLOGICS A range of biologic agents that bind and neutralize TNF are available. One of these is a TNF type II receptor fused to IgG1 (etanercept), the second is a chimeric mouse/human monoclonal antibody to TNF (infliximab), a third is a fully human antibody to TNF (adalimumab), and a fourth is a humanized monoclonal antibody that neutralizes TNF (golimumab). Clinical trials have shown that parenteral administration of any of these TNF-neutralizing agents is remarkably effective at controlling signs and symptoms of RA in patients who have failed DMARD therapy, as well as in DMARD-naïve patients. Repetitive therapy with these agents is effective with or without concomitant methotrexate, although combination therapy with methotrexate or another DMARD appears to provide the greatest benefit. These agents not only are effective in persistently controlling signs and symptoms of RA in a majority of patients, but they have also been shown to slow the rate of progression of joint damage assessed radiographically and to improve disability. Side effects include the potential for an increased risk of serious infections. Particularly notable is the capacity of TNF blockade to increase the risk of developing reactivation of dormant tuberculosis. It is prudent to carry out tuberculin skin testing and, if necessary, further evaluation with chest radiographs before beginning therapy with an anti-TNF agent to limit the chance of inciting reactivation of tuberculosis. Anti-TNF therapy also has the potential to increase the risk of lymphoma and possibly other malignancies in treated patients. TNF-neutralizing therapy can also induce the development of anti-DNA antibodies, but rarely is there associated evidence of signs and symptoms of systemic lupus erythematosus. Other side effects include infusion or injection site reactions and rarely the development of demyelinating central nervous system disease. Although these side effects are uncommon, their occurrence mandates that TNF-neutralizing therapy be supervised by physicians with experience in their use.

Anakinra is a recombinant IL-1 receptor antagonist that competitively blocks the binding of IL-1β and IL-1α to the IL-1 receptor and thereby inhibits the activity of these two related proinflammatory cytokines. Anakinra has been shown to improve the signs and symptoms of RA, to decrease disability, and to slow progression of articular damage assessed radiographically. It can be given as monotherapy or in combination with methotrexate. The major side effects are injection site reactions. In general, the clinical impact of anakinra appears to be less than that of TNF-neutralizing therapy, but it may be used in those in whom TNF-neutralizing therapy is precluded. It is rarely effective in those who have failed TNF-neutralizing therapy. Combining anakinra with a TNF-blocking agent does not increase efficacy and is associated with an increased frequency of infection and, therefore, is not recommended.

Rituximab, a chimeric antibody directed to CD20 that depletes mature B cells, has been approved for treatment of RA patients who have failed anti-TNF therapy. In combination with methotrexate, this therapy can improve signs and symptoms in these patients and also retard the progress of bone damage. The major adverse events relate to transfusion reactions that can be controlled with glucocorticoids. Although the optimal regimen has not been established, therapy can be repeated usually at 6-month intervals when circulating B cells return.

Abatacept is a fusion protein consisting of CTLA4 and the Fc portion of IgG1. It inhibits T cell activation by competitively inhibiting the co-stimulation of T cells that results from interaction of T cell–expressed CD28 and CD80/86 expressed by antigen-presenting cells. It can be used with or without methotrexate, although its efficacy is greater as co-therapy with methotrexate. It has a positive effect on signs and symptoms of RA and also retards progressive bone damage. It is usually reserved for patients who have failed TNF-neutralizing therapy or in those who have contraindications to TNF blockade. Abatacept is tolerated quite well. Combining abatacept with a TNF-blocking agent does not increase efficacy, and is associated with more adverse events, including serious infections, and, therefore, is not recommended.

IMMUNOSUPPRESSIVE THERAPY The immunosuppressive drugs azathioprine, leflunomide, cyclosporine, and cyclophosphamide have been shown to be effective in the treatment of RA and to exert therapeutic effects similar to those of the DMARDs. However, these agents appear to be no more effective than the DMARDs. Moreover, they cause a variety of toxic side effects, and cyclophosphamide appears to predispose patients to the development of malignant neoplasms. Therefore, these drugs have been reserved for patients who have clearly failed therapy with DMARDs and biologics. On occasion, extraarticular disease such as rheumatoid vasculitis may require cytotoxic immunosuppressive therapy.

Leflunomide is metabolized to an active metabolite that acts to inhibit dihydroorotate dehydrogenase, an essential enzyme in the pyrimidine biosynthetic pathway. Its predominant action is to inhibit the proliferation of T lymphocytes. Leflunomide has been shown to control the signs and symptoms of RA and to slow the progression of joint damage as effectively as methotrexate. Leflunomide can be given alone or with methotrexate and is the most frequently employed immunosuppressive agent used to treat patients with RA. It is used as monotherapy in patients who have had adverse reactions to methotrexate or inadequate responses to it. The major side effect is the associated increase in liver function enzymes that occurs in 5% of patients receiving leflunomide alone and in >50% of individuals taking leflunomide with methotrexate.

SURGERY Surgery plays a role in the management of patients with severely damaged joints. Although arthroplasties and total joint replacements can be done on a number of joints, the most successful procedures are carried out on hips, knees, and shoulders. Realistic goals of these procedures are relief of pain and reduction of disability. Reconstructive hand surgery may lead to cosmetic improvement and some functional benefit. Open or arthroscopic synovectomy may be useful in some patients with persistent monarthritis, especially of the knee. Although synovectomy may offer short-term relief of symptoms, it does not appear to retard bone destruction or alter the natural history of the disease. In addition, early tenosynovectomy of the wrist may prevent tendon rupture.

Approach to the Patient:
RHEUMATOID ARTHRITIS

An approach to the medical management of patients with RA is depicted in **Fig. 5-3**. The principles underlying care of these patients reflect the value of early appropriately aggressive intervention, the variability of the disease, the frequent persistent nature of the inflammation and its potential to cause disability, the relationship between sustained inflammation and bone erosions and mortality, and the need to reevaluate

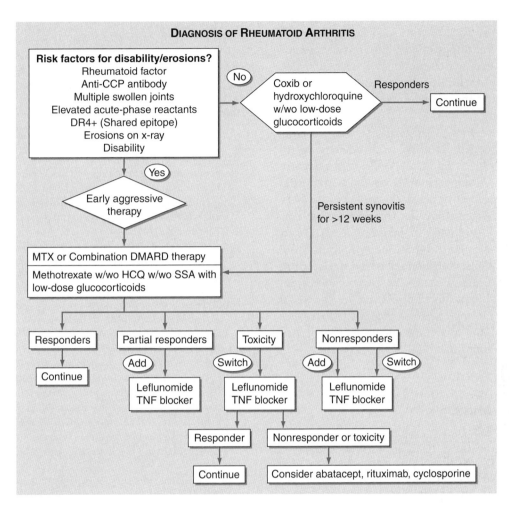

FIGURE 5-3

Algorithm for the medical management of rheumatoid arthritis. Coxib, COX-2 inhibitors; DMARD, disease-modifying anti-rheumatic drug; CCP, cyclic citrullinated polypeptide; MTX, methotrexate; SSA, sulfasalazine; TNF, tumor necrosis factor.

the patient frequently for symptomatic response to therapy, progression of disability and joint damage, and side effects of treatment. At the onset of disease it is difficult to predict the natural history of an individual patient's illness. Therefore, the classic approach was to attempt to alleviate the patient's symptoms with NSAIDs or Coxibs. Some patients may have mild disease that requires no additional therapy. However, most patients will require additional therapy, and the treating physician must be vigilant and prepared to institute appropriate therapy as soon as indicated. Nearly all patients will benefit from a course of low-dose glucocorticoids, and this should be considered routinely. If the patient has any evidence of aggressive disease, as described above, or persistent synovitis for >3 months, initiation of DMARD therapy should be considered as early as feasible. In RA patients there appears to be a window of opportunity early in the course of the disease, during which initiation of aggressive therapy can have a

major impact on subsequent damage to articular structures and disability.

At some time during the course for most patients, the possibility of initiating DMARD therapy is entertained. The presence of risk factors for bone damage or disability or persistent synovitis of >3 months' duration are the usual indications to initiate DMARD therapy. The decision to begin use of a DMARD and/or low-dose oral glucocorticoids requires experience and clinical judgment as well as the ability to assess joint swelling and functional activity and the patient's pain tolerance and expectation of therapy accurately. In this setting, the fully informed patient must play an active role in the decision to begin DMARD and/or low-dose oral glucocorticoid therapy, after careful review of the therapeutic and toxic potential of the various drugs. If DMARD therapy, usually methotrexate, fails to control signs and symptoms of RA, a decision to add or switch to a biologic agent is considered. These are quite potent at controlling signs and symptoms of RA, slowing damage to articular structures, and limiting disability, but are very expensive and associated with serious adverse events. The decision to employ these agents requires considerable experience, judgment, and the agreement of a fully informed patient.

If a patient responds to a DMARD, therapy is continued with careful monitoring to avoid toxicity. All DMARDs provide a suppressive effect and therefore require prolong administration. Even with successful therapy, local injection of glucocorticoids may be necessary to diminish inflammation that may persist in a limited number of joints. In addition, NSAIDs or Coxibs may be necessary to mitigate symptoms. Even after inflammation has totally resolved, symptoms from loss of cartilage and supervening degenerative joint disease or altered joint function may require additional treatment. Surgery may also be necessary to relieve pain or diminish the functional impairment secondary to alterations in joint function.

FURTHER READINGS

ARNETT FC et al: The American Rheumatism Association 1987 Revised Criteria for the Classification of Rheumatoid Arthritis. Arthritis Rheum 31:315, 1988

ASKLING J et al: Risks of solid cancers in patients with rheumatoid arthritis and after treatment with tumour necrosis factor antagonists. Ann Rheum Dis 64(10):1421, 2005

AUGER I et al: Influence of HLA-DR genes on the production of rheumatoid arthritis-specific autoantibodies to citrullinated fibrinogen. Arthritis Rheum 52(11):3424, 2005

BAECKLUND E et al: Lymphoma subtypes in patients with rheumatoid arthritis: Increased proportion of diffuse large B cell lymphoma. Arthritis Rheum 48(6):1543, 2003

———— et al: Association of chronic inflammation, not its treatment, with increased lymphoma risk in rheumatoid arthritis. Arthritis Rheum 54(3):692, 2006

BATHON JM et al: A comparison of etanercept and methotrexate in patients with early rheumatoid arthritis. N Engl J Med 343:1586, 2000

BEGOVICH AB et al: A missense single-nucleotide polymorphism in a gene encoding a protein tyrosine phosphatase (PTPN22) is associated with rheumatoid arthritis. Am J Hum Genet 75(2):330, 2004

BERGLIN E et al: A combination of autoantibodies to cyclic citrullinated peptide (CCP) and HLA-DRB1 locus antigens is strongly associated with future onset of rheumatoid arthritis. Arthritis Res Ther 6(4):R303, 2004

———— et al: Radiological outcome in rheumatoid arthritis is predicted by presence of antibodies against cyclic citrullinated peptide before and at disease onset, and by IgA-RF at disease onset. Ann Rheum Dis 65(4):453, 2006

BONGARTZ T et al: Anti-TNF antibody therapy in rheumatoid arthritis and the risk of serious infections and malignancies: Systematic review and meta-analysis of rare harmful effects in randomized controlled trials. JAMA 295(19):2275, 2006

BORCHERS AT et al: The use of methotrexate in rheumatoid arthritis. Semin Arthritis Rheum 34(1):465, 2004

BREEDVELD FC et al: The PREMIER study: A multicenter, randomized, double-blind clinical trial of combination therapy with adalimumab plus methotrexate versus methotrexate alone or adalimumab alone in patients with early, aggressive rheumatoid arthritis who had not had previous methotrexate treatment. Arthritis Rheum 54(1):26, 2006

BRESNIHAN B et al: Treatment of rheumatoid arthritis with recombinant human interleukin-1 receptor antagonist. Arthritis Rheum 41:2196, 1998

BROWN SL et al: Tumor necrosis factor antagonist therapy and lymphoma development: Twenty-six cases reported to the Food and Drug Administration. Arthritis Rheum 46(12):3151, 2002

BUCH MH et al: Lack of response to anakinra in rheumatoid arthritis following failure of tumor necrosis factor alpha blockade. Arthritis Rheum 50(3):725, 2004

BUKHARI M et al: Rheumatoid factor is the major predictor of increasing severity of radiographic erosions in rheumatoid arthritis: Results from the Norfolk Arthritis Register Study, a large inception cohort. Arthritis Rheum 46(4):906, 2002

CARREIRA PE et al: Polymorphism of the interleukin-1 receptor antagonist gene: A factor in susceptibility to rheumatoid arthritis in a Spanish population. Arthritis Rheum 52(10):3015, 2005

CHOY EH et al: Therapeutic benefit of blocking interleukin-6 activity with an anti-interleukin-6 receptor monoclonal antibody in rheumatoid arthritis: A randomized, double-blind, placebo-controlled, dose-escalation trial. Arthritis Rheum 46(12):53, 2002

COHEN SB et al: A multicentre, double-blind, randomised, placebo-controlled trial of anakinra (Kineret), a recombinant interleukin 1 receptor antagonist, in patients with rheumatoid arthritis treated with background methotrexate. Ann Rheum Dis 63(9):1062, 2004

———— et al: The efficiency of switching from infliximab to etanercept and vice-versa in patients with rheumatoid arthritis. Clin Exp Rheumatol 23(6):795, 2005

COMBE B et al: Prognostic factors for radiographic damage in early rheumatoid arthritis: A multiparameter prospective study. Arthritis Rheum 44(8):1736, 2001

CONAGHAN PG et al: Elucidation of the relationship between synovitis and bone damage: A randomized magnetic resonance imaging study of individual joints in patients with early rheumatoid arthritis. Arthritis Rheum 48(1):64, 2003

COSTENBADER KH et al: Smoking intensity, duration, and cessation, and the risk of rheumatoid arthritis in women. Am J Med 119(6):503, 2006

CRISWELL LA, GREGERSEN PK: Current understanding of the genetic aetiology of rheumatoid arthritis and likely future developments. Rheumatology 44(Suppl. 4):iv13, 2005

DA SILVA JA et al: Safety of low-dose glucocorticoid treatment in rheumatoid arthritis: Published evidence and prospective trial data. Ann Rheum Dis 65(3):285, 2006

DEL RINCON I et al: Association between carotid atherosclerosis and markers of inflammation in rheumatoid arthritis patients and healthy subjects. Arthritis Rheum 48(7):1833, 2003

DE RYCKE L et al: Rheumatoid factor and anticitrullinated protein antibodies in rheumatoid arthritis: Diagnostic value, associations with radiological progression rate, and extra-articular manifestations. Ann Rheum Dis 63(12):1587, 2004

DIEUDE P et al: Rheumatoid arthritis seropositive for the rheumatoid factor is linked to the protein tyrosine phosphatase nonreceptor 22-620W allele. Arthritis Res Ther 7(6):R1200, 2005

DORAN MF et al: Trends in incidence and mortality in rheumatoid arthritis in Rochester, Minnesota, over a forty-year period. Arthritis Rheum 46(3):625, 2002

DRAZEN JM: COX-2 inhibitors-a lesson in unexpected problems. N Engl J Med 352:1131, 2005

DROSSAERS-BAKKER KW et al: Long-term outcome in rheumatoid arthritis: A simple algorithm of baseline parameters can predict radiographic damage, disability, and disease course at 12-year follow-up. Arthritis Rheum 47(4):383, 2002

DU MONTCEL ST et al: New classification of HLA-DRB1 alleles supports the shared epitope hypothesis of rheumatoid arthritis susceptibility. Arthritis Rheum 52(11):3659, 2005

EDWARDS JC et al: Efficacy of B-cell-targeted therapy with rituximab in patients with rheumatoid arthritis. N Engl J Med 350(25):2572, 2004

EMERY P et al: The efficacy and safety of rituximab in patients with active rheumatoid arthritis despite methotrexate treatment. Arthritis Rheum 54(5):1390, 2006

——— et al: Golimumab, a human anti-tumor necrosis factor alpha monoclonal antibody, injected subcutaneously every four weeks in methotrexate-naïve patients with active rheumatoid arthritis: Twenty-four-week results of a phase III, multicenter, randomized, double-blind, placebo-controlled study of golimumab before methotrexate as first-line therapy for early-onset rheumatoid arthritis. Arthritis Rheum 60:2272, 2009

ENZER I et al: An epidemiologic study of trends in prevalence of rheumatoid factor seropositivity in Pima Indians: Evidence of a decline due to both secular and birth-cohort influences. Arthritis Rheum 46(7):1729, 2002

FINCKH A et al: The effectiveness of anti-tumor necrosis factor therapy in preventing progressive radiographic joint damage in rheumatoid arthritis: A population-based study. Arthritis Rheum 54(1):54, 2006

FLEISCHMANN R et al: Long-term safety of etanercept in elderly subjects with rheumatic diseases. Ann Rheum Dis 65(3):379, 2006

GABRIEL SE et al: Survival in rheumatoid arthritis: A population-based analysis of trends over 40 years. Arthritis Rheum 48(1):54, 2003

GEBOREK P et al: Tumour necrosis factor blockers do not increase overall tumour risk in patients with rheumatoid arthritis, but may be associated with an increased risk of lymphomas. Ann Rheum Dis 64(5):699, 2005

GENOVESE MC et al: Etanercept versus methotrexate in patients with early rheumatoid arthritis: Two-year radiographic and clinical outcomes. Arthritis Rheum 46(6):1443, 2002

——— et al: Abatacept for rheumatoid arthritis refractory to tumor necrosis factor alpha inhibition. N Engl J Med 353(11):1114, 2005

——— et al: Long-term safety, efficacy, and radiographic outcome with etanercept treatment in patients with early rheumatoid arthritis. J Rheumatol 32(7):1232, 2005

——— et al: Interleukin-6 receptor inhibition with tocilizumab reduces disease activity in rheumatoid arthritis with inadequate response to disease-modifying antirheumatic drugs: The tocilizumab in combination with traditional disease-modifying antirheumatic drug therapy study. Arthritis Rheum 58:2968, 2008

GERARDS AH et al: Cyclosporin A monotherapy versus cyclosporin A and methotrexate combination therapy in patients with early rheumatoid arthritis: A double-blind randomised placebo-controlled trial. Ann Rheum Dis 62(4):291, 2003

GOEKOOP-RUITERMAN YP et al: Clinical and radiographic outcomes of four different treatment strategies in patients with early rheumatoid arthritis (the BeSt study): A randomized, controlled trial. Arthritis Rheum 52(11):3381, 2005

——— et al: Comparison of treatment strategies in early rheumatoid arthritis: a randomized trial. Ann Intern Med 146:406, 2007

GOLDBACH-MANSKY R, LIPSKY PE: New concepts in the treatment of rheumatoid arthritis. Annu Rev Med 54:197, 2003

——— et al: Comparison of Tripterygium wilfordii Hook F versus sulfasalazine in the treatment of rheumatoid arthritis: A randomized trial. Ann Intern Med 151:229, 2009

GOMEZ-REINO JJ et al: Treatment of rheumatoid arthritis with tumor necrosis factor inhibitors may predispose to significant increase in tuberculosis risk: A multicenter active-surveillance report. Arthritis Rheum 48(8):2122, 2003

GONZALEZ-GAY MA et al: High-grade C-reactive protein elevation correlates with accelerated atherogenesis in patients with rheumatoid arthritis. J Rheumatol 32(7):1219, 2005

——— et al: Rheumatoid arthritis: A disease associated with accelerated atherogenesis. Semin Arthritis Rheum 35(1):8, 2005

HAN S et al: Meta-analysis of the association of CTLA-4 exon-1 +49A/G polymorphism with rheumatoid arthritis. Hum Genet 118(1):123, 2005

HANSEN KE et al: The safety and efficacy of leflunomide in combination with infliximab in rheumatoid arthritis. Arthritis Rheum 51(2):228, 2004

HUIZINGA TW et al: Refining the complex rheumatoid arthritis phenotype based on specificity of the HLA-DRB1 shared epitope for antibodies to citrullinated proteins. Arthritis Rheum 52(11):3433, 2005

JACOBSSON LT et al: Treatment with tumor necrosis factor blockers is associated with a lower incidence of first cardiovascular events in patients with rheumatoid arthritis. J Rheumatol 32(7):1213, 2005

KALDEN JR et al: Use of combination of leflunomide with biological agents in treatment of rheumatoid arthritis. J Rheumatol 32(8):1620, 2005

KAY J et al: Golimumab in patients with active rheumatoid arthritis despite treatment with methotrexate: A randomized, double-blind, placebo-controlled, dose-ranging study. Arthritis Rheum 58:964, 2008

KEANE J et al: Tuberculosis associated with infliximab, a tumor necrosis alpha-neutralizing agent. N Engl J Med 345:1098, 2001

KEYSTONE EC et al: Once-weekly administration of 50 mg etanercept in patients with active rheumatoid arthritis: Results of a multicenter, randomized, double-blind, placebo-controlled trial. Arthritis Rheum 50(2):353, 2004

——— et al: Radiographic, clinical, and functional outcomes of treatment with adalimumab (a human anti-tumor necrosis factor monoclonal antibody) in patients with active rheumatoid arthritis receiving concomitant methotrexate therapy: A randomized, placebo-controlled, 52-week trial. Arthritis Rheum 50:1400, 2004

——— et al: Recent concepts in the inhibition of radiographic progression with biologics. Curr Opin Rheumatol 21:231, 2009

KHANNA D et al: Reduction of the efficacy of methotrexate by the use of folic acid: Post hoc analysis from two randomized controlled studies. Arthritis Rheum 52(10):3030, 2005

KLARESKOG L et al: Therapeutic effect of the combination of etanercept and methotrexate compared with each treatment alone in patients with rheumatoid arthritis: Double-blind, randomised, controlled trial. Lancet 363(9410):675, 2004

——— et al: A new model for an etiology of rheumatoid arthritis: Smoking may trigger HLA-DR (shared epitope)-restricted immune reactions to autoantigens modified by citrullination. Arthritis Rheum 54(1):38, 2006

KREMER J et al: Concomitant leflunomide therapy in patients with active rheumatoid arthritis despite stable doses of methotrexate: A randomized, double-blind, placebo-controlled trial. Ann Intern Med 137(9):726, 2002. Summary for patients in: Ann Intern Med 137(9):I42, 2002

———— et al: Tacrolimus in rheumatoid arthritis patients receiving concomitant methotrexate: A six-month, open-label study. Arthritis Rheum 48(10):2763, 2003

———— et al: Treatment of rheumatoid arthritis by selective inhibition of T-cell activation with fusion protein CTLA4Ig. N Engl J Med 349(20):1907, 2003

———— et al: Combination leflunomide and methotrexate (MTX) therapy for patients with active rheumatoid arthritis failing MTX monotherapy: Open-label extension of a randomized, double-blind, placebo controlled trial. J Rheumatol 31(8):1521, 2004

———— et al: Treatment of rheumatoid arthritis with the selective costimulation modulator abatacept: Twelve-month results of a phase IIb, double-blind, randomized, placebo-controlled trial. Arthritis Rheum 52(8):2263, 2005.

———— et al: Effects of abatacept in patients with methotrexate-resistant active rheumatoid arthritis: A randomized trial. Ann Intern Med 144:865, 2006

Kochi Y et al: A functional variant in FCRL3, encoding Fc receptor-like 3, is associated with rheumatoid arthritis and several autoimmunities. Nat Genet 37(5):478, 2005

Kuhn KA et al: Antibodies against citrullinated proteins enhance tissue injury in experimental autoimmune arthritis. J Clin Invest 116(4):961, 2006

Landewe RB et al: COBRA combination therapy in patients with early rheumatoid arthritis: Long-term structural benefits of a brief intervention. Arthritis Rheum 46(2):347, 2002

Lard LR et al: Early and aggressive treatment of rheumatoid arthritis patients affects the association of HLA class II antigens with progression of joint damage. Arthritis Rheum 46(4):899, 2002

———— et al: Association of the -2849 interleukin-10 promoter polymorphism with autoantibody production and joint destruction in rheumatoid arthritis. Arthritis Rheum 48(7):1841, 2003

Linn-Rasker SP et al: Smoking is a risk factor for anti-CCP antibodies only in rheumatoid arthritis patients who carry HLA-DRB1 shared epitope alleles. Ann Rheum Dis 65(3):366, 2006

Lipsky PE et al: Infliximab and methotrexate in the treatment of rheumatoid arthritis. Anti-Tumor Necrosis Factor Trial in Rheumatoid Arthritis with Concomitant Therapy Study Group. N Engl J Med 343(22):1594, 2000

———— et al: Why does rheumatoid arthritis involve the joints? N Engl J Med 356:2419, 2007

Listing J et al: Infections in patients with rheumatoid arthritis treated with biologic agents. Arthritis Rheum 52(11):3403, 2005

Maddison P et al: Leflunomide in rheumatoid arthritis: Recommendations through a process of consensus. Rheumatology (Oxford) 44(3):280, 2005

Maini RN et al: Sustained improvement over two years in physical function, structural damage, and signs and symptoms among patients with rheumatoid arthritis treated with infliximab and methotrexate. Arthritis Rheum 50(4):1051, 2004

———— et al: Double-blind, randomized, controlled clinical trial of the interleukin-6 receptor antagonist, tocilizumab, in European patients with rheumatoid arthritis who had an incomplete response to methotrexate. Arthritis Rheum 54:2817, 2006

Maradit-Kremers H et al: Cardiovascular death in rheumatoid arthritis: A population-based study. Arthritis Rheum 52(3):722, 2005

———— et al: Increased unrecognized coronary heart disease and sudden deaths in rheumatoid arthritis: A population-based cohort study. Arthritis Rheum 52(2):402, 2005

Messori A et al: New drugs for rheumatoid arthritis. N Engl J Med 351(9):937, 2004

Meyer O et al: Anticitrullinated protein/peptide antibody assays in early rheumatoid arthritis for predicting five year radiographic damage. Ann Rheum Dis 62(2):120, 2003

Mohan N et al: Demyelination occurring during anti-tumor factor alpha therapy for inflammatory arthritides. Arthritis Rheum 44:2862, 2001

Mottonen T et al: Delay to institution of therapy and induction of remission using single-drug or combination-disease-modifying antirheumatic drug therapy in early rheumatoid arthritis. Arthritis Rheum 46(4):894, 2002

Navarro-Cano G et al: Antibodies against cyclic citrullinated peptide and IgA rheumatoid factor predict the development of rheumatoid arthritis. Arthritis Rheum 48(10):2741, 2003

Nicola PJ et al: The risk of congestive heart failure in rheumatoid arthritis: A population-based study over 46 years. Arthritis Rheum 52(2):412, 2005

———— et al: Contribution of congestive heart failure and ischemic heart disease to excess mortality in rheumatoid arthritis. Arthritis Rheum 54(1):60, 2006

Nielen MM et al: Increased levels of C-reactive protein in serum from blood donors before the onset of rheumatoid arthritis. Arthritis Rheum 50(8):2423, 2004

———— et al: Simultaneous development of acute phase response and autoantibodies in preclinical rheumatoid arthritis. Ann Rheum Dis 65(4):535, 2006

Nikas SN et al: Efficacy and safety of switching from infliximab to adalimumab: A comparative controlled study. Ann Rheum Dis 65(2):257, 2006

Nishimoto N et al: Treatment of rheumatoid arthritis with humanized anti-interleukin-6 receptor antibody: A multicenter, double-blind, placebo-controlled trial. Arthritis Rheum 50(6):1761, 2004

Nishimura K et al: Meta-analysis: Diagnostic accuracy of anti-cyclic citrullinated peptide antibody and rheumatoid factor for rheumatoid arthritis. Ann Intern Med 146:797, 2007

O'Dell JR: Therapeutic strategies for rheumatoid arthritis. N Engl J Med 350(25):2591, 2004

———— et al: Treatment of rheumatoid arthritis with methotrexate and hydroxychloroquine, methotrexate and sulfasalazine, or a combination of the three medications: Results of a two-year, randomized, double-blind, placebo-controlled trial. Arthritis Rheum 46:1164, 2002

———— et al: Etanercept in combination with sulfasalazine, hydroxychloroquine, or gold in the treatment of rheumatoid arthritis. J Rheumatol 33(2):213, 2006

Olsen NJ, Stein CM: New drugs for rheumatoid arthritis. N Engl J Med 350(21):2167, 2004

Ozminkowski RJ et al: The impact of rheumatoid arthritis on medical expenditures, absenteeism, and short-term disability benefits. J Occup Environ Med 48(2):135, 2006

Park YB et al: Atherosclerosis in rheumatoid arthritis: Morphologic evidence obtained by carotid ultrasound. Arthritis Rheum 46(7):1714, 2002

Pincus T et al: Patients seen for standard rheumatoid arthritis care have significantly better articular, radiographic, laboratory, and functional status in 2000 than in 1985. Arthritis Rheum 52(4):1009, 2005

Pinheiro GC et al: Anti-cyclic citrullinated peptide antibodies in advanced rheumatoid arthritis. Ann Intern Med 139(3):234, 2003

Plenge RM et al: Replication of putative candidate-gene associations with rheumatoid arthritis in >4,000 samples from North America and Sweden: Association of susceptibility with PTPN22, CTLA4, and PADI4. Am J Hum Genet 77(6):1044, 2005

Poor G et al: Efficacy and safety of leflunomide 10 mg versus 20 mg once daily in patients with active rheumatoid arthritis: Multinational double-blind, randomized trial. Rheumatology (Oxford) 43(6): 744, 2004

PROKUNINA L et al: Association of the PD-1.3A allele of the PDCD1 gene in patients with rheumatoid arthritis negative for rheumatoid factor and the shared epitope. Arthritis Rheum 50(6):1770, 2004

PROTS I et al: Association of the IL4R single-nucleotide polymorphism I50V with rapidly erosive rheumatoid arthritis. Arthritis Rheum 54(5):1491, 2006

PUOLAKKA K et al: Impact of initial aggressive drug treatment with a combination of disease-modifying antirheumatic drugs on the development of work disability in early rheumatoid arthritis: A five-year randomized followup trial. Arthritis Rheum 50(1):55, 2004

QUINN MA et al: Prognostic factors in a large cohort of patients with early undifferentiated inflammatory arthritis after application of a structured management protocol. Arthritis Rheum 48(11):3039, 2003

———— et al: Very early treatment with infliximab in addition to methotrexate in early, poor-prognosis rheumatoid arthritis reduces magnetic resonance imaging evidence of synovitis and damage, with sustained benefit after infliximab withdrawal: Results from a twelve-month randomized, double-blind, placebo-controlled trial. Arthritis Rheum 52(1):27, 2005

RADSTAKE TR et al: Correlation of rheumatoid arthritis severity with the genetic functional variants and circulating levels of macrophage migration inhibitory factor. Arthritis Rheum 52(10):3020, 2005

RANTAPAA-DAHLQVIST S et al: Antibodies against cyclic citrullinated peptide and IgA rheumatoid factor predict the development of rheumatoid arthritis. Arthritis Rheum 48(10):2741, 2003

RASCH EK et al: Prevalence of rheumatoid arthritis in persons 60 years of age and older in the United States: Effect of different methods of case classification. Arthritis Rheum 48(4):917, 2003

RAZA K et al: Early rheumatoid arthritis is characterized by a distinct and transient synovial fluid cytokine profile of T cell and stromal cell origin. Arthritis Res Ther 7(4):R784, 2005

SCHIFF MH et al: The safety of anakinra in high-risk patients with active rheumatoid arthritis: Six-month observations of patients with comorbid conditions. Arthritis Rheum 50(6):1752, 2004

SHARP JT et al: Treatment with leflunomide slows radiographic progression of rheumatoid arthritis: Results from three randomized controlled trials of leflunomide in patients with active rheumatoid arthritis. Arthritis Rheum 43:495, 2000

SMOLEN JS et al: Evidence of radiographic benefit of treatment with infliximab plus methotrexate in rheumatoid arthritis patients who had no clinical improvement: A detailed subanalysis of data from the anti-tumor necrosis factor trial in rheumatoid arthritis with concomitant therapy study. Arthritis Rheum 52(4):1020, 2005

———— et al: Predictors of joint damage in patients with early rheumatoid arthritis treated with high-dose methotrexate with or without concomitant infliximab: Results from the ASPIRE trial. Arthritis Rheum 54(3):702, 2006

SOKKA T et al: Radiographic progression is getting milder in patients with early rheumatoid arthritis. Results of 3 cohorts over 5 years. J Rheumatol 31(6):1073, 2004

ST CLAIR EW et al: Combination of infliximab and methotrexate therapy for early rheumatoid arthritis: A randomized, controlled trial. Arthritis Rheum 50(11):3432, 2004

SUZUKI A et al: Functional haplotypes of PADI4, encoding citrullinating enzyme peptidylarginine deiminase 4, are associated with rheumatoid arthritis. Nat Genet 34(4):395, 2003

SVENSSON B et al: Low-dose prednisolone in addition to the initial disease-modifying antirheumatic drug in patients with early active rheumatoid arthritis reduces joint destruction and increases the remission rate: A two-year randomized trial. Arthritis Rheum 52(11): 3360, 2005

TURESSON C, MATTESON EL: Genetics of rheumatoid arthritis. Mayo Clin Proc 81(1):94, 2006

UHLIG T, KVIEN TK: Is rheumatoid arthritis disappearing? Ann Rheum Dis 64(1):7, 2005

VAN DE PUTTE LB et al: Efficacy and safety of adalimumab as monotherapy in patients with rheumatoid arthritis for whom previous disease modifying antirheumatic drug treatment has failed. Ann Rheum Dis 63(5):508, 2004

VAN DER BIJL AE et al: Infliximab and methotrexate as induction therapy in patients with early rheumatoid arthritis. Arthritis Rheum 56:2129, 2007

VAN DER HEIJDE D et al: Presentation and analysis of data on radiographic outcome in clinical trials: Experience from the TEMPO study. Arthritis Rheum 52(1):49, 2005

VAN DER HELM-VAN MIL AH et al: Antibodies to citrullinated proteins and differences in clinical progression of rheumatoid arthritis. Arthritis Res Ther 7(5):R949, 2005

VAN EVERDINGEN AA et al: Low-dose prednisone therapy for patients with early active rheumatoid arthritis: Clinical efficacy, disease-modifying properties, and side effects: A randomized, double-blind, placebo-controlled clinical trial. Ann Intern Med 136(1):1, 2002

VAN GAALEN FA et al: Autoantibodies to cyclic citrullinated peptides predict progression to rheumatoid arthritis in patients with undifferentiated arthritis: A prospective cohort study. Arthritis Rheum 50(3):709, 2004

VERSTAPPEN SM et al: Five-year followup of rheumatoid arthritis patients after early treatment with disease-modifying antirheumatic drugs versus treatment according to the pyramid approach in the first year. Arthritis Rheum 48(7):1797, 2003

WARRINGTON KJ et al: Rheumatoid arthritis is an independent risk factor for multi-vessel coronary artery disease: A case control study. Arthritis Res Ther 7(5):R984, 2005

WASSENBERG S et al: Very low-dose prednisolone in early rheumatoid arthritis retards radiographic progression over two years: A multicenter, double-blind, placebo-controlled trial. Arthritis Rheum 52(11):3371, 2005

WEINBLATT ME et al: A trial of etanercept, a recombinant tumor necrosis factor receptor: Fc fusion protein, in patients with rheumatoid arthritis receiving methotrexate. N Engl J Med 340:253, 1999

———— et al: Adalimumab, a fully human anti-tumor necrosis factor alpha monoclonal antibody, for the treatment of rheumatoid arthritis in patients taking concomitant methotrexate: The ARMADA trial. Arthritis Rheum 48(1):35, 2003

———— et al: Selective co-stimulation modulation using abatacept in patients with active rheumatoid arthritis while receiving etanercept: A randomized trial. Ann Rheum Dis 66:228, 2007

WELSING PM et al: Is the disease course of rheumatoid arthritis becoming milder? Time trends since 1985 in an inception cohort of early rheumatoid arthritis. Arthritis Rheum 52(9):2616, 2005

WOLFE F et al: Predicting mortality in patients with rheumatoid arthritis. Arthritis Rheum 48(6):1530, 2003

———— et al: Lymphoma in rheumatoid arthritis: The effect of methotrexate and anti-tumor necrosis factor therapy in 18,572 patients. Arthritis Rheum 50(6):1740, 2004

———— et al: Household income and earnings losses among 6,396 persons with rheumatoid arthritis. J Rheumatol 32(10):1875, 2005

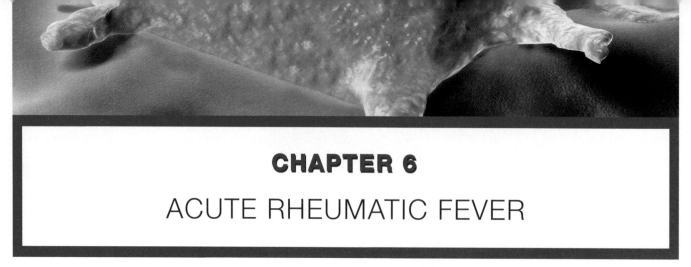

CHAPTER 6

ACUTE RHEUMATIC FEVER

Jonathan R. Carapetis

Acute rheumatic fever (ARF) is a multisystem disease resulting from an autoimmune reaction to infection with group A streptococci. Although many parts of the body may be affected, almost all of the manifestations resolve completely. The exception is cardiac valvular damage [rheumatic heart disease (RHD)], which may persist after the other features have disappeared.

ARF and RHD are diseases of poverty. They were common in all countries until the early twentieth century, when their incidence began to decline in industrialized nations. This decline was largely attributable to improved living conditions—particularly less crowded housing and better hygiene—which resulted in reduced transmission of group A streptococci. The introduction of antibiotics and improved systems of medical care had a supplemental effect. Recurrent outbreaks of ARF began in the 1980s in the Rocky Mountain states of the United States, where elevated rates persist.

The virtual disappearance of ARF and reduction in the incidence of RHD in industrialized countries during the twentieth century unfortunately was not replicated in developing countries, where these diseases continue unabated. RHD is the most common cause of heart disease in children in developing countries and is a major cause of mortality and morbidity in adults as well. It was recently estimated that between 15 and 19 million people worldwide are affected by RHD, with approximately one-quarter of a million deaths occurring each year.

Some 95% of ARF cases and RHD deaths now occur in developing countries.

Although ARF and RHD are relatively common in all developing countries, they occur at particularly elevated rates in certain regions. These "hot spots" are sub-Saharan Africa, Pacific nations, Australasia, and the Indian subcontinent (**Fig. 6-1**).

EPIDEMIOLOGY

ARF is mainly a disease of children aged 5–14 years. Initial episodes become less common in older adolescents and young adults and are rare in persons aged >30 years. By contrast, recurrent episodes of ARF remain relatively common in adolescents and young adults. This pattern contrasts with the prevalence of RHD, which peaks between 25 and 40 years. There is no clear gender association for ARF, but RHD more commonly affects females, sometimes up to twice as frequently as males.

PATHOGENESIS

Organism Factors

Based on currently available evidence, ARF is exclusively caused by infection of the upper respiratory tract with group A streptococci. It is now thought that any strain of group A streptococcus has the potential to cause ARF. The potential role of skin infection and of groups C and G streptococci are currently being investigated.

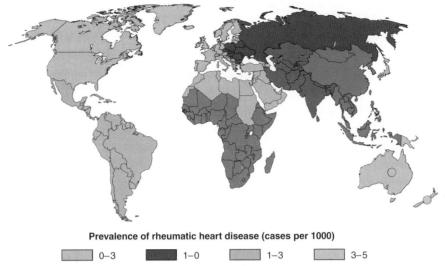

Prevalence of rheumatic heart disease (cases per 1000)

0–3		1–0		1–3		3–5	
0–8		1–8		2–2		5–7	

FIGURE 6-1

Prevalence of rheumatic heart disease in children aged 5–14 years. Circles within Australia and New Zealand represent indigenous populations, and also Pacific Islanders in New Zealand. *(Reprinted with permission from JR Carapetis et al: Lancet Infect Dis.)*

It has been postulated that a series of preceding streptococcal infections is needed to "prime" the immune system prior to the final infection that directly causes disease.

Host Factors

Approximately 3–6% of any population may be susceptible to ARF, and this proportion does not vary dramatically between populations. Findings of familial clustering of cases and concordance in monozygotic twins—particularly for chorea—confirm that susceptibility to ARF is an inherited characteristic. Particular HLA class II alleles appear to be strongly associated with susceptibility. Associations have also been described with high levels of circulating mannose-binding lectin and polymorphisms of transforming growth factor β_1 gene and immunoglobulin genes. High-level expression of a particular alloantigen present on B cells, D8-17, has been found in patients with a history of ARF in many populations, with intermediate-level expression in first-degree family members, suggesting that this may be a marker of inherited susceptibility.

The Immune Response

When a susceptible host encounters a group A streptococcus, an autoimmune reaction results, which leads to damage to human tissues as a result of cross-reactivity between epitopes on the organism and the host (**Fig. 6-2**).

Epitopes present in the cell wall, cell membrane, and the A, B, and C repeat regions of the streptococcal M protein are immunologically similar to molecules in human myosin, tropomyosin, keratin, actin, laminin, vimentin, and N-acetylglucosamine. This molecular mimicry is the basis for the autoimmune response that leads to ARF. It has been hypothesized that human molecules—particularly epitopes in cardiac myosin—result in T cell sensitization. These T cells are then recalled following subsequent exposure to group A streptococci bearing immunologically similar epitopes.

However, myosin cross-reactivity with M protein does not explain the valvular damage that is the hallmark of rheumatic carditis, given that myosin is not present in valvular tissue. The link may be laminin, another α-helical coiled-coil protein like myosin and M protein, which is found in cardiac endothelium and is recognized by anti-myosin, anti-M protein T cells. Moreover, antibodies to cardiac valve tissue cross-react with the N-acetylglucosamine of group A streptococcal carbohydrate, and there is some evidence that these antibodies may be responsible for valvular damage.

CLINICAL FEATURES

There is a latent period of ~3 weeks (1–5 weeks) between the precipitating group A streptococcal infection and the appearance of the clinical features of ARF. The exceptions are chorea and indolent carditis, which may follow prolonged latent periods lasting up to 6 months. Although many patients report a prior sore throat, the preceding group A streptococcal infection is commonly subclinical; in these cases it can only be confirmed using streptococcal antibody testing. The most common clinical presentation of ARF is polyarthritis and fever. Polyarthritis

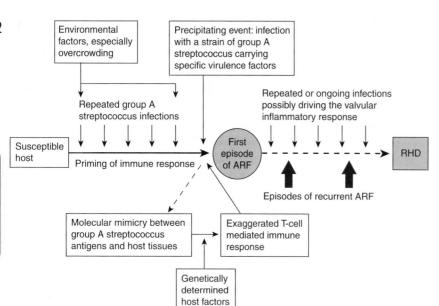

FIGURE 6-2
Pathogenetic pathway for acute rheumatic fever and rheumatic heart disease. *(Reprinted with permission from Lancet 366:155, 2005.)*

is present in 60–75% of cases and carditis in 50–60%. The prevalence of chorea in ARF varies substantially between populations, ranging from <2% to 30%. Erythema marginatum and subcutaneous nodules are now rare, being found in <5% of cases.

Heart Involvement

Up to 60% of patients with ARF progress to RHD. The endocardium, pericardium, or myocardium may be affected. Valvular damage is the hallmark of rheumatic carditis. The mitral valve is almost always affected, sometimes together with the aortic valve; isolated aortic valve involvement is rare. Early valvular damage leads to regurgitation. Over ensuing years, usually as a result of recurrent episodes, leaflet thickening, scarring, calcification, and valvular stenosis may develop. Pericarditis most commonly causes a friction rub or a small effusion on echocardiography and may occasionally cause pleuritic central chest pain. Myocardial involvement is almost never responsible in itself for cardiac failure. Therefore, the characteristic manifestation of carditis in previously unaffected individuals is mitral regurgitation, sometimes accompanied by aortic regurgitation. Myocardial inflammation may affect electrical conduction pathways, leading to P-R interval prolongation (first-degree AV block or rarely higher-level block) and softening of the first heart sound.

Joint Involvement

To qualify as a major manifestation, joint involvement in ARF must be arthritic, i.e., objective evidence of inflammation, with hot, swollen, red and/or tender joints, and involvement of more than one joint (i.e., polyarthritis). The typical arthritis is migratory, moving from one joint to another over a period of hours. ARF almost always affects the large joints—most commonly the knees, ankles, hips, and elbows—and is asymmetric. The pain is severe and usually disabling until anti-inflammatory medication is commenced.

Less severe joint involvement is also relatively common but qualifies only as a minor manifestation. Arthralgia without objective joint inflammation usually affects large joints in the same migratory pattern as polyarthritis. In some populations, aseptic monoarthritis may be a presenting feature of ARF. This may occur because of early commencement of anti-inflammatory medication before the typical migratory pattern is established.

The joint manifestations of ARF are highly responsive to salicylates and other nonsteroidal anti-inflammatory drugs (NSAIDs). Indeed, joint involvement that persists more than 1 or 2 days after starting salicylates is unlikely to be due to ARF. Conversely, if salicylates are commenced early in the illness, before fever and migratory polyarthritis have become manifest, it may be difficult to make a diagnosis of ARF. For this reason, salicylates and other NSAIDs should be withheld—and pain managed with acetaminophen or codeine—until the diagnosis is confirmed.

Chorea

Sydenham's chorea commonly occurs in the absence of other manifestations, follows a prolonged latent period after group A streptococcal infection, and is found mainly in females. The choreiform movements affect particularly the head (causing characteristic darting movements of the tongue) and the upper limbs. They may be generalized or restricted to one side of the body (hemi-chorea). The chorea varies in severity. In mild cases it may be evident only on careful examination, while in the most severe cases the affected individuals are unable to perform activities of daily living and are at risk of injuring themselves. Chorea eventually resolves completely, usually within 6 weeks.

Skin Manifestations

The classic rash of ARF is *erythema marginatum*, which begins as pink macules that clear centrally, leaving a serpiginous, spreading edge. The rash is evanescent, appearing and disappearing before the examiner's eyes. It occurs usually on the trunk, sometimes on the limbs, but almost never on the face.

Subcutaneous nodules occur as painless, small (0.5–2 cm), mobile lumps beneath the skin overlying bony prominences, particularly of the hands, feet, elbows, occiput, and occasionally the vertebrae. They are a delayed manifestation, appearing 2–3 weeks after the onset of disease, last for just a few days up to 3 weeks, and are commonly associated with carditis.

Other Features

Fever occurs in most cases of ARF, although rarely in cases of pure chorea. Although high-grade fever (≥39°C) is the rule, lower grade temperature elevations are not uncommon. Elevated acute-phase reactants are also present in most cases. C-reactive protein (CRP) and erythrocyte sedimentation rate (ESR) are often dramatically elevated. Occasionally the peripheral leukocyte count is mildly elevated.

Evidence of a Preceding Group A Streptococcal Infection

With the exception of chorea and low-grade carditis, both of which may become manifest many months later, evidence of a preceding group A streptococcal infection is essential in making the diagnosis of ARF. As most cases do not have a positive throat swab culture or rapid antigen test, serologic evidence is usually needed. The most common serologic tests are the antistreptolysin O (ASO) and anti-DNase B (ADB) titers. Where possible, age-specific reference ranges should be determined in a local population of healthy people without a recent group A streptococcal infection.

Other Post-Streptococcal Syndromes That May Be Confused with Rheumatic Fever

Post-streptococcal reactive arthritis (PSRA) is differentiated from ARF on the basis of (1) small-joint involvement that is often symmetric; (2) a short latent period following streptococcal infection (usually <1 week); (3) occasional causation by non-group A β-hemolytic streptococcal infection; (4) slower responsiveness to salicylates; and (5) the absence of other features of ARF, particularly carditis.

Pediatric Autoimmune Neuropsychiatric Disorders Associated with Streptococcal infection (PANDAS) is a term that links a range of tic disorders and obsessive-compulsive symptoms with group A streptococcal infections. People with PANDAS are said not to be at risk of carditis, unlike patients with Sydenham's chorea. The diagnoses of PANDAS and PSRA should rarely be made in populations with a high incidence of ARF.

Confirming the Diagnosis

Because there is no definitive test, the diagnosis of ARF relies on the presence of a combination of typical clinical features together with evidence of the precipitating group A streptococcal infection, and the exclusion of other diagnoses. This uncertainty led Dr. T. Duckett Jones in 1944 to develop a set of criteria (subsequently known as the *Jones criteria*) to aid in the diagnosis. An expert panel convened by the World Health Organization (WHO) clarified the use of the Jones criteria in ARF recurrences (Table 6-1). These criteria include a preceding streptococcal type A infection as well as some combination of major and minor manifestations.

℞ Treatment:
ACUTE RHEUMATIC FEVER

Patients with possible ARF should be followed closely to ensure that the diagnosis is confirmed, treatment of heart failure and other symptoms is undertaken, and preventive measures including commencement of secondary prophylaxis, inclusion on an ARF registry, and health education are commenced. Echocardiography should be performed on all possible cases to aid in making the diagnosis and to determine the severity at baseline of any carditis. Other tests that should be performed are listed in Table 6-2.

There is no treatment for ARF that has been proven to alter the likelihood of developing, or the severity of, RHD. With the exception of treatment of heart failure, which may be life-saving in cases of severe carditis, the treatment of ARF is symptomatic.

ANTIBIOTICS All patients with ARF should receive antibiotics sufficient to treat the precipitating group A streptococcal infection. Penicillin is the drug of choice and can be given orally (as penicillin, 500 mg PO twice daily for 10 days) or as a single dose of 1.2 million units IM benzathine penicillin G. Erythromycin, 250 mg bid,

TABLE 6-1

2002–2003 WORLD HEALTH ORGANIZATION CRITERIA FOR THE DIAGNOSIS OF RHEUMATIC FEVER AND RHEUMATIC HEART DISEASE (BASED ON THE 1992 REVISED JONES CRITERIA)

DIAGNOSTIC CATEGORIES	CRITERIA
Primary episode of rheumatic fever[a]	Two major or one major and two minor manifestations plus evidence of preceding group A streptococcal infection
Recurrent attack of rheumatic fever in a patient without established rheumatic heart disease	Two major or one major and two minor manifestations plus evidence of preceding group A streptococcal infection
Recurrent attack of rheumatic fever in a patient with established rheumatic heart disease[b]	Two minor manifestations plus evidence of preceding group A streptococcal infection[c]
Rheumatic chorea	Other major manifestations or evidence of group A streptococcal infection not required
Insidious Onset Rheumatic Carditis[b]	
Chronic valve lesions of rheumatic heart disease (patients presenting for the first time with pure mitral stenosis or mixed mitral valve disease and/or aortic valve disease)[d]	Do not require any other criteria to be diagnosed as having rheumatic heart disease
Major manifestations	Carditis
	Polyarthritis
	Chorea
	Erythema marginatum
	Subcutaneous nodules
Minor manifestations	Clinical: fever, polyarthralgia
	Laboratory: elevated erythrocyte sedimentation rate or leukocyte count[e]
	Electrocardiogram: prolonged P-R interval
Supporting evidence of a preceding streptococcal infection within the last 45 days	Elevated or rising antistreptolysin O or other streptococcal antibody, or
	A positive throat culture, or
	Rapid antigen test for group A streptococcus, or
	Recent scarlet fever[e]

[a]Patients may present with polyarthritis (or with only polyarthralgia or monoarthritis) and with several (3 or more) other minor manifestations, together with evidence of recent group A streptococcal infection. Some of these cases may later turn out to be rheumatic fever. It is prudent to consider them as cases of "probable rheumatic fever" (once other diagnoses are excluded) and advise regular secondary prophylaxis. Such patients require close follow-up and regular examination of the heart. This cautious approach is particularly suitable for patients in vulnerable age groups in high incidence settings.

[b]Infective endocarditis should be excluded.

[c]Some patients with recurrent attacks may not fulfill these criteria.

[d]Congenital heart disease should be excluded.

[e]1992 Revised Jones criteria do not include elevated leukocyte count as a laboratory minor manifestation (but do include elevated C-reactive protein), and do not include recent scarlet fever as supporting evidence of a recent streptococcal infection.

Source: Reprinted with permission from WHO Expert Consultation on Rheumatic Fever and Rheumatic Heart Disease (2001: Geneva, Switzerland): *Rheumatic Fever and Rheumatic Heart Disease: Report of a WHO Expert Consultation* (WHO Tech Rep Ser, 923). Geneva, World Health Organization, 2004.

may be used for patients with penicillin allergy. Because long-term secondary prophylaxis will be needed—and penicillin is the drug of choice for this—reported penicillin allergy should be confirmed, preferably in consultation with an allergist.

SALICYLATES AND NSAIDs These may be used for the treatment of arthritis, arthralgia, and fever, once the diagnosis is confirmed. They are of no value in the treatment of carditis or chorea. Aspirin is the drug of choice. An initial dose of 80–100 mg/kg per day in children (4–8 g/d in adults) in 4–5 divided doses is often needed for the first few days up to 2 weeks. A lower dose should be used if symptoms of salicylate toxicity

emerge, such as nausea, vomiting, or tinnitus. When the acute symptoms are substantially resolved, the dose can be reduced to 60–70 mg/kg per day for a further 2–4 weeks. Fever, joint manifestations, and elevated acute-phase reactants sometimes recur up to 3 weeks after the medication is discontinued. This does not indicate a recurrence and can be managed by recommencing salicylates for a brief period. Although less well studied, naproxen at a dose of 10–20 mg/kg per day has been reported to lead to good symptomatic response.

CONGESTIVE HEART FAILURE

Glucocorticoids The use of glucocorticoids in ARF remains controversial. Two meta-analyses have failed to

TABLE 6-2

RECOMMENDED TESTS IN CASES OF POSSIBLE ACUTE RHEUMATIC FEVER

Recommended for All Cases

White blood cell count
Erythrocyte sedimentation rate
C-reactive protein
Blood cultures if febrile
Electrocardiogram (repeat in 2 weeks and 2 months if prolonged P-R interval or other rhythm abnormality)
Chest x-ray if clinical or echocardiographic evidence of carditis
Echocardiogram (consider repeating after 1 month if negative)
Throat swab (preferably before giving antibiotics)—culture for group A streptococcus
Anti-streptococcal serology: both antistreptolysin O and anti-DNase B titers, if available (repeat 10–14 days later if 1st test not confirmatory)

Tests for Alternative Diagnoses, Depending on Clinical Features

Repeated blood cultures if possible endocarditis
Joint aspirate (microscopy and culture) for possible septic arthritis
Copper, ceruloplasmin, anti-nuclear antibody, drug screen for choreiform movements
Serology and auto-immune markers for arboviral, auto-immune or reactive arthritis

Source: Reprinted with permission from National Heart Foundation of Australia.

---

demonstrate a benefit of glucocorticoids compared to placebo or salicylates in improving the short- or longer-term outcome of carditis. However, the studies included in these meta-analyses all took place >40 years ago and did not use medications in common usage today. Many clinicians treat cases of severe carditis (causing heart failure) with glucocorticoids in the belief that they may reduce the acute inflammation and result in more rapid resolution of failure. However, the potential benefits of this treatment should be balanced against the possible adverse effects, including gastrointestinal bleeding and fluid retention. If used, prednisone or prednisolone are recommended at doses of 1–2 mg/kg per day (maximum, 80 mg). Intravenous methylprednisolone may be used in very severe carditis. Glucocorticoids are often only required for a few days or up to a maximum of 3 weeks.

BED REST Traditional recommendations for long-term bed rest, once the cornerstone of management, are no longer widely practiced. Instead, bed rest should be prescribed as needed while arthritis and arthralgia are present, and for patients with heart failure. Once symptoms are well controlled, gradual mobilization can commence as tolerated.

CHOREA Medications to control the abnormal movements do not alter the duration or outcome of chorea. Milder cases can usually be managed by providing a calm environment. In patients with severe chorea, carbamazepine or sodium valproate are preferred to haloperidol. A response may not be seen for 1–2 weeks, and a successful response may only be to reduce rather than resolve the abnormal movements. Medication should be continued for 1–2 weeks after symptoms subside.

INTRAVENOUS IMMUNOGLOBULIN (IVIg) Small studies have suggested that IVIg may lead to more rapid resolution of chorea but has shown no benefit on the short- or long-term outcome of carditis in ARF without chorea. In the absence of better data, IVIg is *not* recommended except in cases of severe chorea refractory to other treatments.

PROGNOSIS

Untreated, ARF lasts on average 12 weeks. With treatment, patients are usually discharged from hospital within 1–2 weeks. Inflammatory markers should be monitored every 1–2 weeks until they have normalized (usually within 4–6 weeks), and an echocardiogram should be performed after 1 month to determine if there has been progression of carditis. Cases with more severe carditis need close clinical and echocardiographic monitoring in the longer term.

Once the acute episode has resolved, the priority in management is to ensure long-term clinical follow-up and adherence to a regimen of secondary prophylaxis. Patients should be entered onto the local ARF registry (if present) and contact made with primary care practitioners to ensure a plan for follow-up and administration of secondary prophylaxis before the patient is discharged. Patients and their families should also be educated about their disease, emphasizing the importance of adherence to secondary prophylaxis. If carditis is present, they should also be informed of the need for antibiotic prophylaxis against endocarditis for dental and surgical procedures.

PREVENTION

Primary Prevention

Ideally, primary prevention would entail elimination of the major risk factors for streptococcal infection, particularly overcrowded housing and inadequate hygiene infrastructure. This is difficult to achieve in most places where ARF is common.

Therefore, the mainstay of primary prevention for ARF remains primary prophylaxis, i.e., the timely and complete treatment of group A streptococcal sore throat with antibiotics. If commenced within 9 days of sore throat onset, a course of 10 days of penicillin V (500 mg bid PO in adults) or a single IM injection of 1.2 million units of benzathine penicillin G will prevent almost all cases of ARF that would otherwise have developed. This important strategy relies on individuals presenting for medical care when they have a sore throat, the availability of trained health and microbiology staff along with the materials and infrastructure to take throat swabs, and a reliable supply of penicillin. Unfortunately, many of these elements are not available in developing countries. Moreover, the majority of cases of ARF do not follow a sore throat sufficiently severe for the patient to seek medical attention.

Secondary Prevention

The mainstay of controlling ARF and RHD is secondary prevention. Because patients with ARF are at dramatically higher risk than the general population of developing a further episode of ARF after a group A streptococcal infection, they should receive long-term penicillin prophylaxis to prevent recurrences. The best antibiotic for secondary prophylaxis is benzathine penicillin G (1.2 million units, or 600,000 units if <30 kg) delivered every 4 weeks or more frequently (e.g., every 3 weeks or even every 2 weeks) to persons considered to be at particularly high risk. Oral penicillin V (250 mg) can be given twice-daily instead but is somewhat less effective than benzathine penicillin G. Penicillin allergic patients can receive erythromycin (250 mg) twice daily.

The duration of secondary prophylaxis is determined by many factors, in particular the duration since the last episode of ARF (recurrences become less likely with increasing time), age (recurrences are less likely with increasing age), and the severity of RHD (if severe, it may be prudent to avoid even a very small risk of recurrence because of the potentially serious consequences) (**Table 6-3**). Secondary prophylaxis is best delivered as part of a coordinated RHD control program, based around a registry of patients. Registries improve the ability to follow patients and identify those who default from prophylaxis and institute strategies to improve adherence.

TABLE 6-3

SUGGESTED DURATION OF SECONDARY PROPHYLAXIS[a]

CATEGORY OF PATIENT	DURATION OF PROPHYLAXIS
Patient without proven carditis	For 5 years after the last attack or 18 years of age (whichever is longer)
Patient with carditis (mild mitral regurgitation or healed carditis)	For 10 years after the last attack, or 25 years of age (whichever is longer)
More severe valvular disease	Lifelong
Valvular surgery	Lifelong

[a]These are only recommendations and must be modified by individual circumstances as warranted.

Source: Reprinted with permission from WHO Expert Consultation on Rheumatic Fever and Rheumatic Heart Disease (2001: Geneva, Switzerland): *Rheumatic Fever and Rheumatic Heart Disease: Report of a WHO Expert Consultation* (WHO Tech Rep Ser, 923). Geneva, World Health Organization, 2004.

FURTHER READINGS

BRYANT PA et al. Some of the people, some of the time: Susceptibility to acute rheumatic fever. Circulation 119:742, 2009

CARAPETIS JR et al: Acute rheumatic fever. Lancet 366:155, 2005
——— et al: The global burden of group A streptococcal diseases. Lancet Infect Dis 5:685, 2005

CILLIERS AM: Rheumatic fever and its management. BMJ 333:1153, 2006

GERBER MA et al. Prevention of rheumatic fever and diagnosis and treatment of acute streptococcal pharyngitis: A scientific statement from the American Heart Association Rheumatic Fever, Endocarditis, and Kawasaki Disease Committee of the Council on Cardiovascular Disease in the Young, the Interdisciplinary Council on Functional Genomics and Translational Biology, and the Interdisciplinary Council on Quality of Care and Outcomes Research: Endorsed by the American Academy of Pediatrics. Circulation 119:154, 2009

GUILHERME L et al: Molecular mimicry in the autoimmune pathogenesis of rheumatic heart disease. Autoimmunity 39:31, 2006

NATIONAL HEART FOUNDATION OF AUSTRALIA: *Diagnosis and Management of Acute Rheumatic Fever and Rheumatic Heart Disease in Australia: Complete Evidence-Based Review and Guideline.* Melbourne, National Heart Foundation of Australia, 2006

SPECIAL WRITING GROUP OF THE COMMITTEE ON RHEUMATIC FEVER, ENDOCARDITIS, AND KAWASAKI DISEASE OF THE AMERICAN HEART ASSOCIATION: Guidelines for the diagnosis of acute rheumatic fever: Jones criteria, 1992 update. JAMA 268:2069, 1992

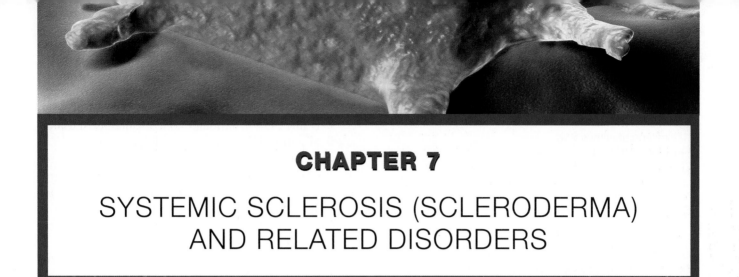

CHAPTER 7

SYSTEMIC SCLEROSIS (SCLERODERMA) AND RELATED DISORDERS

John Varga

DEFINITION

Systemic sclerosis (SSc) is a chronic systemic disorder of unknown etiology. SSc is characterized by thickening of the skin (scleroderma) and distinctive involvement of multiple internal organs, most notably the lungs, gastrointestinal tract, heart, and kidneys. The early stage of the disease, associated with prominent inflammatory features, is followed by the development of widespread functional and structural alterations in multiple vascular beds and progressive visceral organ dysfunction due to fibrosis. The presence of thickened skin (scleroderma) distinguishes SSc from other connective tissue diseases. Scleroderma-like skin induration can occur in various disorders in addition to localized forms of scleroderma (Table 7-1), and it is important to accurately differentiate these conditions from SSc. The disease is highly heterogeneous. Patients with SSc can be classified into two distinct subsets defined by the distribution pattern and extent of skin involvement, as well as other clinical and laboratory manifestations (Table 7-2). Diffuse cutaneous SSc (dcSSc) presents with progressive skin induration, starting in the fingers and ascending from distal to proximal extremities, the face, and the trunk. These patients are at risk for early pulmonary fibrosis and acute renal involvement. In limited cutaneous SSc (lcSSc), patients generally have long-standing Raynaud's phenomenon before other manifestations of SSc appear. Skin induration is limited to the fingers (sclerodactyly), distal extremities, and face, and the trunk is not affected. A subset of patients with lcSSc have prominent calcinosis cutis, Raynaud's phenomenon, esophageal dysmotility, sclerodactyly, and telangiectasia, a constellation termed *CREST syndrome*. However, these features may also be seen in patients with dcSSc. Visceral organ involvement in lcSSc tends to show insidious progression. Although the long-term prognosis of lcSSc is better than that of dcSSc, pulmonary arterial hypertension (PAH), hypothyroidism, and primary biliary cirrhosis may occur in the late stage of the former. In some patients, Raynaud's phenomenon and other typical features of SSc occur in the absence of detectable skin thickening. This syndrome has been termed *SSc sine scleroderma*.

EPIDEMIOLOGY

SSc is an acquired sporadic disease with a worldwide distribution and affecting all races. In the United States, the incidence is 9–19 cases per million per year. The only community-based survey of SSc yielded a prevalence of 286 cases per million population. There are an estimated 100,000 cases of SSc in the United States, although this number may be significantly

TABLE 7-1

CONDITIONS ASSOCIATED WITH SCLERODERMA-LIKE INDURATION

Systemic sclerosis
    Limited cutaneous SSc
    Diffuse cutaneous SSc
Localized scleroderma
    Guttate morphea, diffuse morphea
    Linear scleroderma, coup de sabre, hemifacial atrophy
Overlap syndromes
    Mixed connective tissue disease
    SSc/polymyositis
Undifferentiated connective tissue disease
Scleredema and diabetic scleredema
Scleromyxedema (papular mucinosis)
Nephrogenic fibrosing syndrome (nephrogenic fibrosing
  dermatopathy)
Chronic graft-versus-host disease
Diffuse fasciitis with eosinophilia (Shulman disease,
  eosinophilic fasciitis)
Eosinophilia-myalgia syndrome
Chemically induced scleroderma-like conditions
    Vinyl chloride–induced disease
    Pentazocine-induced skin fibrosis
Paraneoplastic syndrome

higher if patients who do not meet strict classification criteria are also included. Studies from England, Australia, and Japan showed rates of SSc that were lower than in the United States. Age, gender, and ethnicity are important factors determining disease susceptibility. Like other connective tissue diseases, SSc shows a female predominance, greatest in the child-bearing years and declining after menopause. While SSc can present at any age, the most common age of onset is in the range of 30–50 years. African Americans have a higher incidence than whites, and disease onset occurs at an earlier age. Furthermore, African Americans are more likely to have the diffuse cutaneous form of SSc with interstitial lung involvement as well as a worse prognosis.

GENETIC CONSIDERATIONS

SSc shows a non-Mendelian pattern of inheritance. The concordance rate for SSc among twins is low (4.7%), although concordance for the presence of antinuclear antibodies is significantly greater. A genetic contribution to disease susceptibility is indicated by the fact that 1.6% of SSc patients have a first-degree relative with SSc. The risk of other autoimmune diseases, including systemic lupus erythematosus (Chap. 4) and rheumatoid arthritis (Chap. 5), is also increased. Among Choctaw Native Americans, SSc prevalence as high as 4690 per million has been reported. Genetic investigations in SSc to date have focused on polymorphisms of candidate genes, particularly those involved in immunity and inflammation, vascular function, and connective tissue homeostasis. Associations of single nucleotide polymorphism (SNP) with SSc have been reported in the genes encoding angiotensin-converting enzyme (ACE); endothelin-1 and nitric oxide synthase; B cell markers (CD19); chemokines (monocyte chemoattractant protein-1) and chemokine receptors; cytokines [interleukin (IL) 1α, IL-4, and tumor necrosis factor α (TNF-α)]; growth factors and their receptors [connective tissue growth factor (CTGF) and transforming growth factor β (TGF-β)]; and extracellular matrix proteins [fibronectin, fibrillin, and secreted protein acidic-rich in cysteine (SPARC)].

ENVIRONMENTAL FACTORS

Patients with SSc have increased serum antibodies to human cytomegalovirus (hCMV), and antitopoisomerase-I (Scl-70) autoantibodies recognize antigenic epitopes present on the hCMV-derived proteins, suggesting molecular mimicry as a possible mechanistic link between hCMV infection and SSc. Evidence of human parvovirus B19 infection in SSc patients has also been presented; however, the etiologic role of viruses remains unproven. Reports of apparent geographic clustering of SSc cases suggesting shared environmental exposures

TABLE 7-2

SUBSETS OF SYSTEMIC SCLEROSIS (SSc): LIMITED CUTANEOUS SSc VERSUS DIFFUSE CUTANEOUS SSc

FEATURES	LIMITED CUTANEOUS SSc	DIFFUSE CUTANEOUS SSc
Skin involvement	Limited to fingers, distal to elbows, face; slow progression	Diffuse: fingers, extremities, face, trunk; rapid progression
Raynaud's phenomenon	Precedes skin involvement; associated with critical ischemia	Onset contemporaneous with skin involvement
Pulmonary fibrosis	May occur, moderate	Frequent, early and severe
Pulmonary arterial hypertension	Frequent, late, may be isolated	May occur, associated with pulmonary fibrosis
Scleroderma renal crisis	Very rare	Occurs in 15%; early
Calcinosis cutis	Frequent, prominent	May occur, mild
Characteristic autoantibodies	Anticentromere	Antitopoisomerase I (Scl-70)

TABLE 7-3

INTERNAL ORGAN INVOLVEMENT: LIMITED CUTANEOUS AND DIFFUSE CUTANEOUS FORMS OF SYSTEMIC SCLEROSIS

FEATURES	LIMITED CUTANEOUS SSc (%)	DIFFUSE CUTANEOUS SSc (%)
Skin involvement	90[a]	100
Raynaud's phenomenon	99	98
Esophageal involvement	90	80
Pulmonary fibrosis	35	65
Pulmonary arterial hypertension	25	15
Myopathy	11	23
Cardiac involvement	9	12
Scleroderma renal crisis	2	15

[a]10% of lcSSc patients have SSc sine scleroderma.

in its clinical expression from one patient to the next. Patients can be classified into one of two major subsets defined by the degree of clinically involved skin (Table 7-2). In dcSSc, internal organ involvement occurs early and is often progressive. In contrast, lcSSc presents with long-standing Raynaud's phenomenon, is associated with indolent skin and limited internal organ involvement, and carries a better prognosis. While classification of SSc into diffuse and limited cutaneous subsets is useful, disease expression is far more complex, and several distinct phenotypes are recognized within each subset. For example, 10–15% of patients with lcSSc develop severe pulmonary artery hypertension without significant interstitial lung disease (ILD). Other patients have systemic features of SSc without appreciable skin involvement (SSc sine scleroderma). Unique clinical phenotypes of SSc associate with specific autoantibodies (Table 7-4). Patients with "overlap" have typical SSc

TABLE 7-4

AUTOANTIBODIES IN SYSTEMIC SCLEROSIS (SSc)

TARGET ANTIGEN	SSc SUBSET	CHARACTERISTIC CLINICAL ASSOCIATION
Topoisomerase-I	dcSSc	ILD, cardiac involvement, scleroderma renal crisis
Centromere proteins	lcSSc	Digital ischemia, calcinosis, isolated PAH
U3-RNP	dcSSc	PAH, ILD, scleroderma renal crisis, myositis
Th/ T0	lcSSc	ILD, PAH
PM/Scl	lcSSc	Calcinosis, myositis
U1-RNP	MCTD	PAH
RNA polymerase III	dcSSc	Extensive skin, scleroderma renal crisis

Note: dcSSc, diffuse cutaneous SSc; lcSSc, limited cutaneous SSc; ILD, interstitial lung disease; PAH, pulmonary arterial hypertension.

features coexisting with clinical and laboratory evidence of another autoimmune disease such as polymyositis, autoimmune thyroid disease, Sjögren's syndrome, polyarthritis, autoimmune liver disease, or systemic lupus erythematosus.

The term *scleroderma* refers to localized scleroderma and is used to describe a group of localized fibrosing skin disorders that primarily affect children (Table 7-1). In contrast to SSc, localized scleroderma is rarely associated with internal organ involvement. Morphea presents as solitary or multiple circular patches of thickened skin and, less commonly, widespread induration (generalized morphea); the fingers are spared. Linear scleroderma— streaks of thickened skin, typically in one or both lower extremities—may affect the subcutaneous tissues with fibrosis and atrophy of supporting structures, muscle, and bone. In children, the growth of affected long bones can be retarded. When linear scleroderma lesions cross joints, significant contractures can develop.

Initial Clinical Presentation

The initial clinical presentation is quite different in the diffuse and the limited cutaneous forms of the disease. In dcSSc, the interval between Raynaud's phenomenon and appearance of other manifestations is generally brief (weeks to months). Soft tissue swelling and intense pruritus are signs of the early inflammatory "edematous" phase of dcSSc. The skin on the fingers, hands, distal limbs, and face is usually affected first. Patients may note diffuse hyperpigmentation. Carpal tunnel syndrome can occur. Arthralgias are common and may be associated with muscle weakness and decreased joint mobility. During the ensuing weeks to months, the inflammatory edematous phase evolves into the "fibrotic" phase. Fibrosis starts in the dermis and is associated with loss of body hair, reduced production of skin oils, and a decline in sweating capacity. The subcutaneous tissue becomes affected, with fat atrophy and fibrosis of underlying fascia, muscle, and other soft tissue structures. Progressive flexion contractures of the fingers ensue. The wrists, elbows, shoulders, hip girdles, knees, and ankles are also affected due to fibrosis of the supporting joint structures. While advancing skin involvement is the most visible manifestation of early active dcSSc, progressive internal organ involvement occurs during this stage. The initial 4 years of the disease is the period of rapidly evolving systemic involvement; if organ failure does not occur during this period, the systemic process may then stabilize without further progression.

The course of the disease in lcSSc is more indolent and relatively benign. The period between the onset of Raynaud's phenomenon and additional manifestations such as gastroesophageal reflux, telangiectasia, or calcinosis is commonly several years. Raynaud's phenomenon tends to be more severe in lcSSc and is frequently associated with critical digital ischemia, ulcerations, and autoamputation.

Although significant renal involvement or pulmonary fibrosis is uncommon, isolated pulmonary artery hypertension develops in 10–15% of patients with lcSSc. Overlap of SSc with other autoimmune syndromes, including the sicca complex, polyarthritis, cutaneous vasculitis, and biliary cirrhosis, occurs primarily in the lcSSc subset.

ORGAN INVOLVEMENT

Raynaud's Phenomenon

Raynaud's phenomenon, defined as episodic vasoconstriction in the fingers and toes, develops in virtually every patient with SSc. In some, episodes may also affect the tip of the nose and earlobes. Attacks are triggered by exposure to cold, a decrease in temperature, emotional stress, and vibration. In colder climates, patients commonly experience an increase in the frequency and severity of episodes during the winter months. Typical attacks start with pallor, followed by cyanosis of variable duration. Eventually erythema develops spontaneously or with rewarming of the digit. The progression of the three color phases reflects the underlying pathogenic mechanisms of vasoconstriction, ischemia, and reperfusion. Some patients with Raynaud's phenomenon may experience only pallor or cyanosis.

As much as 3–5% of the general population has Raynaud's phenomenon, and it is more frequent in women. In the absence of associated signs or symptoms of an underlying condition, Raynaud's phenomenon is classified as primary, and represents an exaggerated physiological response to cold. Secondary Raynaud's phenomenon occurs as a complication of SSc and other connective tissue diseases, hematological and endocrine conditions, and occupational disorders, as well as in association with the use of beta blockers such as atenolol, anticancer drugs such as cisplatin and bleomycin, and a variety of other medications. Distinguishing primary versus secondary Raynaud's phenomenon can present a diagnostic challenge. The lack of an underlying cause for Raynaud's phenomenon on the basis of the history and physical examination; a positive family history of Raynaud's phenomenon; absence of digital tissue necrosis, ulceration, or gangrene; and a negative test for antinuclear antibodies support the diagnosis of primary Raynaud's phenomenon. Secondary Raynaud's phenomenon tends to develop at an older age (>30 years), is clinically more severe (episodes more frequent, prolonged, and painful), and is frequently associated with ischemic lesions and infarction in the digits (**Fig. 7-3**). The cutaneous capillaries at the nailbed can be viewed under a drop of grade B immersion oil using a low-power stereoscopic microscope. Nailfold microscopy may be helpful in Raynaud's phenomenon; patients with primary Raynaud's phenomenon have normal capillaries that appear as regularly spaced parallel vascular loops, whereas in SSc and other connective tissue diseases, nailfold capillaries are distorted

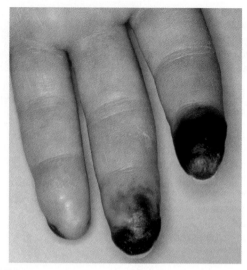

FIGURE 7-3
Digital necrosis. Sharply demarcated necrosis of the fingertip in a patient with limited cutaneous SSc.

with widened and irregular loops, dilated lumen, and areas of vascular "dropout." In patients with SSc, Raynaud's-like abnormal vascular reactivity may involve multiple vascular beds, and cold-induced episodic vasospasm has been documented in the pulmonary, renal, gastrointestinal, and coronary circulations.

Skin Features

Clinically evident skin thickening is the hallmark of SSc that distinguishes it from other connective tissue diseases. The distribution of skin thickening is invariably symmetrical and bilateral. In the early stages of dcSSc, edema is gradually replaced by skin thickening that characteristically advances from distal to proximal extremities in an ascending centripetal fashion. In the affected areas, the skin is firm, coarse, and thickened. The extremities and trunk may be darkly pigmented. In some patients, diffuse tanning in the absence of sun exposure is a very early manifestation of skin involvement. In dark-skinned patients, vitiligo-like hypopigmentation may occur. Because pigment loss spares the perifollicular areas, a "salt-and-pepper" appearance of the skin may be seen; this pattern is most common on the scalp, upper back, and chest. Dermal sclerosis due to collagen accumulation causes obliteration of hair follicles, sweat glands, and sebaceous glands, resulting in hair loss, decreased sweating, and dry skin. Transverse creases on the dorsum of the fingers disappear (**Fig. 7-4**). The fingers develop fixed flexion contractures, causing reduced hand mobility and muscle atrophy. Skin thickening in combination with fibrosis of the subjacent tendons accounts for contractures of the wrists, elbows, and knees. Thick ridges at the neck due to firm adherence of skin to the underlying platysma muscle interfere with neck extension. The face assumes a characteristic "mauskopf"

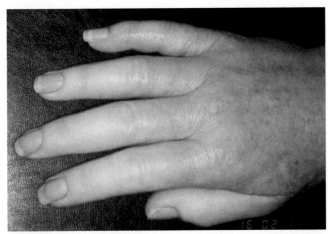

FIGURE 7-4

Sclerodactyly. Note skin induration and fixed flexion contractures at the proximal interphalangeal joints in a patient with limited cutaneous SSc.

appearance with taut and shiny skin, loss of wrinkles, and occasionally an expressionless facies due to reduced mobility of the eyelids, cheeks, and mouth. Thinning of the lips with accentuation of the central incisor teeth and fine wrinkles (radial furrowing) around the mouth complete the picture. The oral aperture may be dramatically reduced; microstomia interferes with eating and oral hygiene. The nose assumes a pinched, beak-like appearance.

In established SSc of long duration, the affected skin is firmly bound to the subcutaneous fat (tethering) and undergoes thinning and atrophy. Macular telangiectasia 2–20 mm in diameter occur frequently, particularly in lcSSc. These skin lesions, which resemble the telangiectasia seen in hereditary hemorrhagic telangiectasia, are prominent on the face, hands, lips, and oral cavity. Breakdown of atrophic skin leads to slow-healing ulcerations that are most common at the extensor surfaces of the proximal interphalangeal joints. Other sites for skin ulcerations include the volar pads of the fingertips and bony prominences such as the elbows and malleoli. Chronic ulcers are painful and may become secondarily infected, resulting in osteomyelitis. Healing of ischemic fingertip ulcerations leaves characteristic digital "pits." Soft tissue loss at the fingertips due to ischemia is frequent and may be associated with striking resorption of the terminal phalanges (acro-osteolysis) (Fig. 7-5).

Calcium deposits occur in the skin and soft tissues, particularly in patients with lcSSc who are positive for anticentromere antibodies. The deposits, varying in size from tiny punctate lesions to large conglomerate masses, are composed of calcium hydroxyapatite crystals and can be readily visualized on plain x-rays. Frequent locations include the finger pads, palms, extensor surfaces of the forearms, and the olecranon and prepatellar bursae (Fig. 7-6). Paraspinal calcifications may cause neurological complications. Calcific deposits are generally noted as persistent firm, nontender subcutaneous lumps and may occasionally

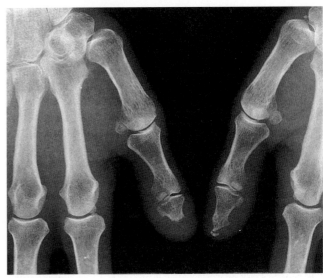

FIGURE 7-5

Acro-osteolysis. Note dissolution of terminal phalanges in a patient with long-standing limited cutaneous SSc.

ulcerate through the overlying skin, producing drainage of chalky white material, pain, and local inflammation.

Pulmonary Features

Pulmonary involvement can be documented in most patients with SSc and is now the leading cause of death. The two main types of significant pulmonary involvement are ILD and PAH; many patients develop some degree of both complications. Less frequent pulmonary manifestations include aspiration pneumonitis complicating gastroesophageal reflux, pulmonary hemorrhage due to endobronchial telangiectasia, obliterative bronchiolitis, pleural reactions, restrictive ventilatory defect due to chest wall fibrosis, and spontaneous pneumothorax. The incidence of lung cancer, particularly bronchoalveolar carcinoma, may be increased in patients with SSc.

Pulmonary involvement may remain asymptomatic until it is advanced. The most frequent presenting symptoms of pulmonary involvement—exertional dyspnea, fatigue, and reduced exercise tolerance—are often subtle

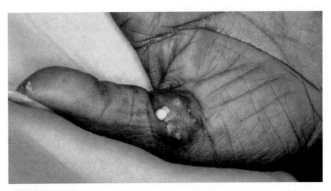

FIGURE 7-6

Calcinosis cutis. Note large calcific deposit breaking through the skin in a patient with limited cutaneous SSc.

and slowly progressive. A chronic dry cough may be present. Physical examination may reveal "Velcro" crackles at the lung bases. Pulmonary function testing (PFT) is a sensitive method for detecting early pulmonary involvement in asymptomatic patients. The most common abnormalities are reductions in forced vital capacity (FVC) or single breath diffusing capacity (DLCO). A reduction in DLCO that is significantly out of proportion to the reduction in FVC suggests pulmonary vascular disease, but may also be due to anemia. With exercise, patients show a decrease in PO_2.

Interstitial Lung Disease (ILD)

Some evidence of ILD can be found at autopsy in up to 90% of patients with SSc and by thin-section high-resolution computed tomography (HRCT) in 85%. ILD and pulmonary fibrosis cause restrictive lung disease with impaired gas exchange, characterized on PFT by decreased FVC and DLCO but unaffected flow rates. Clinically significant ILD develops in 16–43% of patients with SSc, the frequency depending on the detection method used and the characteristics of the patient population. Risk factors include male gender, African-American race, diffuse skin involvement, severe gastroesophageal reflux, and the presence of topoisomerase-I autoantibodies, as well as a low FVC or DLCO at initial presentation. In patients who develop significant ILD, the most rapid progression in lung disease occurs early in the course of the disease (within the first 3 years), when the FVC declines by an average of 32% per year.

Chest radiography is useful for ruling out infection and other causes of pulmonary involvement, but it is relatively insensitive for detection of early ILD. HRCT of the chest is more sensitive and may show reticular linear opacities predominantly in the lower lobes, even in asymptomatic patients (**Fig. 7-7**). Additional findings include mediastinal lymphadenopathy, nodules, and honeycombing. Ground-glass opacification, seen in 50% of patients, is not specific for identifying alveolitis or predicting rapidly progressing lung disease. Bronchoalveolar lavage (BAL) may be useful for identifying inflammation in the lower respiratory tract and ruling out infection. In some studies, an elevated proportion of neutrophils (>2%) and/or eosinophils (>3%) in the BAL fluid was associated with more extensive lung disease, more rapid decline in FVC, and reduced survival. Lung biopsy is indicated only in patients with atypical findings on chest radiographs and should be thoracoscopically guided. The histologic pattern on lung biopsy may be helpful in predicting the risk of progression of ILD. The most common pattern in SSc, nonspecific interstitial pneumonitis, carries a better prognosis than usual interstitial pneumonitis. Recent studies suggest that measurement of serum markers such as KL-6, a glycoprotein found in type II pneumocytes and alveolar macrophages, may have utility in the detection and serial monitoring of ILD in patients with SSc.

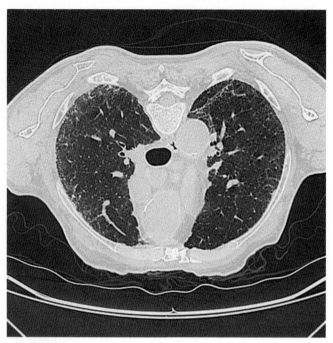

FIGURE 7-7

High-resolution CT scan of the lungs. Note peripheral bilateral reticulonodular opacifications in the lower lobes of the lungs in a patient with diffuse cutaneous SSc.

Pulmonary Arterial Hypertension (PAH)

PAH, defined as a mean pulmonary arterial pressure >25 mmHg at rest, as determined by right heart catheterization, is increasingly recognized as a major complication of SSc. Approximately 12–25% of SSc patients have evidence of PAH. In these patients, PAH may occur in association with ILD or as an isolated pulmonary abnormality. The natural history of SSc-associated PAH is variable, but in many patients it follows a relentlessly downhill course with development of right heart failure and significant mortality. Risk factors for PAH include limited cutaneous disease with anticentromere antibodies, late age at disease onset, severe Raynaud's phenomenon, and the presence of U1-RNP, U3-RNP (fibrillarin), and B23 antibodies.

Patients with early PAH are generally asymptomatic. The initial symptom is typically exertional dyspnea and reduced exercise capacity. With progression, angina, exertional near-syncope, and symptoms and signs of right-sided heart failure appear. Physical examination shows tachypnea, a prominent pulmonic S2 heart sound, palpable right ventricular heave, elevated jugular venous pressure, and dependent edema. Doppler echocardiography provides an estimate of pulmonary arterial systolic pressures and also indicates the presence of valvular abnormalities or left ventricular systolic or diastolic dysfunction that could cause pulmonary hypertension due to elevated pulmonary venous pressures. Echocardiogram-derived estimates of pulmonary arterial systolic pressures exceeding 40 mmHg

TABLE 8-1

ASSOCIATION OF SJÖGREN'S SYNDROME WITH OTHER AUTOIMMUNE DISEASES
Rheumatoid arthritis
Systemic lupus erythematosus
Scleroderma
Mixed connective tissue disease
Primary biliary cirrhosis
Vasculitis
Chronic active hepatitis

apoptotic mechanisms. Finally, they inappropriately produce proinflammatory cytokines and lymphoattractant chemokines necessary for sustaining the autoimmune lesion and progressing to more sophisticated ectopic germinal center formation. Recent studies have shown that, similar to T cells, CD40+ B cells also have a tendency to be resistant to apoptosis. B cell activating factor (BAFF) has been found to be elevated in patients with Sjögren's syndrome, especially those with hypergammaglobulinemia, and probably accounts for this antiapoptotic effect. Interestingly, glandular epithelial cells seem to have an active role in the production of BAFF. The triggering factor for epithelial activation appears to be a persistent enteroviral infection (possibly by Coxsackievirus strains).

A defect in cholinergic activity mediated through the M3 receptor, which leads to neuroepithelial dysfunction and diminished glandular secretions, has been proposed. Finally, the observation that the water-channel protein aquaporin-5 redistributes from the apical membranes to the cytoplasm of acinar epithelial cells offers another alternative theory for Sjögren's syndrome pathogenesis.

Immunogenetic studies have demonstrated that HLA-B8, -DR3, and -DRw52 are prevalent in patients with primary Sjögren's syndrome. Molecular analysis of HLA class II genes has revealed that patients with Sjögren's syndrome, regardless of their ethnic origin, are highly associated with the HLA DQA1*0501 allele, pointing out that genetic predisposition may play an important role.

CLINICAL MANIFESTATIONS

The majority of Sjögren's syndrome patients have symptoms related to diminished lacrimal and salivary gland function. In most patients, the primary syndrome runs a slow and benign course. The initial manifestations can be mucosal or nonspecific dryness, and 8–10 years may elapse from the initial symptoms to full-blown development of the disease.

The principal oral symptom of Sjögren's syndrome is dryness (xerostomia). Patients complain of difficulty in swallowing dry food, inability to speak continuously, a burning sensation, increase in dental caries, and problems in wearing complete dentures. Physical examination shows a dry, erythematous, sticky oral mucosa. There is atrophy of the filiform papillae on the dorsum of the tongue, and saliva from the major glands is either not expressible or cloudy. Enlargement of the parotid or other major salivary glands occurs in two-thirds of patients with primary Sjögren's syndrome but is uncommon in those with the secondary syndrome. Diagnostic tests include sialometry, sialography, and scintigraphy. The labial minor salivary gland biopsy permits histopathologic confirmation of the focal lymphocytic infiltrates.

Ocular involvement is the other major manifestation of Sjögren's syndrome. Patients usually complain of a sandy or gritty feeling under the eyelids. Other symptoms include burning, accumulation of thick strands at the inner canthi, decreased tearing, redness, itching, eye fatigue, and increased photosensitivity. These symptoms are attributed to the destruction of corneal and bulbar conjunctival epithelium, defined as *keratoconjunctivitis sicca*. Diagnostic evaluation of keratoconjunctivitis sicca includes measurement of tear flow by Schirmer's I test and tear composition as assessed by the tear breakup time or tear lysozyme content. Slit-lamp examination of the cornea and conjunctiva after rose Bengal staining reveals punctuate corneal ulcerations and attached filaments of corneal epithelium.

Involvement of other exocrine glands occurs less frequently and includes a decrease in mucous gland secretions of the upper and lower respiratory tree, resulting in dry nose, throat, and trachea (xerotrachea), and diminished secretion of the exocrine glands of the gastrointestinal tract, leading to esophageal mucosal atrophy, atrophic gastritis, and subclinical pancreatitis. Dyspareunia due to dryness of the external genitalia and dry skin also may occur.

Extraglandular (systemic) manifestations are seen in one-third of patients with Sjögren's syndrome (Table 8-2),

TABLE 8-2

INCIDENCE OF EXTRAGLANDULAR MANIFESTATIONS IN PRIMARY SJÖGREN'S SYNDROME	
CLINICAL MANIFESTATION	**PERCENT**
Arthralgias/arthritis	60
Raynaud's phenomenon	37
Lymphadenopathy	14
Lung involvement	14
Vasculitis	11
Kidney involvement	9
Liver involvement	6
Lymphoma	6
Splenomegaly	3
Peripheral neuropathy	2
Myositis	1

while they are very rare in patients with Sjögren's syndrome associated with rheumatoid arthritis. These patients complain more often of easy fatigability, low-grade fever, Raynaud's phenomenon, myalgias, and arthralgias. Most patients with primary Sjögren's syndrome experience at least one episode of nonerosive arthritis during the course of their disease. Manifestations of pulmonary involvement are frequently evident histologically but rarely clinically important. Dry cough is the major manifestation that is attributed to small airway disease. Renal involvement includes interstitial nephritis, clinically manifested by hyposthenuria and renal tubular dysfunction with or without acidosis. Untreated acidosis may lead to nephrocalcinosis. Glomerulonephritis is a rare finding that occurs in patients with mixed cryoglobulinemia, or systemic lupus erythematosus overlapping with Sjögren's syndrome. Vasculitis affects small- and medium-sized vessels. The most common clinical features are purpura, recurrent urticaria, skin ulcerations, glomerulonephritis, and mononeuritis multiplex. Sensorineural hearing loss was found in one-half of patients with Sjögren's syndrome and correlated with the presence of anticardiolipin antibodies, while anti–Ro/SS-A positivity is associated with congenital heart block.

It has been suggested that primary Sjögren's syndrome with vasculitis may also present with multifocal, recurrent, and progressive nervous system disease, such as hemiparesis, transverse myelopathy, hemisensory deficits, seizures, and movement disorders. Aseptic meningitis and multiple sclerosis also have been reported in these patients.

Lymphoma is a well-known manifestation of Sjögren's syndrome that usually presents later in the illness. Persistent parotid gland enlargement, purpura, leukopenia, cryoglobulinemia, and low C4 complement levels are manifestations suggesting the development of lymphoma. Interestingly, the same risk factors account for glomerulonephritis and are those that confer increased mortality. Most lymphomas are extranodal, low-grade marginal zone B cell lymphomas and are usually detected incidentally upon evaluating the labial biopsy. The affected lymph nodes are usually peripheral. Survival is decreased in patients with B symptoms, lymph node mass >7 cm in diameter, and high or intermediate histologic grade.

Routine laboratory tests reveal mild normochromic, normocytic anemia. An elevated erythrocyte sedimentation rate is found in approximately 70% of patients.

DIAGNOSIS AND DIFFERENTIAL DIAGNOSIS

The diagnosis of primary Sjögren's syndrome is obtained if the patient presents with eye and/or mouth dryness, the eye tests disclose keratoconjunctivitis sicca, the mouth evaluation reveals the classic manifestations of the syndrome, and the patient's serum reacts with Ro/SS-A and/or La/SS-B autoantigens. Labial biopsy is needed when the diagnosis is uncertain or to rule out other conditions that may cause dry mouth or eyes or parotid gland enlargement (Tables 8-3 and 8-4). Validated diagnostic criteria have been established by a European study and have now been further improved by a European-American study group (Table 8-5). Hepatitis C virus infection should be ruled out since, apart from serologic tests, the remainder of the clinicopathologic picture is almost identical to that of Sjögren's syndrome.

TABLE 8-3

DIFFERENTIAL DIAGNOSIS OF SICCA SYMPTOMS

XEROSTOMIA	DRY EYE	BILATERAL PAROTID GLAND ENLARGEMENT
Viral infections	Inflammation	Viral infections
Drugs	Stevens-Johnson syndrome	Mumps
Psychotherapeutic	Pemphigoid	Influenza
Parasympatholytic	Chronic conjunctivitis	Epstein-Barr
Antihypertensive	Chronic blepharitis	Coxsackievirus A
Psychogenic	Sjögren's syndrome	Cytomegalovirus
Irradiation	Toxicity	HIV
Diabetes mellitus	Burns	Sarcoidosis
Trauma	Drugs	Amyloidosis
Sjögren's syndrome	Neurologic conditions	Sjögren's syndrome
	Impaired lacrimal gland function	Metabolic
	Impaired eyelid function	Diabetes mellitus
	Miscellaneous	Hyperlipoproteinemias
	Trauma	Chronic pancreatitis
	Hypovitaminosis A	Hepatic cirrhosis
	Blink abnormality	Endocrine
	Anesthetic cornea	Acromegaly
	Lid scarring	Gonadal hypofunction
	Epithelial irregularity	

TABLE 8-4

DIFFERENTIAL DIAGNOSIS OF SJÖGREN'S SYNDROME

HIV INFECTION AND SICCA SYNDROME	SJÖGREN'S SYNDROME	SARCOIDOSIS
Predominant in young males	Predominant in middle-aged women	Invariable
Lack of autoantibodies to Ro/SS-A and/or La/SS-B	Presence of autoantibodies	Lack of autoantibodies to Ro/SS-A and/or La/SS-B
Lymphoid infiltrates of salivary glands by CD8+ lymphocytes	Lymphoid infiltrates of salivary glands by CD4+ lymphocytes	Granulomas in salivary glands
Association with HLA-DR5	Association with HLA-DR3 and -DRw52	Unknown
Positive serologic tests for HIV	Negative serologic tests for HIV	Negative serologic tests for HIV

℞ **Treatment:**
SJÖGREN'S SYNDROME

Treatment of Sjögren's syndrome is aimed at symptomatic relief and limiting the damaging local effects of chronic xerostomia and keratoconjunctivitis sicca by substituting or simulating the missing secretions (Fig. 8-1).

To replace deficient tears, there are several readily available ophthalmic preparations (Tearisol; Liquifilm; 0.5% methylcellulose; Hypo Tears). If corneal ulcerations are present, eye patching and boric acid ointments are recommended. Certain drugs that may decrease lacrimal and salivary secretion such as diuretics, antihypertensive drugs, anticholinergics, and antidepressants should be avoided.

For xerostomia the best replacement is water. Propionic acid gels may be used to treat vaginal dryness. To stimulate secretions, pilocarpine (5 mg thrice daily) or cevimeline (30 mg thrice daily) administered orally appears to improve sicca manifestations, and both are well tolerated. Hydroxychloroquine (200 mg) is helpful for arthralgias.

TABLE 8-5

REVISED INTERNATIONAL CLASSIFICATION CRITERIA FOR SJÖGREN'S SYNDROME[a,b,c]

I. Ocular symptoms: a positive response to at least one of three validated questions.
  1. Have you had daily, persistent, troublesome dry eyes for more than 3 months?
  2. Do you have a recurrent sensation of sand or gravel in the eyes?
  3. Do you use tear substitutes more than three times a day?
II. Oral symptoms: a positive response to at least one of three validated questions.
  1. Have you had a daily feeling of dry mouth for more than 3 months?
  2. Have you had recurrent or persistently swollen salivary glands as an adult?
  3. Do you frequently drink liquids to aid in swallowing dry foods?
III. Ocular signs: objective evidence of ocular involvement defined as a positive result to at least one of the following two tests:
  1. Shirmer's I test, performed without anesthesia (≤5 mm in 5 min)
  2. Rose Bengal score or other ocular dye score (≥4 according to van Bijsterveld's scoring system)
IV. Histopathology: in minor salivary glands focal lymphocytic sialoadenitis, with a focus score ≥1.
V. Salivary gland involvement: objective evidence of salivary gland involvement defined by a positive result to at least one of the following diagnostic tests:
  1. Unstimulated whole salivary flow (≤1.5 mL in 15 min)
  2. Parotid sialography
  3. Salivary scintigraphy
VI. Antibodies in the serum to Ro/SS-A or La/SS-B antigens, or both

[a]Exclusion criteria: past head and neck radiation treatment, hepatitis C infection, AIDS, preexisting lymphoma, sarcoidosis, graft versus host disease, use of anticholinergic drugs.
[b]Primary Sjögren's syndrome: any four of the six items, as long as item IV (histopathology) or VI (serology) is positive, or any three of the four objective criteria items (items III, IV, V, VI).
[c]In patients with a potentially associated disease (e.g., another well-defined connective tissue disease), the presence of item I or item II plus any two from among items III, IV, and V may be considered as indicative of secondary Sjögren's syndrome.
Source: From Vitali C et al.

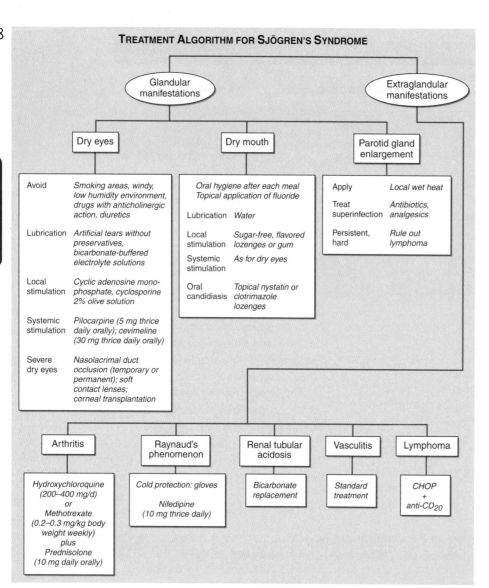

FIGURE 8-1
Treatment algorithm for Sjögren's syndrome.

Patients with renal tubular acidosis should receive sodium bicarbonate orally (0.5–2.0 mmol/kg in four divided doses). Glucocorticoids (1 mg/kg per day) and/or immunosuppressive agents (e.g., cyclophosphamide) are indicated only for the treatment of systemic vasculitis. Anti–tumor necrosis factor agents appear ineffective, while anti-CD20 monoclonal antibody therapy in combination with a classic cyclophosphamide, doxorubicin, vincristine, prednisone (CHOP) regimen leads to increased survival in patients with lymphoma.

FURTHER READINGS

CAPORALI R et al: Safety and usefulness of minor salivary gland biopsy: Retrospective analysis of 502 procedures performed at a single center. Arthritis Rheum 59:714, 2008

DAWSON L et al: Antimuscarinic antibodies in Sjögren's syndrome: Where are we, and where are we going? Arthritis Rheum 52:2984, 2005

EKSTRÖM Smedby K et al: Autoimmune disorders and risk of non-Hodgkin lymphoma subtypes: A pooled analysis within the InterLymph Consortium. Blood 111:4029, 2008

FOULKS GN: Treatment of dry eye disease by the non-ophthalmologist. Rheum Dis Clin North Am 34:987, 2008

KASSAN S, Moutsopoulos HM: Clinical manifestations and early diagnosis of Sjögren syndrome. Arch Intern Med 164:1275, 2004

MAVRAGANI CP et al: The management of Sjögren's syndrome. Nat Clin Pract Rheum 2:252, 2006

MITSIAS DI et al: The role of epithelial cells in the initiation and perpetuation of autoimmune lesions: Lessons from Sjögren's syndrome (autoimmune epithelitis). Lupus 15:255, 2006

PIJPE J et al: Rituximab treatment in patients with primary Sjögren's syndrome: An open-label phase II study. Arthritis Rheum 52:2740, 2005

RAMOS-CASALS M et al: Primary Sjögren syndrome in Spain: Clinical and immunologic expression in 1010 patients. Medicine 87:210, 2008.

SZODORAY P et al: Programmed cell death of peripheral blood B cells determined by laser scanning cytometry in Sjögren's syndrome with a special emphasis on BAFF. J Clin Immunol 24:600, 2004

TRIANTAFYLLOPOULOU A et al: Evidence for Coxsackievirus infection in primary Sjögren's syndrome. Arthritis Rheum 50:2897, 2004

VITALI C et al: Classification criteria for Sjögren's syndrome: A revised version of the European criteria proposed by the American-European Consensus Group. Ann Rheum Dis 61:554, 2002

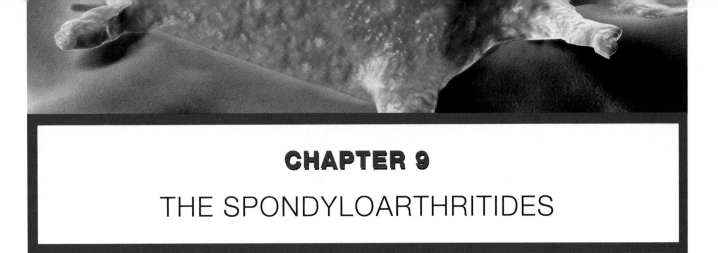

CHAPTER 9

THE SPONDYLOARTHRITIDES

Joel D. Taurog

The spondyloarthritides are a group of disorders that share certain clinical features and genetic associations. These disorders include ankylosing spondylitis, reactive arthritis, psoriatic arthritis and spondylitis, enteropathic arthritis and spondylitis, juvenile-onset spondyloarthritis, and undifferentiated spondyloarthritis. The similarities in clinical manifestations and genetic predisposition suggest that these disorders share pathogenic mechanisms.

ANKYLOSING SPONDYLITIS

Ankylosing spondylitis (AS) is an inflammatory disorder of unknown cause that primarily affects the axial skeleton; peripheral joints and extraarticular structures are also frequently involved. The disease usually begins in the second or third decade; male to female prevalence is between 2:1 and 3:1. Older names include *Marie-Strümpell disease* or *Bechterew's disease*.

EPIDEMIOLOGY

AS shows a striking correlation with the histocompatibility antigen HLA-B27 and occurs worldwide roughly in proportion to the prevalence of this antigen (Chap. 2). In North American Caucasians, the prevalence of B27 is 7%, whereas it is 90% in patients with AS, independent of disease severity.

In population surveys, AS is present in 1–6% of adults inheriting B27, whereas the prevalence is 10–30% among B27+ adult first-degree relatives of AS probands. The concordance rate in identical twins is approximately 65%. It appears that susceptibility to AS is determined largely by genetic factors, with B27 comprising about one-third of the genetic component. Probable linkage has been found to the interleukin 1 (IL-1) gene cluster on chromosome 2 and to several other genomic regions.

PATHOLOGY

The sites of axial inflammation in AS are inaccessible to routine biopsy and are rarely approached surgically. Knowledge of the axial histopathology is therefore based on a limited number of mostly advanced cases. Sacroiliitis is often the earliest manifestations of AS. Synovitis, pannus, myxoid marrow, subchondral granulation tissue and marrow edema, enthesitis, and chondroid differentiation are found. Macrophages, T cells, and osteoclasts are prevalent. Eventually the eroded joint margins are gradually replaced by fibrocartilage regeneration and then by ossification. The joint may become totally obliterated.

In the spine, early in the process there is inflammatory granulation tissue at the junction of annulus fibrosus and vertebral bone. The outer annular fibers are eroded and eventually replaced by bone, forming the beginning of a bony syndesmophyte, which then grows by continued enchondral ossification, ultimately bridging the adjacent vertebral bodies. Ascending progression of this process leads to the "bamboo spine." Other lesions in the spine include diffuse osteoporosis, erosion of vertebral bodies at the disk margin, "squaring" of vertebrae, and inflammation and destruction of the disk-bone border. Inflammatory arthritis of the apophyseal joints is common, with erosion of cartilage by pannus, often followed by bony ankylosis.

Bone mineral density is diminished in the spine and proximal femur early in the course of the disease, before the advent of significant immobilization.

Peripheral synovitis in AS shows marked vascularity, lining layer hyperplasia, lymphoid infiltration, and pannus formation. Central cartilaginous erosions caused by proliferation of subchondral granulation tissue are common.

Inflammation in the fibrocartilaginous enthesis, the region where a tendon, ligament, or joint capsule attaches to bone, is a characteristic lesion in AS and other SpA, both at axial and peripheral sites. Enthesitis is associated with prominent edema of the adjacent bone marrow and is often characterized by erosive lesions that eventually undergo ossification.

PATHOGENESIS

The pathogenesis of AS is incompletely understood but is almost certainly immune mediated. There is lively controversy regarding the primary site of disease initiation. A unifying concept is that the AS disease process begins at sites where articular cartilage, ligaments, and other structures attach to bone. The dramatic response of the disease to therapeutic blockade of tumor necrosis factor α (TNF-α) indicates that this cytokine plays a central role in the immunopathogenesis of AS. The inflamed sacroiliac joint is infiltrated with CD4+ and CD8+ T cells and macrophages and shows high levels of TNF-α, particularly early in the disease course. Abundant transforming growth factor β (TGF-β) has been found in more advanced lesions. Peripheral synovitis in AS and the other spondyloarthritides is characterized by neutrophils, macrophages expressing CD68 and CD163, CD4+ and CD8+ T cells, and B cells. There is prominent staining for intercellular adhesion molecule 1 (ICAM-1), vascular cell adhesion molecule 1 (VCAM-1), matrix metalloproteinase-3 (MMP-3), and myeloid-related proteins 8 and 14 (MRP-8 and MRP-14). Unlike rheumatoid arthritis (RA) synovium, citrullinated proteins and cartilage gp39 peptide-MHC complexes are absent.

No specific event or exogenous agent that triggers the onset of disease has been identified, although overlapping features with reactive arthritis and inflammatory bowel disease (IBD) suggest that enteric bacteria may play a role. Elevated serum titers of antibodies to certain enteric bacteria are common in AS patients, but no role for these antibodies in the pathogenesis of AS has been identified. Strong evidence that B27 plays a direct role is provided by genetic epidemiology studies and by the finding that rats transgenic for B27 spontaneously develop dramatic arthritis and spondylitis. It has yet to be determined whether the role of B27 involves classical peptide antigen presentation to CD8+ T cells or some other mechanism, or both. More generally, the relative degree of participation of innate and adaptive immunity remains to be determined.

CLINICAL MANIFESTATIONS

The symptoms of the disease are usually first noticed in late adolescence or early adulthood; the median age in Western countries is 23. In 5% of patients, symptoms begin after age 40. The initial symptom is usually dull pain, insidious in onset, felt deep in the lower lumbar or gluteal region, accompanied by low-back morning stiffness of up to a few hours' duration that improves with activity and returns following periods of inactivity. Within a few months of onset, the pain has usually become persistent and bilateral. Nocturnal exacerbation of pain that forces the patient to rise and move around may be frequent.

In some patients, bony tenderness (presumably reflecting enthesitis) may accompany back pain or stiffness, while in others it may be the predominant complaint. Common sites include the costosternal junctions, spinous processes, iliac crests, greater trochanters, ischial tuberosities, tibial tubercles, and heels. Occasionally, bony chest pain is the presenting complaint. Arthritis in the hips and shoulders ("root" joints) occurs in 25–35% of patients, in many cases early in the disease course. Arthritis of peripheral joints other than the hips and shoulders, usually asymmetric, occurs in up to 30% of patients and can occur at any stage of the disease. Neck pain and stiffness from involvement of the cervical spine are usually relatively late manifestations. Occasional patients, particularly in the older age group, present with predominantly constitutional symptoms.

AS often has a juvenile onset in developing countries. Peripheral arthritis and enthesitis usually predominate, with axial symptoms supervening in late adolescence.

Initially, physical findings mirror the inflammatory process. The most specific findings involve loss of spinal mobility, with limitation of anterior and lateral flexion and extension of the lumbar spine and of chest expansion. Limitation of motion is usually out of proportion to the degree of bony ankylosis, reflecting muscle spasm secondary to pain and inflammation. Pain in the sacroiliac joints may be elicited either with direct pressure or with maneuvers that stress the joints. In addition, there is commonly tenderness upon palpation at the sites of symptomatic bony tenderness and paraspinous muscle spasm.

The Schober test is a useful measure of lumbar spine flexion. The patient stands erect, with heels together, and marks are made directly over the spine 5 cm below and 10 cm above the lumbosacral junction (identified by a horizontal line between the posterosuperior iliac spines). The patient then bends forward maximally, and the distance between the two marks is measured. The distance between the two marks increases by ≥5 cm in the case of normal mobility and by <4 cm in the case of decreased mobility. Chest expansion is measured as the difference between maximal inspiration and maximal forced expiration in the fourth intercostal space in males or just below the breasts in females. Normal chest expansion is ≥5 cm.

Limitation or pain with motion of the hips or shoulders is usually present if either of these joints is involved. It should be emphasized that early in the course of mild cases, symptoms may be subtle and nonspecific, and the physical examination may be completely normal.

The course of the disease is extremely variable, ranging from the individual with mild stiffness and radiographically equivocal sacroiliitis to the patient with a totally fused spine and severe bilateral hip arthritis, accompanied by severe peripheral arthritis and extraarticular manifestations. Pain tends to be persistent early in the disease and then becomes intermittent, with alternating exacerbations and quiescent periods. In a typical severe untreated case with progression of the spondylitis to syndesmophyte formation, the patient's posture undergoes characteristic changes, with obliterated lumbar lordosis, buttock atrophy, and accentuated thoracic kyphosis. There may be a forward stoop of the neck or flexion contractures at the hips, compensated by flexion at the knees. Disease progression can be estimated clinically from loss of height, limitation of chest expansion and spinal flexion, and occiput-to-wall distance. Occasional individuals are encountered with advanced physical findings who report having never had significant symptoms.

For a given patient, the rate of progression of radiographically demonstrable damage is linear over decades. In some but not all studies, onset of the disease in adolescence and early hip involvement correlate with a worse prognosis. The disease in women tends to progress less frequently to total spinal ankylosis, although there is some evidence for an increased prevalence of isolated cervical ankylosis and peripheral arthritis in women. In industrialized countries, peripheral arthritis (distal to hips and shoulders) occurs overall in less than half of patients with AS, usually as a late manifestation, whereas in developing countries, the prevalence is much higher, with onset typically early in the disease course. Pregnancy has no consistent effect on AS, with symptoms improving, remaining the same, or deteriorating in about one-third of pregnant patients, respectively.

The most serious complication of the spinal disease is spinal fracture, which can occur with even minor trauma to the rigid, osteoporotic spine. The lower cervical spine is most commonly involved. These fractures are often displaced and cause spinal cord injury. A recent survey suggested a >10% lifetime risk of fracture. Occasionally, fracture through a diskovertebral junction and adjacent neural arch, termed *pseudoarthrosis* and occurring most commonly in the thoracolumbar spine, can be an unrecognized source of persistent localized pain and/or neurologic dysfunction. Wedging of thoracic vertebrae is common and correlates with accentuated kyphosis.

The most common extraarticular manifestation is acute anterior uveitis, which occurs in 40% of patients and can antedate the spondylitis. Attacks are typically unilateral, causing pain, photophobia, and increased lacrimation. These tend to recur, often in the opposite eye. Cataracts and secondary glaucoma are not uncommon sequelae. Up to 60% of patients have inflammation in the colon or ileum. This is usually asymptomatic, but frank IBD occurs in 5–10% of patients with AS (see "Enteropathic Arthritis" later in the chapter). About 10% of patients meeting criteria for AS have psoriasis (see "Psoriatic Arthritis" later in the chapter). Aortic insufficiency, sometimes producing symptoms of congestive heart failure, occurs in a few percent of patients, occasionally early in the course of the spinal disease but usually after prolonged disease. Third-degree heart block may occur alone or together with aortic insufficiency. Subclinical pulmonary lesions and cardiac dysfunction may be relatively common. Cauda equina syndrome and upper pulmonary lobe fibrosis are rare late complications. Retroperitoneal fibrosis is a rare associated condition. Prostatitis has been reported to have an increased prevalence. Amyloidosis is rare (Chap. 15).

Several validated measures of disease activity and functional outcome have recently been developed for AS. Despite the persistence of the disease, most patients remain gainfully employed. Some but not all studies of survival in AS have suggested that AS shortens life span, compared with the general population. Mortality attributable to AS is largely the result of spinal trauma, aortic insufficiency, respiratory failure, amyloid nephropathy, or complications of therapy such as upper gastrointestinal hemorrhage.

LABORATORY FINDINGS

No laboratory test is diagnostic of AS. In most ethnic groups, B27 is present in approximately 90% of patients. Erythrocyte sedimentation rate (ESR) and C-reactive protein (CRP) are often, but not always, elevated. Mild anemia may be present. Patients with severe disease may show an elevated alkaline phosphatase level. Elevated serum IgA levels are common. Rheumatoid factor, anti-CCP, and antinuclear antibodies are largely absent unless caused by a coexistent disease, although the latter may appear with anti–TNF therapy. Synovial fluid from peripheral joints in AS is nonspecifically inflammatory. In cases with restriction of chest wall motion, decreased vital capacity and increased functional residual capacity are common, but airflow measurements are normal and ventilatory function is usually well maintained.

RADIOGRAPHIC FINDINGS

Radiographically demonstrable sacroiliitis is usually present in AS. The earliest changes by standard radiography are blurring of the cortical margins of the subchondral bone, followed by erosions and sclerosis. Progression of the erosions leads to "pseudowidening" of the joint space; as fibrous and then bony ankylosis supervene, the joints may become obliterated. The changes and progression of the lesions are usually symmetric.

In the lumbar spine, progression of the disease leads to straightening, caused by loss of lordosis, and reactive sclerosis, caused by osteitis of the anterior corners of the vertebral bodies with subsequent erosion, leading to "squaring" of the vertebral bodies. Progressive ossification leads to eventual formation of marginal syndesmophytes, visible on plain films as bony bridges connecting successive vertebral bodies anteriorly and laterally.

In mild cases, years may elapse before unequivocal sacroiliac abnormalities are evident on plain radiographs. Computed tomography (CT) and magnetic resonance imaging (MRI) can detect abnormalities reliably at an earlier stage than plain radiography. Dynamic MRI with fat saturation, either short tau inversion recovery (STIR) sequence or T1-weighted images with contrast enhancement, is highly sensitive and specific for identifying early intraarticular inflammation, cartilage changes, and underlying bone marrow edema in sacroiliitis (**Fig. 9-1**). These techniques are also highly sensitive for evaluation of acute and chronic spinal changes (**Fig. 9-2**).

Reduced bone mineral density can be detected by dual-energy x-ray absorptiometry of the femoral neck and the lumbar spine. Falsely elevated readings related to spinal ossification can be avoided by using a lateral projection of the L3 vertebral body.

DIAGNOSIS

It is important to establish the diagnosis of early AS before the development of irreversible deformity. This

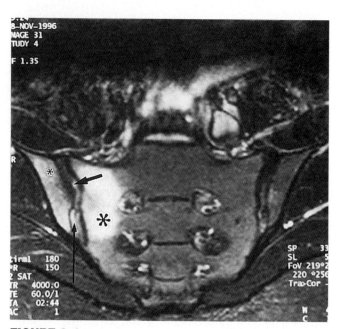

FIGURE 9-1

Early sacroiliitis in a patient with AS, indicated by prominent sacral bone marrow edema (asterisks) on a coronal oblique STIR (short tau inversion recovery) magnetic resonance image. (*From DS Levine et al: Clin Radiol 59:400, 2004.*)

goal presents a challenge for several reasons: (1) back pain is very common, but AS is much less common; (2) an early presumptive diagnosis often relies on clinical grounds requiring considerable expertise; and (3) young individuals with early AS are often reluctant to seek medical care. The widely used modified New York criteria

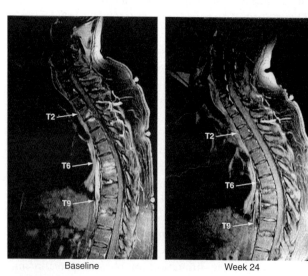

Baseline   Week 24

FIGURE 9-2

Spinal inflammation (spondylodiscitis) in a patient with AS and its dramatic response to treatment with infliximab. Gadolinium-enhanced T1-weighted magnetic resonance images, with fat saturation, at baseline and after 24 weeks of infliximab therapy. (*From J Braun et al: Arthritis Rheum 54(5):1646, 2006.*)

(1984) are classification rather than diagnostic criteria, and they are insensitive in early or mild cases. These consist of the following: (1) a history of inflammatory back pain (see below), (2) limitation of motion of the lumbar spine in both the sagittal and frontal planes, (3) limited chest expansion, and (4) definite radiographic sacroiliitis. Criterion 4 plus any one of the other three criteria is sufficient for a diagnosis of definite AS. Dynamic MRI is definitely more sensitive than plain radiography. Although its exact sensitivity and specificity remain to be defined, it is recommended in suspected cases in which plain radiography either fails to show definite changes or is undesirable (e.g., in young women or children).

The presence of B27 is neither necessary nor sufficient for the diagnosis. However, in accord with Bayes' theorem, the presence or absence of B27 greatly increases or decreases, respectively, the probability of AS in patients with equivocal clinical findings lacking radiographic abnormalities. Moreover, the absence of B27 in a typical case of AS significantly increases the probability of coexistent IBD.

AS must be differentiated from numerous other causes of low-back pain, some far more common than AS. For several decades, the following five features have been used to distinguish the inflammatory back pain of AS: (1) age of onset below 40, (2) insidious onset, (3) duration >3 months before medical attention is sought, (4) morning stiffness, and (5) improvement with exercise or activity. The most common causes of back pain other than AS are primarily mechanical or degenerative rather than primarily inflammatory and do not show clustering of these features. A recent reassessment has led to the following proposed criteria for inflammatory back pain in adults ≤50 years old: (1) morning stiffness >30 min, (2) improvement with exercise but not with rest, (3) awakening from back pain during only the second half of the night, and (4) alternating buttock pain.

Less-common metabolic, infectious, and malignant causes of back pain must also be differentiated from AS, including infectious spondylitis, spondylodiscitis, and sacroiliitis. Ochronosis can produce a phenotype that is clinically and radiographically similar to AS. Calcification and ossification of paraspinous ligaments occur in *diffuse idiopathic skeletal hyperostosis* (DISH), which occurs in the middle-aged and elderly and is usually not symptomatic. Ligamentous calcification gives the appearance of "flowing wax" on the anterior bodies of the vertebrae. Intervertebral disk spaces are preserved, and sacroiliac and apophyseal joints appear normal, helping to differentiate DISH from spondylosis and from AS, respectively.

℞ Treatment:
ANKYLOSING SPONDYLITIS

Any management of AS should include an exercise program designed to maintain posture and range of motion. Until recently, nonsteroidal anti-inflammatory drugs (NSAIDs) have been the mainstay of pharmacologic therapy for AS. These agents reduce pain and tenderness and increase mobility in many patients with AS. Moreover, in a recent 2-year randomized controlled study, radiographic progression of AS was significantly slower in patients taking daily NSAIDs than in those taking them only as needed for severe pain or stiffness. However, many patients with AS have continued symptoms and develop deformity despite NSAID therapy. Beginning in 2000, dramatic responses to anti–TNF-α therapy were reported in patients with AS and other spondyloarthritides. Patients with AS treated with either infliximab (chimeric human/mouse anti–TNF-α monoclonal antibody), etanercept (soluble p75 TNF-α receptor–IgG fusion protein), or adalimumab (human anti–TNF-α monoclonal antibody) have shown rapid, profound, and sustained reductions in all clinical and laboratory measures of disease activity. Patients with long-standing disease and even some with complete spinal ankylosis have shown striking improvement in both objective and subjective indicators of disease activity and function, including morning stiffness, pain, spinal mobility, peripheral joint swelling, CRP, and ESR. MRI studies indicate substantial resolution of bone marrow edema, enthesitis, and joint effusions in the sacroiliac joints, spine, and peripheral joints (Fig. 9-2). Similar results have been obtained in large randomized controlled trials of all three agents and many open label studies. About half of the patients achieve a >50% reduction in the Bath Ankylosing Spondylitis Disease Activity Index (BASDAI), the most commonly used measure of disease activity. Increased bone mineral density is found as early as 24 weeks after onset of therapy. Whether radiographic disease progression is slowed has not yet been determined definitively.

The dosages of these agents used in AS patients have usually been similar to those in RA. Infliximab is given as an intravenous infusion, typically at a dose of 3–5 mg/kg body weight, and then repeated 2 weeks later, again 6 weeks later, and then at 8-week intervals. Some success has been achieved with longer intervals, including infusion only upon recurrence of symptoms. Etanercept is given by subcutaneous injection in a dose of 25 mg twice weekly or 50 mg once weekly. Adalimumab is given by subcutaneous injection in a dose of 40 mg biweekly.

Although these potent immunosuppressive agents have so far been relatively safe, seven types of side effects are not rare: (1) serious infections, including disseminated tuberculosis; (2) hematologic disorders, such as pancytopenia; (3) demyelinating disorders; (4) exacerbation of congestive heart failure; (5) systemic lupus erythematosus–related autoantibodies and clinical features; (6) hypersensitivity infusion or injection site reactions; and (7) severe liver disease. Increased incidence of malignancy is of theoretical concern but has not been observed in AS patients treated for up to 5 years.

Because of the expense, potentially serious side effects, and unknown long-term effects of these agents, their use should be restricted to patients with a definite diagnosis and active disease (BASDAI ≥4 out of 10 and expert opinion) that is inadequately responsive to therapy with at least two different NSAIDs. Before initiation of anti-TNF therapy, all patients should be tested for tuberculin reactivity, and reactors (≥5 mm) should be treated with anti-tuberculous agents. Contraindications include active infection or high risk of infection; malignancy or premalignancy; and history of systemic lupus erythematosus, multiple sclerosis, or related autoimmunity. Pregnancy and breast-feeding are relative contraindications. Continuation beyond 12 weeks of therapy requires a 50% reduction in BASDAI (or absolute reduction of 2 out of 10) and favorable expert opinion. Sulfasalazine, in doses of 2–3 g/d, has been shown to be of modest benefit, primarily for peripheral arthritis. A therapeutic trial of this agent should precede any use of anti-TNF agents in patients with predominantly peripheral arthritis. Methotrexate, although widely used, has not been shown to be of benefit in AS, nor has any therapeutic role for gold or oral glucocorticoids been documented. Potential benefit in AS has been reported for thalidomide, 200 mg/d, perhaps acting through inhibition of TNF-α.

The most common indication for surgery in patients with AS is severe hip joint arthritis, the pain and stiffness of which are usually dramatically relieved by total hip arthroplasty. A small number of patients may benefit from surgical correction of extreme flexion deformities of the spine or of atlantoaxial subluxation.

Attacks of uveitis are usually managed effectively with local glucocorticoid administration in conjunction with mydriatic agents, although systemic glucocorticoids or even immunosuppressive drugs and rarely infliximab may be required in some cases. TNF inhibitors reduce the frequency of attacks of uveitis in patients with AS. A few individuals have developed new or recurrent uveitis subsequent to the use of a TNF inhibitor, especially etanercept.

Coexistent cardiac disease may require pacemaker implantation and/or aortic valve replacement. Management of osteoporosis of the axial skeleton is at present similar to that used for primary osteoporosis, since data specific for AS are not available.

REACTIVE ARTHRITIS

Reactive arthritis (ReA) refers to acute nonpurulent arthritis complicating an infection elsewhere in the body. In recent years, the term has been used primarily to refer to spondyloarthritis following enteric or urogenital infections.

Other forms of reactive and infection-related arthritis not associated with B27 and showing a spectrum of clinical features different from spondyloarthritis, such as rheumatic fever or Lyme disease, are discussed in Chaps. 6 and 20.

HISTORIC BACKGROUND

The association of acute arthritis with episodes of diarrhea or urethritis has been recognized for centuries. A large number of cases during World Wars I and II focused attention on the triad of arthritis, urethritis, and conjunctivitis, which became known as *Fiessenger-Leroy-Reiter syndrome*, often with additional mucocutaneous lesions. These eponyms are now of historic interest only.

The identification of bacterial species capable of triggering the clinical syndrome and the finding that many patients possess the B27 antigen have led to the unifying concept of ReA as a clinical syndrome triggered by specific etiologic agents in a genetically susceptible host. A similar spectrum of clinical manifestations can be triggered by enteric infection with any of several *Shigella*, *Salmonella*, *Yersinia*, and *Campylobacter* species; by genital infection with *Chlamydia trachomatis*; and by other agents as well. The triad of arthritis, urethritis, and conjunctivitis represents part of the spectrum of the clinical manifestations of ReA. For the purposes of this chapter, the use of the term *ReA* will be restricted to those cases of spondyloarthritis in which there is at least presumptive evidence for a related antecedent infection. Patients with clinical features of ReA who lack evidence of an antecedent infection will be considered to have *undifferentiated spondyloarthritis*, discussed below.

EPIDEMIOLOGY

Following the first reports of association of ReA with HLA-B27, in most hospital-based series in which *Shigella*, *Yersinia*, or *Chlamydia* were the triggering infectious agents, 60–85% of patients were found to be B27 positive, with a lower prevalence in ReA triggered by *Salmonella* and *Campylobacter*. In more recent community-based or common source epidemic studies, the prevalence of B27 has often been below 50%, and in some instances not elevated at all. The most common age range is 18–40 years, but ReA can occur both in children over 5 years of age and in older adults.

The gender ratio in ReA following enteric infection is nearly 1:1, whereas venereally acquired ReA occurs predominantly in men. The overall prevalence and incidence of ReA are difficult to assess because of the variable prevalence of the triggering infections and genetic susceptibility factors in different populations. In Scandinavian countries, an annual incidence of 10–28/100,000 has been reported. The spondyloarthritides were formerly almost unknown in sub-Saharan Africa. However, ReA and other peripheral spondyloarthritides have now become the most common rheumatic diseases in Africans in the wake of the AIDS epidemic, without association to B27, which is very rare in these populations. Spondyloarthritis in Africans with HIV infection usually occurs in individuals with stage I disease (as classified by the World Health Organization). It is often the first manifestation of infection and often remits with disease progression. In contrast, Western Caucasian patients with HIV and spondyloarthritis are predominantly B27 positive, and the arthritis flares as AIDS advances.

PATHOLOGY

Synovial histology is similar to that of other spondyloarthritides. Enthesitis shows increased vascularity and macrophage infiltration of fibrocartilage. Microscopic histopathologic evidence of inflammation has occasionally been noted in the colon and ileum of patients with postvenereal ReA, but much less commonly than in postenteric ReA. The skin lesions of keratoderma blenorrhagica, which is associated mainly with venereally acquired ReA, are histologically indistinguishable from psoriatic lesions.

ETIOLOGY AND PATHOGENESIS

Of the four *Shigella* species, *S. sonnei*, *S. boydii*, *S. flexneri*, and *S. dysenteriae*, *S. flexneri* has most often been implicated in cases of ReA, both sporadic and epidemic. Recent data suggest that *S. sonnei* and *S. dysenteriae* trigger some cases of ReA.

Other bacteria identified definitively as triggers of ReA include several *Salmonella* spp., *Yersinia enterocolitica*, *Yersinia pseudotuberculosis*, *Campylobacter jejuni*, and *C. trachomatis*. There is also increasing evidence implicating *Clostridium difficile*, *Campylobacter coli*, certain toxigenic *Escherichia coli*, and possibly *Ureaplasma urealyticum* and *Mycoplasma genitalium*. Respiratory infection with *Chlamydia pneumoniae* has also been implicated. There are numerous isolated reports of acute arthritis preceded by other bacterial, viral, or parasitic infections, but whether the microorganisms involved are actual triggers of ReA remains to be determined.

It has not been determined whether ReA occurs by the same pathogenic mechanism following infection with each of these microorganisms, nor has the mechanism been fully elucidated in the case of any one of the known bacterial triggers. Most, if not all, of the triggering organisms produce lipopolysaccharide (LPS) and share a capacity to attack mucosal surfaces, to invade host cells, and to survive intracellularly. Antigens from *Chlamydia*, *Yersinia*, *Salmonella*, and *Shigella* have been shown to be present in the synovium and/or synovial fluid leukocytes of patients with ReA for long periods following the acute attack. In ReA triggered by *Y. enterocolitica*, bacterial LPS and heat shock protein antigens have been found in peripheral blood cells years after the triggering infection. *Yersinia* DNA and *C. trachomatis* DNA and RNA have been detected in synovial tissue from ReA patients, suggesting the presence of viable organisms despite uniform failure to culture the organism from these specimens. The dormant form of *C. trachomatis* that persists in synovium transcriptionally upregulates many genes orthologous to genes upregulated in persistent *M. tuberculosis* infection.

T cells that specifically respond to antigens of the inciting organism have been found in inflamed synovium but not in peripheral blood of patients with ReA. These T cells are predominantly CD4+, but CD8+ B27-restricted bacteria-specific cytolytic T cells have also been isolated in *Yersinia*- and *C. trachomatis*–induced ReA. A unique conserved T cell antigen receptor sequence has been identified in B27-restricted synovial T cells in ReA. Unlike the synovial CD4 T cells in RA, which are predominantly of the TH1 phenotype, those in ReA also show a TH2 phenotype. A T regulatory 1 (Tr1) phenotype with elevated IL-10 and TGF-β in T, B, and macrophage lineages has also been found in ReA synovium. IL-10 promoter haplotypes have been found to be significantly different in ReA patients than in B27+ controls.

HLA-B27 seems to be associated with more severe and chronic forms of ReA, but its pathogenic role remains to be determined. HLA-B27 significantly prolongs the intracellular survival of *Y. enterocolitica* and *Salmonella enteritidis* in human and mouse cell lines. Prolonged intracellular bacterial survival, promoted by B27, other factors, or both, may permit trafficking of infected leukocytes from the site of primary infection to joints, where a T cell response to persistent bacterial antigens may then promote arthritis.

CLINICAL FEATURES

The clinical manifestations of ReA constitute a spectrum that ranges from an isolated, transient monarthritis to severe multisystem disease. A careful history will usually elicit evidence of an antecedent infection 1–4 weeks before onset of symptoms of the reactive disease. However, in a sizable minority, no clinical or laboratory evidence of an antecedent infection can be found. In many cases of presumed venereally acquired reactive disease, there is a history of a recent new sexual partner, even in the absence of laboratory evidence of infection.

Constitutional symptoms are common, including fatigue, malaise, fever, and weight loss. The musculoskeletal symptoms are usually acute in onset. Arthritis is usually asymmetric and additive, with involvement of new joints occurring over a period of a few days to 1–2 weeks. The joints of the lower extremities, especially the knee, ankle, and subtalar, metatarsophalangeal, and toe interphalangeal joints, are the most common sites of involvement, but the wrist and fingers can be involved as well. The arthritis is usually quite painful, and tense joint effusions are not uncommon, especially in the knee. Patients often cannot walk without support. Dactylitis, or "sausage digit," a diffuse swelling of a solitary finger or toe, is a distinctive feature of ReA and other peripheral spondyloarthritides but can be seen in polyarticular gout and sarcoidosis. Tendinitis and fasciitis are particularly characteristic lesions, producing pain at multiple insertion sites (entheses), especially the Achilles insertion, the plantar fascia, and sites along the axial skeleton. Spinal and low-back pain are quite common and may be caused by insertional inflammation, muscle spasm, acute sacroiliitis, or, presumably, arthritis in intervertebral articulations.

Urogenital lesions may occur throughout the course of the disease. In males, urethritis may be marked or relatively asymptomatic and may be either an accompaniment of the triggering infection or a result of the reactive phase of the disease. Prostatitis is also common. Similarly, in females, cervicitis or salpingitis may be caused either by the infectious trigger or by the sterile reactive process.

Ocular disease is common, ranging from transient, asymptomatic conjunctivitis to an aggressive anterior uveitis that occasionally proves refractory to treatment and may result in blindness.

Mucocutaneous lesions are frequent. Oral ulcers tend to be superficial, transient, and often asymptomatic. The characteristic skin lesions, *keratoderma blenorrhagica*, consist of vesicles that become hyperkeratotic, ultimately forming a crust before disappearing. They are most common on the palms and soles but may occur elsewhere as well. In patients with HIV infection, these lesions are often extremely severe and extensive, sometimes dominating the clinical picture. Lesions on the glans penis, termed *circinate balanitis*, are common; these consist of vesicles that quickly rupture to form painless superficial erosions, which in circumcised individuals can form crusts similar to those of keratoderma blenorrhagica. Nail changes are common and consist of onycholysis, distal yellowish discoloration, and/or heaped-up hyperkeratosis.

Less-frequent or rare manifestations of ReA include cardiac conduction defects, aortic insufficiency, central or peripheral nervous system lesions, and pleuropulmonary infiltrates.

Arthritis typically persists 3–5 months, but courses up to 1 year can occur. Chronic joint symptoms persist in about 15% of patients and in up to 60% in hospital-based series. Recurrences of the acute syndrome are also common. Work disability or forced change in occupation are common in those with persistent joint symptoms. Chronic heel pain is often particularly distressing. Low-back pain, sacroiliitis, and frank AS are also common sequelae. In most studies, HLA-B27–positive patients have shown a worse outcome than B27-negative patients. Patients with *Yersinia*-induced arthritis have less chronic disease than those whose initial episode follows epidemic shigellosis.

LABORATORY AND RADIOGRAPHIC FINDINGS

The ESR is usually elevated during the acute phase of the disease. Mild anemia may be present, and acute-phase reactants tend to be increased. Synovial fluid is non-specifically inflammatory. In most ethnic groups, about half the patients are B27 positive. It is unusual for the triggering infection to persist at the site of primary mucosal infection through the time of onset of the reactive disease, but it may occasionally be possible to culture the organism, e.g., in the case of *Yersinia*- or *Chlamydia*-induced disease. Serologic evidence of a recent infection may be present, such as a marked elevation of antibodies to *Yersinia*, *Salmonella*, or *Chlamydia*. Polymerase chain reaction (PCR) of first-voided urine specimens for chlamydial DNA is said to have high sensitivity.

In early or mild disease, radiographic changes may be absent or confined to juxtaarticular osteoporosis. With long-standing persistent disease, marginal erosions and loss of joint space can be seen in affected joints. Periostitis with reactive new bone formation is characteristic of the disease, as it is with all the spondyloarthritides. Spurs at the insertion of the plantar fascia are common.

Sacroiliitis and spondylitis may be seen as late sequelae. The sacroiliitis is more commonly asymmetric than in AS, and the spondylitis, rather than ascending symmetrically from the lower lumbar segments, can begin anywhere along the lumbar spine. The syndesmophytes may be coarse and nonmarginal, arising from the middle of a vertebral body, a pattern rarely seen in primary AS. Progression to spinal fusion is uncommon.

DIAGNOSIS

ReA is a clinical diagnosis with no definitively diagnostic laboratory test or radiographic finding. The diagnosis should be entertained in any patient with an acute inflammatory, asymmetric, additive arthritis or tendinitis. The evaluation should include questioning regarding possible triggering events such as an episode of diarrhea or dysuria. On physical examination, attention must be paid to the distribution of the joint and tendon involvement and to possible sites of extraarticular involvement, such as the eyes, mucous membranes, skin, nails, and genitalia. Synovial fluid analysis may be helpful in excluding septic or crystal-induced arthritis. Culture, serology, or molecular methods may help to identify a triggering infection.

Although typing for B27 is not needed to secure the diagnosis in clear-cut cases, it may have prognostic significance in terms of severity, chronicity, and the propensity for spondylitis and uveitis. Furthermore, if positive, it can be helpful diagnostically in atypical cases, but a negative test is of little diagnostic value. HIV testing is often indicated and may be necessary in order to select appropriate therapy.

It is important to differentiate ReA from disseminated gonococcal disease, both of which can be venereally acquired and associated with urethritis. Unlike ReA, gonococcal arthritis and tenosynovitis tend to involve both upper and lower extremities equally, to lack back symptoms, and to be associated with characteristic vesicular skin lesions. A positive gonococcal culture from the urethra or cervix does not exclude a diagnosis of ReA; however, culturing gonococci from blood, skin lesion, or synovium establishes the diagnosis of disseminated gonococcal disease. PCR assay for *Neisseria gonorrhoeae* and *C. trachomatis* may be helpful. Occasionally, only a therapeutic trial of antibiotics can distinguish the two.

ReA shares many features in common with psoriatic arthropathy. However, psoriatic arthritis is usually gradual in onset; the arthritis tends to affect primarily the upper extremities; there is less associated periarthritis; and there are usually no associated mouth ulcers, urethritis, or bowel symptoms.

℞ Treatment:
REACTIVE ARTHRITIS

Most patients with ReA benefit to some degree from NSAIDs, although acute symptoms are rarely completely ameliorated, and some patients fail to respond at all. Indomethacin, 75–150 mg/d in divided doses, is the initial treatment of choice, but other NSAIDs may be tried.

Prompt, appropriate antibiotic treatment of acute chlamydial urethritis or enteric infection may prevent the emergence of ReA. However, several controlled trials have failed to demonstrate any benefit for antibiotic therapy that is initiated after onset of arthritis. One long-term follow-up study suggested that although antibiotic therapy had no effect on the acute episode of ReA, it helped prevent subsequent chronic spondyloarthritis. Another such study failed to demonstrate any long-term benefit.

Multicenter trials have suggested that sulfasalazine, up to 3 g/d in divided doses, may be beneficial to patients with persistent ReA.[1] Patients with persistent disease may respond to azathioprine, 1–2 mg/kg per d, or to methotrexate, up to 20 mg per week. Although no trials of anti–TNF-α in ReA have been reported, anecdotal evidence supports the use of these agents in severe chronic cases, although lack of response has also been observed.[1]

Tendinitis and other enthesitic lesions may benefit from intralesional glucocorticoids. Uveitis may require aggressive treatment with glucocorticoids to prevent serious sequelae. Skin lesions ordinarily require only symptomatic treatment. In patients with HIV infection and ReA, many of whom have severe skin lesions, the skin lesions in particular respond to antiretroviral therapy. Cardiac complications are managed conventionally; management of neurologic complications is symptomatic.

---

[1] Azathioprine, methotrexate, sulfasalazine, pamidronate, and thalidomide have not been approved for this purpose by the U.S. Food and Drug Administration at the time of publication.

Comprehensive management includes counseling of patients in the avoidance of sexually transmitted disease and exposure to enteropathogens, as well as appropriate use of physical therapy, vocational counseling, and continued surveillance for long-term complications such as ankylosing spondylitis.

PSORIATIC ARTHRITIS

Psoriatic arthritis (PsA) refers to an inflammatory arthritis that characteristically occurs in individuals with psoriasis.

HISTORIC BACKGROUND

The association between arthritis and psoriasis was noted in the nineteenth century. In the 1960s, on the basis of epidemiologic and clinical studies, it became clear that unlike RA the arthritis associated with psoriasis was usually seronegative, often involved the distal interphalangeal (DIP) joints of the fingers and the spine and sacroiliac joints, had distinctive radiographic features, and showed considerable familial aggregation. In the 1970s, PsA was included in the broader category of the spondyloarthritides because of features similar to those of AS and ReA.

EPIDEMIOLOGY

Estimates of the prevalence of PsA among individuals with psoriasis range from 5 to 30%. In Caucasian populations, psoriasis is estimated to have a prevalence of 1–3%. Psoriasis and PsA are less common in other races in the absence of HIV infection. First-degree relatives of PsA patients have an elevated risk for psoriasis, for PsA itself, and for other forms of spondyloarthritis. Of patients with psoriasis, 30% have an affected first-degree relative. In monozygotic twins, the concordance for psoriasis is ≥65%, and for PsA ≥30%. A variety of HLA associations have been found. The HLA-Cw6 gene is directly associated with psoriasis, particularly familial juvenile onset (type I) psoriasis. HLA-B27 is associated with psoriatic spondylitis (see below). HLA-DR7, -DQ3, and -B57 are associated with PsA because of linkage disequilibrium with Cw6. Other associations include HLA-B13, -B37, -B38, -B39, and DR4. The MIC-A-A9 allele at the HLA-B-linked MIC-A locus has also recently been reported associated with PsA, as have certain killer immunoglobulin-like receptor (KIR) alleles. The complex inheritance patterns of psoriasis and PsA suggest that several unlinked allelic loci are required for susceptibility. However, only the MHC has shown consistent linkage from study to study.

PATHOLOGY

The inflamed synovium in PsA resembles that of RA, although with somewhat less hyperplasia and cellularity than in RA, and somewhat greater vascularity. Some studies have indicated a higher tendency to synovial fibrosis in PsA. Unlike RA, PsA shows prominent enthesitis, with histology similar to that of the other spondyloarthritides.

PATHOGENESIS

PsA is almost certainly immune mediated and probably shares pathogenic mechanisms with psoriasis. PsA synovium shows infiltration with T cells, B cells, macrophages, and natural killer (NK) receptor–expressing cells, with upregulation of leukocyte homing receptors. Clonally expanded CD8+ T cells are frequent in PsA. Cytokine production in the synovium in PsA resembles that in psoriatic skin lesions and in RA synovium, having predominantly a TH1 pattern. Interleukin (IL) 2, interferon γ, TNF-α, and IL-1β, -6, -8, -10, -12, -13, and -15 are found in PsA synovium or synovial fluid. Consistent with the extensive bone lesions in PsA, patients with PsA have been found to have a marked increase in osteoclastic precursors in peripheral blood and upregulation of RANKL (receptor activator of NF-κβ ligand) in the synovial lining layer.

CLINICAL FEATURES

In 60–70% of cases, psoriasis precedes joint disease. In 15–20%, the two manifestations appear within 1 year of each other. In about 15–20% of cases, the arthritis precedes the onset of psoriasis and can present a diagnostic challenge. The frequency in men and women is almost equal, although the frequency of disease patterns differs somewhat in the two sexes. The disease can begin in childhood or late in life but typically begins in the fourth or fifth decade, at an average age of 37 years.

The spectrum of arthropathy associated with psoriasis is quite broad. Many classification schemes have been proposed. In the original scheme of Wright and Moll, five patterns are described: (1) arthritis of the DIP joints; (2) asymmetric oligoarthritis; (3) symmetric polyarthritis similar to RA; (4) axial involvement (spine and sacroiliac joints); and (5) arthritis mutilans, a highly destructive form of disease. These patterns are not fixed, and the pattern that persists chronically often differs from that of the initial presentation. A simpler scheme in recent use contains three patterns: oligoarthritis, polyarthritis, and axial arthritis.

Nail changes in the fingers or toes occur in 90% of patients with PsA, compared with 40% of psoriatic patients without arthritis, and pustular psoriasis is said to be associated with more severe arthritis. Several articular features distinguish PsA from other joint disorders. Dactylitis occurs in >30%; enthesitis and tenosynovitis are also common and are probably present in most patients although often not appreciated on physical examination. Shortening of digits because of underlying osteolysis is particularly characteristic of PsA, and there

is a much greater tendency than in RA for both fibrous and bony ankylosis of small joints. Rapid ankylosis of one or more proximal interphalangeal (PIP) joints early in the course of disease is not uncommon. Back and neck pain and stiffness are also common in PsA.

Arthropathy confined to the DIP joints predominates in about 15% of cases. Accompanying nail changes in the affected digits are almost always present. These joints are also often affected in the other patterns of PsA. Approximately 30% of patients have asymmetric oligoarthritis. This pattern commonly involves a knee or another large joint with a few small joints in the fingers or toes, often with dactylitis. Symmetric polyarthritis occurs in about 40% of PsA patients at presentation. It may be indistinguishable from RA in terms of the joints involved, but other features characteristic of PsA are usually also present. In general, peripheral joints in PsA tend to be somewhat less tender than in RA, although signs of inflammation are usually present. Almost any peripheral joint can be involved. Axial arthropathy without peripheral involvement is found in about 5% of PsA patients. It may be indistinguishable from idiopathic AS, although more neck involvement and less thoracolumbar spinal involvement is characteristic, and nail changes are not found in idiopathic AS. About 5% of PsA patients have arthritis mutilans, in which there can be widespread shortening of digits ("telescoping"), sometimes coexisting with ankylosis and contractures in other digits.

Six patterns of nail involvement are identified: pitting, horizontal ridging, onycholysis, yellowish discoloration of the nail margins, dystrophic hyperkeratosis, and combinations of these findings. Other extraarticular manifestations of the spondyloarthritides are common. Eye involvement, either conjunctivitis or uveitis, is reported in 7–33% of PsA patients. Unlike the uveitis associated with AS, the uveitis in PsA is more often bilateral, chronic, and/or posterior. Aortic valve insufficiency has been found in <4% of patients, usually after long-standing disease.

Widely varying estimates of clinical outcome have been reported in PsA. At its worst, severe PsA with arthritis mutilans is at least as crippling and ultimately fatal as severe RA. Unlike RA, however, many patients with PsA experience temporary remissions. Overall, erosive disease develops in the majority of patients, progressive disease with deformity and disability is common, and in some large published series, mortality was found to be significantly increased compared with the general population.

The psoriasis and associated arthropathy seen with HIV infection both tend to be severe and can occur in populations with very little psoriasis in noninfected individuals. Severe enthesopathy, dactylitis, and rapidly progressive joint destruction are seen, but axial involvement is very rare. This condition is prevented by or responds well to antiretroviral therapy.

LABORATORY AND RADIOGRAPHIC FINDINGS

There are no diagnostic laboratory tests for PsA. ESR and CRP are often elevated. A small percentage of patients may have low titers of rheumatoid factor or antinuclear antibodies. Uric acid may be elevated in the presence of extensive psoriasis. HLA-B27 is found in 50–70% of patients with axial disease, but ≤15–20% in patients with only peripheral joint involvement.

The peripheral and axial arthropathies in PsA show a number of radiographic features that distinguish them from RA and AS, respectively. Characteristics of peripheral PsA include DIP involvement, including the classic "pencil-in-cup" deformity; marginal erosions with adjacent bony proliferation ("whiskering"); small-joint ankylosis; osteolysis of phalangeal and metacarpal bone, with telescoping of digits; and periostitis and proliferative new bone at sites of enthesitis (Fig. 9-3). Characteristics of axial PsA include asymmetric sacroiliitis; compared with idiopathic AS, less zygoapophyseal joint arthritis, fewer and less symmetric and delicate syndesmophytes; fluffy hyperperiostosis on anterior vertebral bodies; severe cervical spine involvement, with a tendency to atlantoaxial subluxation but relative sparing of the thoracolumbar spine; and paravertebral ossification. Ultrasound and MRI both readily demonstrate enthesitis and tendon sheath effusions that can be difficult to assess on physical examination. A recent MRI study of 68 PsA patients found sacroiliitis in 35%, unrelated to B27 but correlated with restricted spinal movement.

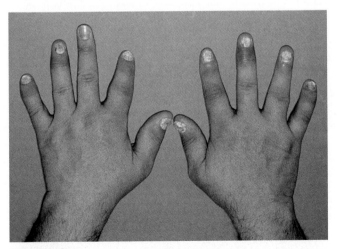

FIGURE 9-3

Characteristic lesions of psoriatic arthritis. Inflammation is prominent in the DIP joints (left 5th, 4th, 2nd; right 3rd and 5th) and PIP joints (left 2nd, right 2nd, 4th, and 5th). There is dactylitis in the left 2nd finger and thumb, with pronounced telescoping of the left 2nd finger. Nail dystrophy (hyperkeratosis and onycholysis) affects each of the fingers except the left 3rd finger, the only finger without arthritis. (*Courtesy of Donald Raddatz, MD; with permission.*)

DIAGNOSIS

The diagnosis of PsA is primarily clinical, based on the presence of psoriasis and characteristic peripheral or spinal joint symptoms, signs, and imaging. Diagnosis can be challenging when the arthritis precedes psoriasis, the psoriasis is undiagnosed or obscure, or the joint involvement closely resembles another form of arthritis. A high index of suspicion is needed in any patient with an undiagnosed inflammatory arthropathy. The history should include inquiry about psoriasis in the patient and family members. Patients should be asked to disrobe for the physical examination, and psoriasiform lesions should be sought in the scalp, ears, umbilicus, and gluteal folds in addition to more accessible sites; the finger and toe nails should also be carefully examined. Axial symptoms or signs, dactylitis, enthesitis, ankylosis, the pattern of joint involvement, and characteristic radiographic changes can be helpful clues. The differential diagnosis of isolated DIP involvement is short. Osteoarthritis (Heberden's nodes) is usually not inflammatory; gout involving more than one DIP joint often involves other sites and is accompanied by tophi; the very rare entity multicentric reticulohistiocytosis involves other joints and has characteristic small pearly periungual skin nodules; and the uncommon entity inflammatory osteoarthritis, like the others, lacks the nail changes of PsA. Radiography can be helpful in all of these cases and in distinguishing between psoriatic spondylitis and idiopathic AS. A history of trauma to an affected joint preceding the onset of arthritis is said to occur more frequently in PsA than in other types of arthritis, perhaps reflecting the Koebner phenomenon in which psoriatic skin lesions can arise at sites of the skin trauma.

℞ Treatment:
PSORIATIC ARTHRITIS

Ideally, coordinated therapy is directed at both the skin and joints in PsA. As described above for AS, use of the anti–TNF-α agents has revolutionized the treatment of PsA. Prompt and dramatic resolution of both arthritis and skin lesions has been observed in large, randomized controlled trials of etanercept, infliximab, and adalimumab. Many of the responding patients had long-standing disease that was resistant to all previous therapy, as well as extensive skin disease. The clinical response is more dramatic than in RA, and delay of disease progression has been demonstrated radiographically. The anti–T cell biologic agent Alefacept, in combination with methotrexate, has also been proven effective in both psoriatic arthritis and psoriasis.

Other treatment for PsA has been based on drugs that have efficacy in RA and/or in psoriasis. Although methotrexate in doses of 15–25 mg/week and sulfasalazine (usually given in doses of 2–3 g/d) have each been found to have clinical efficacy in controlled trials, neither effectively halts progression of erosive joint disease. Other agents with efficacy in psoriasis reported to benefit PsA are cyclosporine, retinoic acid derivatives, and psoralen plus ultraviolet light (PUVA). There is controversy regarding the efficacy in PsA of gold and antimalarials, which have been widely used in RA. The pyrimidine synthetase inhibitor leflunomide has been shown in a randomized controlled trial to be beneficial in both psoriasis and psoriatic arthritis.

All of these treatments require careful monitoring. Immunosuppressive therapy may be used cautiously in HIV-associated PsA if the HIV infection is well controlled.

In one large prospective series, 7% of patients with PsA required musculoskeletal surgery beginning at a mean of 13 years' disease duration. Indications for surgery are similar to those in RA, although there is an impression that outcomes in PsA may be less satisfactory.

UNDIFFERENTIATED AND JUVENILE-ONSET SPONDYLOARTHRITIS

Many patients, usually young adults, present with some features of one or more of the spondyloarthritides discussed above but lack criteria for these diagnoses. For example, a patient may present with inflammatory synovitis of one knee, Achilles tendinitis, and dactylitis of one digit, or sacroiliitis in the absence of other criteria for AS. Such patients are said to have undifferentiated spondyloarthritis, or simply spondyloarthritis, as defined by the European Spondyloarthropathy Study Group (ESSG criteria, **Fig. 9-4**). Some of these patients may have ReA in which the triggering infection remains clinically silent. In other cases, the patient subsequently develops IBD or psoriasis or the process eventually meets criteria for AS. Approximately half the patients with undifferentiated spondyloarthritis are HLA-B27

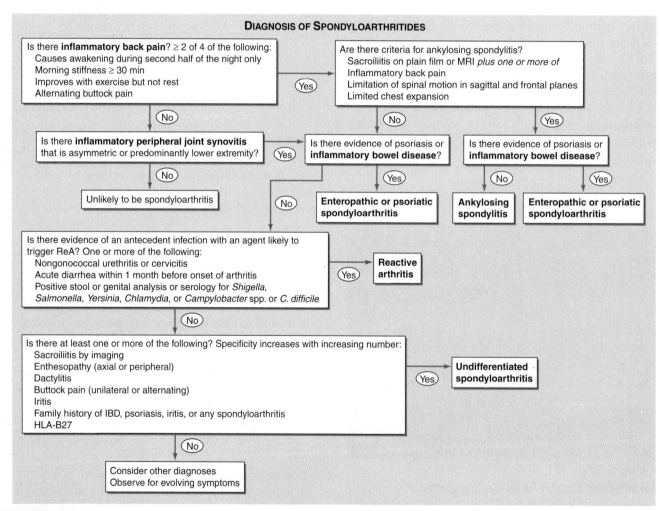

FIGURE 9-4

Algorithm for diagnosis of the spondyloarthritides, adapted from the European Spondyloarthropathy Study Group criteria and the Amor criteria (*M Dougados et al: Arthritis Rheum 34:1218, 1991; B Amor: Rev Rhum Mal Ostéoartic 57:85, 1990*). Sensitivity and specificity for any given decision arm

are approximately 80%. If a diagnosis of psoriatic arthropathy, reactive arthritis, or undifferentiated spondyloarthritis is made on the basis of peripheral arthropathy, then HIV infection needs to be considered.

positive, and thus the absence of B27 is not useful in establishing or excluding the diagnosis. In familial cases, which are much more frequently B27 positive, there is often eventual progression to AS.

In juvenile-onset spondyloarthritis, which begins between ages 7 and 16, most commonly in boys (60–80%), an asymmetric, predominantly lower-extremity oligoarthritis and enthesitis without extraarticular features is the typical mode of presentation. The prevalence of B27 in this condition, which has been termed the seronegative, enthesopathy, arthropathy (SEA) syndrome, is approximately 80%. Many, but not all, of these patients go on to develop AS in late adolescence or adulthood.

Management of undifferentiated spondyloarthritis is similar to that of the other spondyloarthritides. Response to anti–TNF-α therapy has been documented, and this therapy is indicated in severe, persistent cases not responsive to other treatment. One recent study reported significant benefit in patients with long-standing undifferentiated spondyloarthropathy treated for 9 months with doxycycline and rifampin. These data await confirmation.

Current pediatric textbooks and journals should be consulted for information on management of juvenile-onset spondyloarthritis. An algorithm for the diagnosis of the spondyloarthritides in adults is presented in Fig. 9-4.

ENTEROPATHIC ARTHRITIS

HISTORIC BACKGROUND

A relationship between arthritis and IBD was observed in the 1930s. The relationship was further defined by the epidemiologic studies in the 1950s and 1960s and included in the concept of the spondyloarthritides in the 1970s.

EPIDEMIOLOGY

Both of the common forms of IBD, ulcerative colitis (UC) and Crohn's disease (CD), are associated with spondyloarthritis. UC and CD both have an estimated prevalence of 0.05–0.1%, and the incidence of each is thought to have increased in recent decades. AS and peripheral arthritis are both associated with UC and with CD. Wide variations have been reported in the estimated frequencies of these associations. In recent series, AS was diagnosed in 1–10%, and peripheral arthritis in 10–50%, of patients with IBD. Inflammatory back pain and enthesopathy are common, and many patients have sacroiliitis on imaging studies.

The prevalence of UC or CD in patients with AS is thought to be 5–10%. However, investigation of unselected spondyloarthritis patients by ileocolonoscopy has revealed that from one-third to two-thirds of patients with AS have subclinical intestinal inflammation that is evident either macroscopically or histologically. These lesions have also been found in patients with undifferentiated

spondyloarthritis or ReA (both enterically and urogenitally acquired).

Both UC and CD have a tendency to familial aggregation, more so for CD. HLA associations have been weak and inconsistent. HLA-B27 is found in up to 70% of patients with IBD and AS, but in ≤15% of patients with IBD and peripheral arthritis or IBD alone. Three alleles of the *NOD2/CARD15* gene on chromosome 16 have been found in approximately half of patients with CD. These alleles are not associated with the spondyloarthritides per se. However, they are found significantly more often in (1) CD patients with sacroiliitis than in those without sacroiliitis, and (2) SpA patients with chronic inflammatory gut lesions than in those with normal gut histology. These associations are independent of HLA-B27.

PATHOLOGY

Available data for IBD-associated peripheral arthritis suggest a synovial histology similar to other spondyloarthritides. Association with arthropathy does not affect the gut histology of UC or CD. The subclinical inflammatory lesions in the colon and distal ileum associated with spondyloarthritis have been classified as either acute or chronic. The former resemble acute bacterial enteritis, with largely intact architecture and neutrophilic infiltration in the lamina propria. The latter resemble the lesions of CD, with distortion of villi and crypts, aphthoid ulceration, and mononuclear cell infiltration in the lamina propria.

PATHOGENESIS

Both IBD and the spondyloarthropathies are immune mediated, but the specific pathogenic mechanisms are poorly understood, and the connection between the two is obscure. IBD is a common phenotype in a number of rodent lines with transgenic overexpression or targeted deletion of genes involved in immune processes. Arthritis is an accompanying prominent feature in two of these IBD models, HLA-B27 transgenic rats and mice with constitutive overexpression of TNF-α, and immune dysregulation is prominent in both. Several lines of evidence indicate trafficking of leukocytes between the gut and the joint. Mucosal leukocytes from IBD patients have been shown to bind avidly to synovial vasculature through several different adhesion molecules. Macrophages expressing CD163 are prominent in the inflammatory lesions of both gut and synovium in the spondyloarthritides.

CLINICAL FEATURES

AS associated with IBD is clinically indistinguishable from idiopathic AS. It runs a course independent of the bowel disease, and in many patients it precedes the onset of IBD, sometimes by many years. Peripheral arthritis not infrequently begins before onset of overt bowel disease. The spectrum of peripheral arthritis includes acute self-limited attacks of oligoarthritis that often coincide with relapses of IBD, and more chronic and symmetric polyarticular arthritis that runs a course independent of IBD activity. The patterns of joint involvement are similar in UC and CD. In general, erosions and deformities are infrequent in IBD-associated peripheral arthritis, and joint surgery is rarely required. Dactylitis and enthesopathy are occasionally found. In addition to the ~20% of IBD patients with spondyloarthritis, a comparable percentage have arthralgias or fibromyalgia symptoms.

Other extraintestinal manifestations of IBD are seen in addition to arthropathy, including uveitis, pyoderma gangrenosum, erythema nodosum, and finger clubbing, all somewhat more common in CD than UC. The uveitis shares the features described above for PsA-associated uveitis.

LABORATORY AND RADIOGRAPHIC FINDINGS

Laboratory findings reflect the inflammatory and metabolic manifestations of IBD. Joint fluid is usually at least mildly inflammatory. Of patients with AS and IBD, 30–70% carry the HLA-B27 gene, compared with >90% of patients with AS alone and 50–70% of those with AS and psoriasis. Hence, definite or probable AS in a B27-negative individual in the absence of psoriasis should prompt a search for occult IBD. Radiographic changes in the axial skeleton are the same as in uncomplicated AS. Erosions are uncommon in peripheral arthritis but may occur, particularly in the metatarsophalangeal joints. Isolated destructive hip disease has been described.

DIAGNOSIS

Diarrhea and arthritis are both common conditions that can coexist for a variety of reasons. When etiopathogenically related, reactive arthritis and IBD-associated arthritis are the most common causes. Rare causes include celiac disease, blind loop syndromes, and Whipple's disease. In most cases, diagnosis depends upon investigation of the bowel disease.

℞ Treatment:
ENTEROPATHIC ARTHRITIS

As with the spondyloarthritides, treatment of CD has been revolutionized by therapy with anti-TNF agents. Infliximab and adalimumab are effective for induction and maintenance of clinical remission in CD, and infliximab has been shown to be effective in fistulizing CD.

IBD-associated arthritis also responds to these agents. Other treatment for IBD, including sulfasalazine and related drugs, systemic glucocorticoids, and immunosuppressive drugs, are also usually of benefit for associated peripheral arthritis. NSAIDs are generally helpful and well tolerated, but they can precipitate flares of IBD.

SAPHO SYNDROME

The syndrome of synovitis, acne, pustulosis, hyperostosis, and osteitis (SAPHO) is characterized by a variety of skin and musculoskeletal manifestations. Dermatologic manifestations include palmoplantar pustulosis, acne conglobata, acne fulminans, and hidradenitis suppurativa. The main musculoskeletal findings are sternoclavicular and spinal hyperostosis, chronic recurrent foci of sterile osteomyelitis, and axial or peripheral arthritis. Cases with one or a few manifestations are probably the rule. The ESR is usually elevated, sometimes dramatically. In some cases, bacteria, most often *Propionibacterium acnes*, have been cultured from bone biopsy specimens and occasionally other sites. Inflammatory bowel disease was coexistent in 8% of patients in one large series. B27 is found in only a small minority of patients. Either bone scan or CT scan is helpful diagnostically. High-dose NSAIDs may provide relief from bone pain. A number of uncontrolled series and case reports of successful therapy with pamidronate or other bisphosphonates have appeared recently. Response to anti–TNF-α therapy has also been observed, although in a few cases this has been associated with a flare of skin manifestations. Successful prolonged antibiotic therapy has also been reported.

WHIPPLE'S DISEASE

Whipple's disease is a rare chronic bacterial infection, mostly of middle-aged Caucasian men, caused by *Tropheryma whippelii*. At least 75% of affected individuals develop an oligo- or polyarthritis. The joint manifestations usually precede other symptoms of the disease by 5 years or more; they are thus particularly important because antibiotic therapy is curative, whereas the untreated disease is fatal. Large and small peripheral joints and sacroiliac joints may be involved. The arthritis is abrupt in onset, migratory, usually lasts hours to a few days, and then resolves completely. Chronic polyarthritis and joint space loss, visible on x-ray, can occur but are not typical. Eventually prolonged diarrhea, malabsorption, and weight loss occur. Other manifestations of systemic disease include fever, edema, serositis, endocarditis, pneumonia, hypotension, lymphadenopathy, hyperpigmentation, subcutaneous nodules, clubbing, and uveitis. Central nervous system involvement eventually develops in 80% of untreated patients, with cognitive changes, headache, diplopia, and

℞ Treatment:
CHURG-STRAUSS SYNDROME

The prognosis of untreated Churg-Strauss syndrome is poor, with a reported 5-year survival of 25%. With treatment, prognosis is favorable, with one study finding a 78-month actuarial survival rate of 72%. Myocardial involvement is the most frequent cause of death and is responsible for 39% of patient mortality. Glucocorticoids alone appear to be effective in many patients. Dosage tapering is often limited by asthma, and many patients require low-dose prednisone for persistent asthma many years after clinical recovery from vasculitis. In glucocorticoid failure or in patients who present with fulminant multisystem disease, the treatment of choice is a combined regimen of daily cyclophosphamide and prednisone (see "Wegener's Granulomatosis" for a detailed description of this therapeutic regimen).

POLYARTERITIS NODOSA

Definition

PAN, also referred to as *classic PAN*, was described in 1866 by Kussmaul and Maier. It is a multisystem, necrotizing vasculitis of small- and medium-sized muscular arteries in which involvement of the renal and visceral arteries is characteristic. *PAN* does not involve pulmonary arteries, although bronchial vessels may be involved; granulomas, significant eosinophilia, and an allergic diathesis are not observed.

Incidence and Prevalence

It is difficult to establish an accurate incidence of PAN because previous reports have included PAN and microscopic polyangiitis as well as other related vasculitides. PAN, as currently defined, is felt to be a very uncommon disease.

Pathology and Pathogenesis

The vascular lesion in PAN is a necrotizing inflammation of small- and medium-sized muscular arteries. The lesions are segmental and tend to involve bifurcations and branchings of arteries. They may spread circumferentially to involve adjacent veins. However, involvement of venules is not seen in PAN and, if present, suggests microscopic polyangiitis (see below). In the acute stages of disease, polymorphonuclear neutrophils infiltrate all layers of the vessel wall and perivascular areas, which results in intimal proliferation and degeneration of the vessel wall. Mononuclear cells infiltrate the area as the lesions progress to the subacute and chronic stages. Fibrinoid necrosis of the vessels ensues with compromise of the lumen, thrombosis, infarction of the tissues supplied by the involved vessel, and, in some cases, hemorrhage. As the lesions heal, there is collagen deposition, which may lead to further occlusion of the vessel lumen. Aneurysmal dilatations up to 1 cm in size along the involved arteries are characteristic of PAN. Granulomas and substantial eosinophilia with eosinophilic tissue infiltrations are not characteristically found and suggest Churg-Strauss syndrome (see above).

Multiple organ systems are involved, and the clinicopathologic findings reflect the degree and location of vessel involvement and the resulting ischemic changes. As mentioned above, pulmonary arteries are not involved in PAN, and bronchial artery involvement is uncommon. The pathology in the kidney in classic PAN is that of arteritis without glomerulonephritis. In patients with significant hypertension, typical pathologic features of glomerulosclerosis may be seen. In addition, pathologic sequelae of hypertension may be found elsewhere in the body.

The presence of hepatitis B antigenemia in ~10–30% of patients with systemic vasculitis, particularly of the PAN type, together with the isolation of circulating immune complexes composed of hepatitis B antigen and immunoglobulin, and the demonstration by immunofluorescence of hepatitis B antigen, IgM, and complement in the blood vessel walls, strongly suggest the role of immunologic phenomena in the pathogenesis of this disease. Hairy cell leukemia can be associated with PAN; the pathogenic mechanisms of this association are unclear.

Clinical and Laboratory Manifestations

Nonspecific signs and symptoms are the hallmarks of PAN. Fever, weight loss, and malaise are present in over one-half of cases. Patients usually present with vague symptoms such as weakness, malaise, headache, abdominal pain, and myalgias that can rapidly progress to a fulminant illness. Specific complaints related to the vascular involvement within a particular organ system may also dominate the presenting clinical picture as well as the entire course of the illness (Table 10-5). In PAN, renal involvement most commonly manifests as hypertension, renal insufficiency, or hemorrhage due to microaneurysms.

There are no diagnostic serologic tests for PAN. In >75% of patients, the leukocyte count is elevated with a predominance of neutrophils. Eosinophilia is seen only rarely and, when present at high levels, suggests the diagnosis of Churg-Strauss syndrome. The anemia of chronic disease may be seen, and an elevated ESR is almost always present. Other common laboratory findings reflect the particular organ involved. Hypergammaglobulinemia may be present, and up to 30% of patients have a positive test for hepatitis B surface antigen. Antibodies against myeloperoxidase or proteinase-3 (ANCA) are rarely found in patients with PAN.

TABLE 10-5

CLINICAL MANIFESTATIONS RELATED TO ORGAN SYSTEM INVOLVEMENT IN CLASSIC POLYARTERITIS NODOSA

ORGAN SYSTEM	PERCENT INCIDENCE	CLINICAL MANIFESTATIONS
Renal	60	Renal failure, hypertension
Musculoskeletal	64	Arthritis, arthralgia, myalgia
Peripheral nervous system	51	Peripheral neuropathy, mononeuritis multiplex
Gastrointestinal tract	44	Abdominal pain, nausea and vomiting, bleeding, bowel infarction and perforation, cholecystitis, hepatic infarction, pancreatic infarction
Skin	43	Rash, purpura, nodules, cutaneous infarcts, livedo reticularis, Raynaud's phenomenon
Cardiac	36	Congestive heart failure, myocardial infarction, pericarditis
Genitourinary	25	Testicular, ovarian, or epididymal pain
Central nervous system	23	Cerebral vascular accident, altered mental status, seizure

Source: From TR Cupps, AS Fauci: *The Vasculitides.* Philadelphia, Saunders, 1981.

Diagnosis

The diagnosis of PAN is based on the demonstration of characteristic findings of vasculitis on biopsy material of involved organs. In the absence of easily accessible tissue for biopsy, the angiographic demonstration of involved vessels, particularly in the form of aneurysms of small- and medium-sized arteries in the renal, hepatic, and visceral vasculature, is sufficient to make the diagnosis. Aneurysms of vessels are not pathognomonic of PAN; furthermore, aneurysms need not always be present, and angiographic findings may be limited to stenotic segments and obliteration of vessels. Biopsy of symptomatic organs such as nodular skin lesions, painful testes, and nerve/muscle provides the highest diagnostic yields.

℞ Treatment: POLYARTERITIS NODOSA

The prognosis of untreated PAN is extremely poor, with a reported 5-year survival rate between 10 and 20%. Death usually results from gastrointestinal complications, particularly bowel infarcts and perforation, and cardiovascular causes. Intractable hypertension often compounds dysfunction in other organ systems, such as the kidneys, heart, and CNS, leading to additional late morbidity and mortality in PAN. With the introduction of treatment, survival rate has increased substantially. Favorable therapeutic results have been reported in

PAN with the combination of prednisone and cyclophosphamide (see "Wegener's Granulomatosis" for a detailed description of this therapeutic regimen). In less severe cases of PAN, glucocorticoids alone have resulted in disease remission. Favorable results have also been reported in the treatment of PAN related to hepatitis B virus with antiviral therapy in combination with glucocorticoids and plasma exchange. Careful attention to the treatment of hypertension can lessen the acute and late morbidity and mortality associated with renal, cardiac, and CNS complications of PAN. Following successful treatment, relapse of PAN has been estimated to occur in only 10% of patients.

MICROSCOPIC POLYANGIITIS

Definition

The term *microscopic polyarteritis* was introduced into the literature by Davson in 1948 in recognition of the presence of glomerulonephritis in patients with PAN. In 1992, the Chapel Hill Consensus Conference on the Nomenclature of Systemic Vasculitis adopted the term *microscopic polyangiitis* to connote a necrotizing vasculitis with few or no immune complexes affecting small vessels (capillaries, venules, or arterioles). Glomerulonephritis is very common in microscopic polyangiitis, and pulmonary capillaritis often occurs. The absence of granulomatous inflammation in microscopic polyangiitis is said to differentiate it from Wegener's granulomatosis.

Incidence and Prevalence

The incidence of microscopic polyangiitis has not yet been reliably established due to its previous inclusion as part of PAN. The mean age of onset is ~57 years of age, and males are slightly more frequently affected than females.

Pathology and Pathogenesis

The vascular lesion in microscopic polyangiitis is histologically similar to that in PAN. Unlike PAN, the vasculitis seen in microscopic polyangiitis has a predilection to involve capillaries and venules in addition to small- and medium-sized arteries. Immunohistochemical staining reveals a paucity of immunoglobulin deposition in the vascular lesion of microscopic polyangiitis, suggesting that immune complex formation does not play a role in the pathogenesis of this syndrome. The renal lesion seen in microscopic polyangiitis is identical to that of Wegener's granulomatosis. Like Wegener's granulomatosis, microscopic polyangiitis is highly associated with the presence of ANCA, which may play a role in pathogenesis of this syndrome (see above).

Clinical and Laboratory Manifestations

Because of its predilection to involve the small vessels, microscopic polyangiitis and Wegener's granulomatosis share similar clinical features. Disease onset may be gradual with initial symptoms of fever, weight loss, and musculoskeletal pain; however, it is often acute. Glomerulonephritis occurs in at least 79% of patients and can be rapidly progressive, leading to renal failure. Hemoptysis may be the first symptom of alveolar hemorrhage, which occurs in 12% of patients. Other manifestations include mononeuritis multiplex and gastrointestinal tract and cutaneous vasculitis. Upper airways disease and pulmonary nodules are not typically found in microscopic polyangiitis and, if present, suggest Wegener's granulomatosis.

Features of inflammation may be seen, including an elevated ESR, anemia, leukocytosis, and thrombocytosis. ANCA are present in 75% of patients with microscopic polyangiitis, with antimyeloperoxidase antibodies being the predominant ANCA associated with this disease.

Diagnosis

The diagnosis is based on histologic evidence of vasculitis or pauci-immune glomerulonephritis in a patient with compatible clinical features of multisystem disease. Although microscopic polyangiitis is strongly ANCA-associated, no studies have as yet established the sensitivity and specificity of ANCA in this disease.

 Treatment:
MICROSCOPIC POLYANGIITIS

The 5-year survival rate for patients with treated microscopic polyangiitis is 74%, with disease-related mortality occurring from alveolar hemorrhage or gastrointestinal, cardiac, or renal disease. To date there has been limited disease-specific information on the treatment of microscopic polyangiitis. Available data together with a predilection for this disease to affect the small vessels support a therapeutic approach similar to that used in Wegener's granulomatosis. Patients with immediately life-threatening disease should be treated with the combination of prednisone and cyclophosphamide (see "Wegener's Granulomatosis" for a detailed description of this therapeutic regimen). Disease relapse has been observed in at least 34% of patients. Treatment for such relapses would be similar to that used at the time of initial presentation and based upon site and severity of disease.

GIANT CELL ARTERITIS AND POLYMYALGIA RHEUMATICA

Definition

Giant cell arteritis, also referred to as *cranial arteritis* or *temporal arteritis,* is an inflammation of medium- and large-sized arteries. It characteristically involves one or more branches of the carotid artery, particularly the temporal artery. However, it is a systemic disease that can involve arteries in multiple locations, particularly the aorta and its main branches.

Giant cell arteritis is closely associated with *polymyalgia rheumatica,* which is characterized by stiffness, aching, and pain in the muscles of the neck, shoulders, lower back, hips, and thighs. Most commonly, polymyalgia rheumatica occurs in isolation, but it may be seen in 40–50% of patients with giant cell arteritis. In addition, ~10–20% of patients who initially present with features of isolated polymyalgia rheumatica later go on to develop giant cell arteritis. This strong clinical association together with data from pathophysiologic studies has increasingly supported that giant cell arteritis and polymyalgia rheumatica represent differing clinical spectrums of a single disease process.

Incidence and Prevalence

Giant cell arteritis occurs almost exclusively in individuals >50 years. It is more common in women than in men and is rare in blacks. The incidence of giant cell arteritis varies widely in different studies and in different geographic regions. A high incidence has been found in Scandinavia and in regions of the United States with large Scandinavian populations, compared to a lower incidence in southern Europe. The annual incidence rates in individuals ≥50 years range from 6.9–32.8 per 100,000 population. Familial aggregation has been reported, as has an association with HLA-DR4. In addition, genetic linkage studies have demonstrated an association of giant cell arteritis with alleles at the HLA-DRB1 locus, particularly HLA-DRB1*04 variants. In Olmsted County, Minnesota, the annual incidence of polymyalgia rheumatica in individuals ≥50 years is 58.7 per 100,000 population.

Pathology and Pathogenesis

Although the temporal artery is most frequently involved in giant cell arteritis, patients often have a systemic vasculitis of multiple medium- and large-sized arteries, which may go undetected. Histopathologically, the disease is a panarteritis with inflammatory mononuclear cell infiltrates within the vessel wall with frequent giant cell formation. There is proliferation of the intima and fragmentation of the internal elastic lamina. Pathophysiologic findings in organs result from the ischemia related to the involved vessels.

Experimental data support that giant cell arteritis is an antigen-driven disease in which activated T lymphocytes, macrophages, and dendritic cells play a critical role in the disease pathogenesis. Sequence analysis of the T cell receptor of tissue-infiltrating T cells in lesions of giant cell arteritis indicates restricted clonal expansion, suggesting the presence of an antigen residing in the arterial wall. Giant cell arteritis is believed to be initiated in the adventitia where CD4+ T cells become activated and orchestrate macrophage differentiation. T cells recruited to vasculitic lesions in patients with giant cell arteritis produce predominantly IL-2 and IFN-γ, and the latter has been suggested to be involved in the progression to overt arteritis.

Clinical and Laboratory Manifestations

Giant cell arteritis is characterized clinically by the complex of fever, anemia, high ESR, and headaches in a patient over the age of 50 years. Other manifestations include malaise, fatigue, anorexia, weight loss, sweats, arthralgias, and associated polymyalgia rheumatica.

In patients with involvement of the temporal artery, headache is the predominant symptom and may be associated with a tender, thickened, or nodular artery, which may pulsate early in the disease but may become occluded later. Scalp pain and claudication of the jaw and tongue may occur. A well-recognized and dreaded complication of giant cell arteritis, particularly in untreated patients, is ischemic optic neuropathy, which may lead to serious visual symptoms, even sudden blindness in some patients. However, most patients have complaints relating to the head or eyes before visual loss. Attention to such symptoms with institution of appropriate therapy (see below) will usually avoid this complication. Claudication of the

extremities, strokes, myocardial infarctions, and infarctions of visceral organs have been reported. Of note, giant cell arteritis is associated with an increased risk of aortic aneurysm, which is usually a late complication and may lead to dissection and death.

Characteristic laboratory findings in addition to the elevated ESR include a normochromic or slightly hypochromic anemia. Liver function abnormalities are common, particularly increased alkaline phosphatase levels. Increased levels of IgG and complement have been reported. Levels of enzymes indicative of muscle damage such as serum creatine kinase are not elevated.

Diagnosis

The diagnosis of giant cell arteritis and its associated clinicopathologic syndrome can often be suggested clinically by the demonstration of the complex of fever, anemia, and high ESR with or without symptoms of polymyalgia rheumatica in a patient >50 years. The diagnosis is confirmed by biopsy of the temporal artery. Since involvement of the vessel may be segmental, positive yield is increased by obtaining a biopsy segment of 3–5 cm together with serial sectioning of biopsy specimens. Ultrasonography of the temporal artery has been reported to be helpful in diagnosis. A temporal artery biopsy should be obtained as quickly as possible in the setting of ocular signs and symptoms, and under these circumstances therapy should not be delayed pending a biopsy. In this regard, it has been reported that temporal artery biopsies may show vasculitis even after ~14 days of glucocorticoid therapy. A dramatic clinical response to a trial of glucocorticoid therapy can further support the diagnosis.

Isolated polymyalgia rheumatica is a clinical diagnosis made by the presence of typical symptoms of stiffness, aching, and pain in the muscles of the hip and shoulder girdle, an increased ESR, the absence of clinical features suggestive of giant cell arteritis, and a prompt therapeutic response to low dose prednisone.

℞ Treatment:
GIANT CELL ARTERITIS AND POLYMYALGIA RHEUMATICA

Disease-related mortality from giant cell arteritis is very uncommon with fatalities occurring from cerebrovascular events, myocardial infarction, or aortic aneurysm rupture.

The goals of treatment in giant cell arteritis are to reduce symptoms and, most importantly, to prevent visual loss. Giant cell arteritis and its associated symptoms are exquisitely sensitive to glucocorticoid therapy. Treatment should begin with prednisone, 40–60 mg/d for ~1 month, followed by a gradual tapering. When ocular signs and symptoms occur, it is important that therapy be initiated or adjusted to control them. Although the optimal duration of glucocorticoid therapy has not been established, most series have found that patients require treatment for ≥2 years. Symptom recurrence during prednisone tapering develops in 60–85% of patients with giant cell arteritis, requiring a dosage increase. The ESR can serve as a useful indicator of inflammatory disease activity in monitoring and tapering therapy and can be used to judge the pace of the tapering schedule. However, minor increases in the ESR can occur as glucocorticoids are being tapered and do not necessarily reflect an exacerbation of arteritis, particularly if the patient remains symptom-free. Under these circumstances, the tapering should continue with caution. Glucocorticoid toxicity occurs in 35–65% of patients and represents an important cause of patient morbidity. Aspirin has been found to reduce the occurrence of cranial ischemic complications in giant cell arteritis and should be given in addition to glucocorticoids in patients who do not have contraindications. The use of weekly methotrexate as a glucocorticoid-sparing agent has been examined in two randomized placebo-controlled trials that reached conflicting conclusions. In two randomized trials, infliximab was found to provide no benefit and had a higher rate of infection in patients with giant cell arteritis and in polymyalgia rheumatica.

Patients with isolated polymyalgia rheumatica respond promptly to prednisone, which can be started at a lower dose of 10–20 mg/d. Similar to giant cell arteritis, the ESR can serve as a useful indicator in monitoring and prednisone reduction. Recurrent polymyalgia symptoms develop in the majority of patients during prednisone tapering. One study of weekly methotrexate found that the use of this drug reduced the prednisone dose on average by only 1 mg and did not decrease prednisone-related side effects.

TAKAYASU'S ARTERITIS

Definition

Takayasu's arteritis is an inflammatory and stenotic disease of medium- and large-sized arteries characterized by a strong predilection for the aortic arch and its branches. For this reason, it is often referred to as the *aortic arch syndrome*.

Incidence and Prevalence

Takayasu's arteritis is an uncommon disease with an estimated annual incidence rate of 1.2–2.6 cases per million. It is most prevalent in adolescent girls and young women. Although it is more common in Asia, it is neither racially nor geographically restricted.

Pathology and Pathogenesis

The disease involves medium- and large-sized arteries, with a strong predilection for the aortic arch and its branches; the pulmonary artery may also be involved. The most commonly affected arteries seen by angiography are listed in Table 10-6. The involvement of the major branches of the aorta is much more marked at their origin than distally. The disease is a panarteritis with inflammatory mononuclear cell infiltrates and occasionally giant cells. There are marked intimal proliferation and fibrosis, scarring and vascularization of the media, and disruption and degeneration of the elastic lamina. Narrowing of the lumen occurs with or without thrombosis. The vasa vasorum are frequently involved. Pathologic changes in various organs reflect the compromise of blood flow through the involved vessels.

Immunopathogenic mechanisms, the precise nature of which is uncertain, are suspected in this disease. As with several of the vasculitis syndromes, circulating immune complexes have been demonstrated, but their pathogenic significance is unclear.

Clinical and Laboratory Manifestations

Takayasu's arteritis is a systemic disease with generalized as well as vascular symptoms. The generalized symptoms include malaise, fever, night sweats, arthralgias, anorexia, and weight loss, which may occur months before vessel involvement is apparent. These symptoms may merge into those related to vascular compromise and organ ischemia. Pulses are commonly absent in the involved vessels, particularly the subclavian artery. The frequency of arteriographic abnormalities and the potentially associated clinical manifestations are listed in Table 10-6. Hypertension occurs in 32 to 93% of patients and contributes to renal, cardiac, and cerebral injury.

Characteristic laboratory findings include an elevated ESR, mild anemia, and elevated immunoglobulin levels.

Diagnosis

The diagnosis of Takayasu's arteritis should be suspected strongly in a young woman who develops a decrease or absence of peripheral pulses, discrepancies in blood pressure, and arterial bruits. The diagnosis is confirmed by the characteristic pattern on arteriography, which includes irregular vessel walls, stenosis, poststenotic dilatation, aneurysm formation, occlusion, and evidence of increased collateral circulation. Complete aortic arteriography by catheter-directed dye arteriography, magnetic resonance arteriography, or computerized tomography arteriography should be obtained, in order to fully delineate the distribution and degree of arterial disease. Histopathologic demonstration of inflamed vessels adds confirmatory data; however, tissue is rarely readily available for examination.

TABLE 10-6

FREQUENCY OF ARTERIOGRAPHIC ABNORMALITIES AND POTENTIAL CLINICAL MANIFESTATIONS OF ARTERIAL INVOLVEMENT IN TAKAYASU'S ARTERITIS

ARTERY	PERCENT OF ARTERIOGRAPHIC ABNORMALITIES	POTENTIAL CLINICAL MANIFESTATIONS
Subclavian	93	Arm claudication, Raynaud's phenomenon
Common carotid	58	Visual changes, syncope, transient ischemic attacks, stroke
Abdominal aorta[a]	47	Abdominal pain, nausea, vomiting
Renal	38	Hypertension, renal failure
Aortic arch or root	35	Aortic insufficiency, congestive heart failure
Vertebral	35	Visual changes, dizziness
Coeliac axis[a]	18	Abdominal pain, nausea, vomiting
Superior mesenteric[a]	18	Abdominal pain, nausea, vomiting
Iliac	17	Leg claudication
Pulmonary	10–40	Atypical chest pain, dyspnea
Coronary	<10	Chest pain, myocardial infarction

[a]Arteriographic lesions at these locations are usually asymptomatic but may potentially cause these symptoms.
Source: Kerr et al.

℞ Treatment:
TAKAYASU'S ARTERITIS

The long-term outcome of patients with Takayasu's arteritis has varied widely between studies. Although two North American reports found overall survival to be ≥94%, the 5-year mortality rate from other studies has ranged from 0–35%. Disease-related mortality most often occurs from congestive heart failure, cerebrovascular events, myocardial infarction, aneurysm rupture, or renal failure. Even in the absence of life-threatening disease Takayasu's arteritis can be associated with significant morbidity. The course of the disease is variable, and although spontaneous remissions may occur, Takayasu's arteritis is most often chronic and relapsing. Although glucocorticoid therapy in doses of 40–60 mg prednisone per day alleviates symptoms, there are no convincing studies that indicate that they increase survival. The combination of glucocorticoid therapy for acute signs and symptoms and an aggressive surgical and/or angioplastic approach to stenosed vessels has markedly improved outcome and decreased morbidity by lessening the risk of stroke, correcting hypertension due to renal artery stenosis, and improving blood flow to ischemic viscera and limbs. Unless it is urgently required, surgical correction of stenosed arteries should be undertaken only when the vascular inflammatory process is well controlled with medical therapy. In individuals who are refractory to or unable to taper glucocorticoids, methotrexate in doses up to 25 mg/week has

yielded encouraging results. Open-label studies have suggested that anti-TNF therapies may provide benefit, although efficacy cannot be determined in the absence of a randomized trial.

HENOCH-SCHÖNLEIN PURPURA

Definition

Henoch-Schönlein purpura, also referred to as *anaphylactoid purpura*, is a distinct systemic vasculitis syndrome that is characterized by palpable purpura (most commonly distributed over the buttocks and lower extremities), arthralgias, gastrointestinal signs and symptoms, and glomerulonephritis. It is a small-vessel vasculitis.

Incidence and Prevalence

Henoch-Schönlein purpura is usually seen in children; most patients range in age from 4–7 years; however, the disease may also be seen in infants and adults. It is not a rare disease; in one series it accounted for between 5 and 24 admissions per year at a pediatric hospital. The male-to-female ratio is 1.5:1. A seasonal variation with a peak incidence in spring has been noted.

Pathology and Pathogenesis

The presumptive pathogenic mechanism for Henoch-Schönlein purpura is immune-complex deposition. A number of inciting antigens have been suggested including upper respiratory tract infections, various drugs, foods, insect bites, and immunizations. IgA is the antibody class most often seen in the immune complexes and has been demonstrated in the renal biopsies of these patients.

Clinical and Laboratory Manifestations

In pediatric patients, palpable purpura is seen in virtually all patients; most patients develop polyarthralgias in the absence of frank arthritis. Gastrointestinal involvement, which is seen in almost 70% of pediatric patients, is characterized by colicky abdominal pain usually associated with nausea, vomiting, diarrhea, or constipation and is frequently accompanied by the passage of blood and mucus per rectum; bowel intussusception may occur. Renal involvement occurs in 10–50% of patients and is usually characterized by mild glomerulonephritis leading to proteinuria and microscopic hematuria, with red blood cell casts in the majority of patients; it usually resolves spontaneously without therapy. Rarely, a progressive glomerulonephritis will develop. In adults, presenting symptoms are most frequently related to the skin and joints, while initial complaints related to the gut are less common. Although certain studies have found that renal disease is more frequent and more severe in adults, this has not been a consistent finding. However, the course of renal disease in adults may be more insidious and thus requires close follow-up. Myocardial involvement can occur in adults but is rare in children.

Laboratory studies generally show a mild leukocytosis, a normal platelet count, and occasionally eosinophilia. Serum complement components are normal, and IgA levels are elevated in about one-half of patients.

Diagnosis

The diagnosis of Henoch-Schönlein purpura is based on clinical signs and symptoms. Skin biopsy specimen can be useful in confirming leukocytoclastic vasculitis with IgA and C3 deposition by immunofluorescence. Renal biopsy is rarely needed for diagnosis but may provide prognostic information in some patients.

℞ Treatment: HENOCH-SCHÖNLEIN PURPURA

The prognosis of Henoch-Schönlein purpura is excellent. Mortality is exceedingly rare, and 1–5% of children progress to end-stage renal disease. Most patients recover completely, and some do not require therapy. Treatment is similar for adults and children. When glucocorticoid therapy is required, prednisone, in doses of 1 mg/kg per d and tapered according to clinical response, has been shown to be useful in decreasing tissue edema,

arthralgias, and abdominal discomfort; however, it has not proven beneficial in the treatment of skin or renal disease and does not appear to shorten the duration of active disease or lessen the chance of recurrence. Patients with rapidly progressive glomerulonephritis have been anecdotally reported to benefit from intensive plasma exchange combined with cytotoxic drugs. Disease recurrences have been reported in 10–40% of patients.

IDIOPATHIC CUTANEOUS VASCULITIS

Definition

The term *cutaneous vasculitis* is defined broadly as inflammation of the blood vessels of the dermis. Due to its heterogeneity, cutaneous vasculitis has been described by a variety of terms including *hypersensitivity vasculitis* and *cutaneous leukocytoclastic angiitis*. However, cutaneous vasculitis is not one specific disease but a manifestation that can be seen in a variety of settings. In >70% of cases, cutaneous vasculitis occurs either as part of a primary systemic vasculitis or as a secondary vasculitis related to an inciting agent or an underlying disease (see "Secondary Vasculitis" later in the chapter). In the remaining 30% of cases, cutaneous vasculitis occurs idiopathically.

Incidence and Prevalence

Cutaneous vasculitis represents the most commonly encountered vasculitis in clinical practice. The exact incidence of idiopathic cutaneous vasculitis has not been determined due to the predilection for cutaneous vasculitis to be associated with an underlying process and the variability of its clinical course.

Pathology and Pathogenesis

The typical histopathologic feature of cutaneous vasculitis is the presence of vasculitis of small vessels. Postcapillary venules are the most commonly involved vessels; capillaries and arterioles may be involved less frequently. This vasculitis is characterized by a leukocytoclasis, a term that refers to the nuclear debris remaining from the neutrophils that have infiltrated in and around the vessels during the acute stages. In the subacute or chronic stages, mononuclear cells predominate; in certain subgroups, eosinophilic infiltration is seen. Erythrocytes often extravasate from the involved vessels, leading to palpable purpura.

Clinical and Laboratory Manifestations

The hallmark of idiopathic cutaneous vasculitis is the predominance of skin involvement. Skin lesions may appear typically as palpable purpura; however, other cutaneous manifestations of the vasculitis may occur, including macules, papules, vesicles, bullae, subcutaneous nodules, ulcers, and recurrent or chronic urticaria. The skin lesions may be pruritic or even quite painful, with a burning or stinging sensation. Lesions most commonly occur in the lower extremities in ambulatory patients or in the sacral area in bedridden patients due to the effects of hydrostatic forces on the postcapillary venules. Edema may accompany certain lesions, and hyperpigmentation often occurs in areas of recurrent or chronic lesions.

There are no specific laboratory tests diagnostic of idiopathic cutaneous vasculitis. A mild leukocytosis with or without eosinophilia is characteristic, as is an elevated ESR. Laboratory studies should be aimed towards ruling out features to suggest an underlying disease or a systemic vasculitis.

Diagnosis

The diagnosis of cutaneous vasculitis is made by the demonstration of vasculitis on biopsy. An important diagnostic principle in patients with cutaneous vasculitis is to search for an etiology of the vasculitis—be it an exogenous agent, such as a drug or an infection, or an endogenous condition, such as an underlying disease (Fig. 10-1). In addition, a careful physical and laboratory examination should be performed to rule out the possibility of systemic vasculitis. This should start with the least invasive diagnostic approach and proceed to the more invasive only if clinically indicated.

℞ Treatment:
IDIOPATHIC CUTANEOUS VASCULITIS

When an antigenic stimulus is recognized as the precipitating factor in the cutaneous vasculitis, it should be removed; if this is a microbe, appropriate antimicrobial therapy should be instituted. If the vasculitis is associated with another underlying disease, treatment of the latter often results in resolution of the former. In situations where disease is apparently self-limited, no therapy, except possibly symptomatic therapy, is indicated. When cutaneous vasculitis persists and when there is no evidence of an inciting agent, an associated disease, or an underlying systemic vasculitis, the decision to treat should be based on weighing the balance between the degree of symptoms and the risk of treatment. Some cases of idiopathic cutaneous vasculitis resolve spontaneously, while others remit and relapse. In those patients with persistent vasculitis, a variety of therapeutic regimens have been tried with variable results. In general, the treatment of idiopathic cutaneous vasculitis has not been satisfactory. Fortunately, since the disease is generally limited to the skin, this lack of consistent

response to therapy usually does not lead to a life-threatening situation. Glucocorticoids are often used in the treatment of idiopathic cutaneous vasculitis. Therapy is usually instituted as prednisone, 1 mg/kg per d, with rapid tapering where possible, either directly to discontinuation or by conversion to an alternate-day regimen followed by ultimate discontinuation. In cases that prove refractory to glucocorticoids, a trial of a cytotoxic agent may be indicated. Patients with chronic vasculitis isolated to cutaneous venules rarely respond dramatically to any therapeutic regimen, and cytotoxic agents should be used only as a last resort in these patients. Methotrexate and azathioprine have been used in such situations in anecdotal reports. Although cyclophosphamide is the most effective therapy for the systemic vasculitides, it should almost never be used for idiopathic cutaneous vasculitis because of the potential toxicity. Other agents with which there have been anecdotal reports of success include dapsone, colchicine, and nonsteroidal anti-inflammatory agents.

ESSENTIAL MIXED CRYOGLOBULINEMIA

Definition

Cryoglobulins are cold-precipitable monoclonal or polyclonal immunoglobulins. Cryoglobulinemia may be associated with a systemic vasculitis characterized by palpable purpura, arthralgias, weakness, neuropathy, and glomerulonephritis. Although this can be observed in association with a variety of underlying disorders including multiple myeloma, lymphoproliferative disorders, connective tissue diseases, infection, and liver disease, in many instances it appears to be idiopathic. Because of the apparent absence of an underlying disease and the presence of cryoprecipitate containing oligoclonal/polyclonal immunoglobulins, this entity was referred to as *essential mixed cryoglobulinemia*. Since the discovery of hepatitis C, it has been established that in the vast majority of patients, essential mixed cryoglobulinemia is related to an aberrant immune response to chronic hepatitis C infection.

Incidence and Prevalence

The incidence of essential mixed cryoglobulinemia has not been established. It has been estimated, however, that 5% of patients with chronic hepatitis C will develop the syndrome of essential mixed cryoglobulinemia.

Pathology and Pathogenesis

Skin biopsies in essential mixed cryoglobulinemia reveal an inflammatory infiltrate surrounding and involving blood vessel walls, with fibrinoid necrosis, endothelial cell hyperplasia, and hemorrhage. Deposition of immunoglobulin and complement is common. Abnormalities of uninvolved skin including basement membrane alterations and deposits in vessel walls may be found. Membranoproliferative glomerulonephritis is responsible for 80% of all renal lesions in essential mixed cryoglobulinemia.

The association between hepatitis C and essential mixed cryoglobulinemia has been supported by the high frequency of documented hepatitis C infection, the presence of hepatitis C RNA and anti–hepatitis C antibodies in serum cryoprecipitates, evidence of hepatitis C antigens in vasculitic skin lesions, and the effectiveness of antiviral therapy (see below). Current evidence suggests that in the majority of cases, essential mixed cryoglobulinemia occurs when an aberrant immune response to hepatitis C infection leads to the formation of immune complexes consisting of hepatitis C antigens, polyclonal hepatitis C–specific IgG, and monoclonal IgM rheumatoid factor. The deposition of these immune complexes in blood vessel walls triggers an inflammatory cascade that results in the clinical syndrome of essential mixed cryoglobulinemia.

Clinical and Laboratory Manifestations

The most common clinical manifestations of essential mixed cryoglobulinemia are cutaneous vasculitis, arthritis, peripheral neuropathy, and glomerulonephritis. Renal disease develops in 10–30% of patients. Life-threatening rapidly progressive glomerulonephritis or vasculitis of the CNS, gastrointestinal tract, or heart occurs infrequently.

The presence of circulating cryoprecipitates is the fundamental finding in essential mixed cryoglobulinemia. Rheumatoid factor is almost always found and may be a useful clue to the disease when cryoglobulins are not detected. Hypocomplementemia occurs in 90% of patients. An elevated ESR and anemia occur frequently. Evidence for hepatitis C infection must be sought in all patients by testing for hepatitis C antibodies and hepatitis C RNA.

℞ **Treatment:**
ESSENTIAL MIXED CRYOGLOBULINEMIA

Acute mortality from essential mixed cryoglobulinemia is uncommon, but the presence of glomerulonephritis is a poor prognostic sign for overall outcome. In such patients, 15% progress to end-stage renal disease, with 40% later experiencing fatal cardiovascular disease, infection, or liver failure. As indicated above, the majority of cases are associated with hepatitis C infection. In such patients, treatment with IFN-α and ribavirin can prove beneficial. Clinical improvement with antiviral therapy is dependent on the virologic response. Patients who clear hepatitis C from the blood have objective improvement

in their vasculitis along with significant reductions in levels of circulating cryoglobulins, IgM, and rheumatoid factor. However, substantial portions of patients with hepatitis C do not have a sustained virologic response to such therapy, and the vasculitis typically relapses with the return of viremia. While transient improvement can be observed with glucocorticoids, a complete response is seen in only 7% of patients. Plasmapheresis and cytotoxic agents have been used in anecdotal reports. These observations have not been confirmed, and such therapies carry significant risks.

BEHÇET'S SYNDROME

Behçet's syndrome is a clinicopathologic entity characterized by recurrent episodes of oral and genital ulcers, iritis, and cutaneous lesions. The underlying pathologic process is a leukocytoclastic venulitis, although vessels of any size and in any organ can be involved. This disorder is described in detail in Chap. 11.

ISOLATED VASCULITIS OF THE CENTRAL NERVOUS SYSTEM

Isolated vasculitis of the CNS, which is also called *primary angiitis of the CNS* (PACNS), is an uncommon clinicopathologic entity characterized by vasculitis restricted to the vessels of the CNS without other apparent systemic vasculitis. Although the arteriole is most commonly affected, vessels of any size can be involved. The inflammatory process is usually composed of mononuclear cell infiltrates with or without granuloma formation.

Patients may present with severe headaches, altered mental function, and focal neurologic defects. Systemic symptoms are generally absent. Devastating neurologic abnormalities may occur depending on the extent of vessel involvement. The diagnosis can be suggested by abnormal MRI of the brain, an abnormal lumbar puncture, and/or demonstration of characteristic vessel abnormalities on arteriography (Fig. 10-4), but it is confirmed by biopsy of the brain parenchyma and leptomeninges. In the absence of a brain biopsy, care should be taken not to misinterpret as true primary vasculitis angiographic abnormalities that might actually be related to another cause, in particular reversible cerebral vasoconstriction syndrome. The differential diagnosis includes infection, atherosclerosis, emboli, connective tissue disease, sarcoidosis, malignancy, vasospasm, and drug-associated causes. The prognosis of this disease is poor; however, some reports indicate that glucocorticoid therapy, alone or together with cyclophosphamide administered as described above, has induced sustained clinical remissions in a small number of patients.

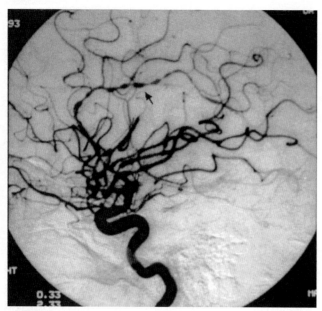

FIGURE 10-4
Cerebral angiogram from a 32-year-old male with central nervous system vasculitis. Dramatic beading (*arrow*) typical of vasculitis is seen.

COGAN'S SYNDROME

Cogan's syndrome is characterized by interstitial keratitis together with vestibuloauditory symptoms. It may be associated with a systemic vasculitis, particularly aortitis with involvement of the aortic valve. Glucocorticoids are the mainstay of treatment. Initiation of treatment as early as possible after the onset of hearing loss improves the likelihood of a favorable outcome.

KAWASAKI DISEASE

Kawasaki disease, also referred to as *mucocutaneous lymph node syndrome*, is an acute, febrile, multisystem disease of children. Some 80% of cases occur prior to the age of 5, with the peak incidence occurring at ≤2 years. It is characterized by nonsuppurative cervical adenitis and changes in the skin and mucous membranes such as edema; congested conjunctivae; erythema of the oral cavity, lips, and palms; and desquamation of the skin of the fingertips. Although the disease is generally benign and self-limited, it is associated with coronary artery aneurysms in ~25% of cases, with an overall case-fatality rate of 0.5–2.8%. These complications usually occur between the third and fourth weeks of illness during the convalescent stage. Vasculitis of the coronary arteries is seen in almost all the fatal cases that have been autopsied. There is typical intimal proliferation and infiltration of the vessel wall with mononuclear cells. Beadlike aneurysms and thromboses may be seen along the artery.

Other manifestations include pericarditis, myocarditis, myocardial ischemia and infarction, and cardiomegaly.

Apart from the up to 2.8% of patients who develop fatal complications, the prognosis of this disease for uneventful recovery is excellent. High-dose IV γ globulin (2 g/kg as a single infusion over 10 h) together with aspirin (100 mg/kg per d for 14 days followed by 3–5 mg/kg per d for several weeks) have been shown to be effective in reducing the prevalence of coronary artery abnormalities when administered early in the course of the disease.

POLYANGIITIS OVERLAP SYNDROMES

Some patients with systemic vasculitis manifest clinico-pathologic characteristics that do not fit precisely into any specific disease but have overlapping features of different vasculitides. Active systemic vasculitis in such settings has the same potential for causing irreversible organ system damage as when it occurs in one of the defined syndromes listed in Table 10-1. The diagnostic and therapeutic considerations as well as the prognosis for these patients depend on the sites and severity of active vasculitis. Patients with vasculitis that could potentially cause irreversible damage to a major organ system should be treated as described under "Wegener's granulomatosis."

SECONDARY VASCULITIS

DRUG-INDUCED VASCULITIS

Vasculitis associated with drug reactions usually presents as palpable purpura that may be generalized or limited to the lower extremities or other dependent areas; however, urticarial lesions, ulcers, and hemorrhagic blisters may also occur. Signs and symptoms may be limited to the skin, although systemic manifestations such as fever, malaise, and polyarthralgias may occur. Although the skin is the predominant organ involved, systemic vasculitis may result from drug reactions. Drugs that have been implicated in vasculitis include allopurinol, thiazides, gold, sulfonamides, phenytoin, and penicillin.

An increasing number of drugs have been reported to cause vasculitis associated with antimyeloperoxidase ANCA. Of these, the best evidence of causality exists for hydralazine and propylthiouracil. The clinical manifestations in ANCA-positive drug-induced vasculitis can range from cutaneous lesions to glomerulonephritis and pulmonary hemorrhage. Outside of drug discontinuation, treatment should be based on the severity of the vasculitis. Patients with immediately life-threatening small-vessel vasculitis should initially be treated with glucocorticoids and cyclophosphamide as described for Wegener's granulomatosis. Following clinical improvement, consideration may be given for tapering such agents along a more rapid schedule.

SERUM SICKNESS AND SERUM SICKNESS–LIKE REACTIONS

These reactions are characterized by the occurrence of fever, urticaria, polyarthralgias, and lymphadenopathy 7–10 days after primary exposure and 2–4 days after secondary exposure to a heterologous protein (classic serum sickness) or a nonprotein drug such as penicillin or sulfa (serum sickness–like reaction). Most of the manifestations are not due to a vasculitis; however, occasional patients will have typical cutaneous venulitis that may progress rarely to a systemic vasculitis.

VASCULITIS ASSOCIATED WITH OTHER UNDERLYING PRIMARY DISEASES

Certain *infections* may directly trigger an inflammatory vasculitic process. For example, rickettsias can invade and proliferate in the endothelial cells of small blood vessels causing a vasculitis. In addition, the inflammatory response around blood vessels associated with certain systemic fungal diseases such as histoplasmosis may mimic a primary vasculitic process. A leukocytoclastic vasculitis predominantly involving the skin with occasional involvement of other organ systems may be a minor component of many other infections. These include *subacute bacterial endocarditis, Epstein-Barr virus infection, HIV infection,* as well as a number of other infections.

Vasculitis can be associated with certain *malignancies,* particularly lymphoid or reticuloendothelial neoplasms. Leukocytoclastic venulitis confined to the skin is the most common finding; however, widespread systemic vasculitis may occur. Of particular note is the association of *hairy cell leukemia* with PAN.

A number of *connective tissue diseases* have vasculitis as a secondary manifestation of the underlying primary process. Foremost among these are *systemic lupus erythematosus* (Chap. 4), *rheumatoid arthritis* (Chap. 5), *inflammatory myositis* (Chap. 16), *relapsing polychondritis* (Chap. 12), and *Sjögren's syndrome* (Chap. 8). The most common form of vasculitis in these conditions is the small-vessel venulitis isolated to the skin. However, certain patients may develop a fulminant systemic necrotizing vasculitis.

Secondary vasculitis has also been observed in association with *ulcerative colitis, congenital deficiencies of various complement components, retroperitoneal fibrosis, primary biliary cirrhosis, α_1-antitrypsin deficiency,* and *intestinal bypass surgery.*

PRINCIPLES OF TREATMENT

Once a diagnosis of vasculitis has been established, a decision regarding therapeutic strategy must be made (Fig. 10-1). The vasculitis syndromes represent a wide spectrum of diseases with varying degrees of severity. Since the potential toxic side effects of certain therapeutic regimens may be substantial, the risk-versus-benefit ratio of any therapeutic approach should be weighed carefully. Specific therapeutic regimens are discussed above for the individual vasculitis syndromes; however, certain general principles regarding therapy should be considered. On the one hand, glucocorticoids and/or cytotoxic therapy should be instituted immediately in diseases where irreversible organ system dysfunction and high morbidity and mortality have been clearly established. Wegener's granulomatosis is the prototype of a severe systemic vasculitis requiring such a therapeutic approach (see above). On the other hand, when feasible, aggressive therapy should be avoided for vasculitic manifestations that rarely result in irreversible organ system dysfunction and that usually do not respond to such therapy. For example, idiopathic cutaneous vasculitis usually resolves with symptomatic treatment, and prolonged courses of glucocorticoids uncommonly result in clinical benefit. Cytotoxic agents have not proved to be beneficial in idiopathic cutaneous vasculitis, and their toxic side effects generally outweigh any potential beneficial effects. Glucocorticoids should be initiated in those systemic vasculitides that cannot be specifically categorized or for which there is no established standard therapy; cytotoxic therapy should be added in these diseases only if an adequate response does not result or if remission can only be achieved and maintained with an unacceptably toxic regimen of glucocorticoids. When remission is achieved, one should continually attempt to taper glucocorticoids and discontinue when possible. When using cytotoxic regimens, one should base the choice of agent upon the available therapeutic data supporting efficacy in that disease, the site and severity of organ involvement, and the toxicity profile of the drug.

Physicians should be thoroughly aware of the toxic side effects of therapeutic agents employed (**Table 10-7**). Many of the side effects of glucocorticoid therapy are markedly decreased in frequency and duration in patients on alternate-day regimens compared to daily regimens. When cyclophosphamide is administered chronically in doses of 2 mg/kg per d for substantial periods of time (one to several years), the incidence of cystitis is at least 30% and the incidence of bladder cancer is at least 6%. Bladder cancer can occur several years after discontinuation of cyclophosphamide therapy; therefore, monitoring for bladder cancer should continue indefinitely in patients who have received prolonged courses of daily cyclophosphamide. Instructing the patient to take cyclophosphamide all at once in the morning with a large amount of fluid throughout the day in order to maintain a dilute urine can reduce the risk of bladder injury. Significant alopecia is unusual in the chronically administered, low-dose regimen. Permanent infertility can occur in both men and women. Bone marrow suppression is an important toxicity of cyclophosphamide and can be observed during glucocorticoid tapering or over time, even after periods of stable measurements.

TABLE 10-7

MAJOR TOXIC SIDE EFFECTS OF DRUGS COMMONLY USED IN THE TREATMENT OF SYSTEMIC VASCULITIS

Glucocorticoids

Osteoporosis	Growth suppression in children
Cataracts	Hypertension
Glaucoma	Avascular necrosis of bone
Diabetes mellitus	Myopathy
Electrolyte abnormalities	Alterations in mood
Metabolic abnormalities	Psychosis
Suppression of inflammatory and immune responses leading to opportunistic infections	Pseudotumor cerebri
	Peptic ulcer diathesis
Cushingoid features	Pancreatitis

Cyclophosphamide

Bone marrow suppression	Hypogammaglobulinemia
Cystitis	Pulmonary fibrosis
Bladder carcinoma	Myelodysplasia
Gonadal suppression	Oncogenesis
Gastrointestinal intolerance	Teratogenicity
	Opportunistic infections

Methotrexate

Gastrointestinal intolerance	Pneumonitis
Stomatitis	Teratogenicity
Bone marrow suppression	Opportunistic infections
Hepatotoxicity (may lead to fibrosis or cirrhosis)	

Monitoring of the complete blood count every 1–2 weeks for as long as the patient receives cyclophosphamide can effectively prevent cytopenias. When the absolute neutrophil count is maintained at >1500/μL, and the patient is not receiving daily glucocorticoids, the incidence of life-threatening opportunistic infections is low. However, the WBC is not an accurate predictor of risk of all opportunistic infections, and infections with *Pneumocystis jiroveci* and certain fungi can be seen in the face of WBCs that are within normal limits, particularly in patients receiving glucocorticoids. All vasculitis patients who are not allergic to sulfa and who are receiving daily glucocorticoids in combination with a cytotoxic drug should receive TMP-SMX as prophylaxis against *P. jiroveci* infection.

Finally, it should be emphasized that each patient is unique and requires individual decision making. The above outline should serve as a framework to guide therapeutic approaches; however, flexibility should be practiced in order to provide maximal therapeutic efficacy with minimal toxic side effects in each patient.

FURTHER READINGS

ACHKAR AA et al: How does previous corticosteroid treatment affect the biopsy findings in giant cell (temporal) arteritis? Ann Intern Med 120:987, 1994

CALABRESE LH et al: Narrative review: Reversible cerebral vasoconstriction syndromes. Ann Intern Med 146:34, 2007

DEGROOT K et al: Randomized trial of cyclophosphamide versus methotrexate for induction of remission in early systemic antineutrophil cytoplasmic antibody-associated vasculitis. Arthritis Rheum 52:2461, 2005

——— et al: Pulse versus daily oral cyclophosphamide for induction of remission in antineutrophil cytoplasmic antibody-associated vasculitis: A randomized trial. Ann Intern Med 150(10):670, 2009

EVANS JM et al: Increased incidence of aortic aneurysm and dissection in giant cell (temporal) arteritis. A population-based study. Ann Intern Med 122:502, 1995

FAUCI A, WOLFF S: Wegener's granulomatosis: Studies in eighteen patients and a review of the literature. Medicine 52:535, 1973

FINKIELMAN JD et al: Antiproteinase 3 antineutrophil cytoplasmic antibodies and disease activity in Wegener granulomatosis. Ann Intern Med 147:611, 2007

GOLBIN JM, Specks U: Targeting B lymphocytes as therapy for ANCA-associated vasculitis. Rheum Dis Clin North Am 33:741, 2007

GUILLEVIN L et al: Treatment of polyarteritis nodosa related to hepatitis B virus with interferon-alpha and plasma exchanges. Ann Rheum Dis 53:334, 1994

——— et al: Churg-Strauss syndrome. Clinical study and long-term follow-up of 96 patients. Medicine (Baltimore) 78:26, 1999

——— et al: Microscopic polyangiitis. Clinical and laboratory findings in eighty-five patients. Arthritis Rheum 42:421, 1999

HOFFMAN GS, Specks U: Antineutrophil cytoplasmic antibodies. Arthritis Rheum 41:1521, 1998

——— et al: Wegener's granulomatosis: An analysis of 158 patients. Ann Intern Med 116:488, 1992

——— et al: Treatment of glucocorticoid-resistant or relapsing Takayasu arteritis with methotrexate. Arthritis Rheum 37:578, 1994

TABLE 12-1

DISORDERS ASSOCIATED WITH RELAPSING POLYCHONDRITIS[a]

Systemic vasculitis
Rheumatoid arthritis
Systemic lupus erythematosus
Sjögren's syndrome
Spondyloarthritides
Behçet's syndrome
Inflammatory bowel disease
Primary biliary cirrhosis
Myelodysplastic syndrome

[a]Systemic vasculitis is the most common association followed by rheumatoid arthritis, systemic lupus erythematosus, and Sjögren's syndrome.
Source: Modified from Michet.

Immunofluorescence studies have shown immunoglobulins and complement at sites of involvement. Extracellular granular material observed in the degenerating cartilage matrix by electron microscopy has been interpreted to be enzymes, immunoglobulins, or proteoglycans.

Immunologic mechanisms play a role in the pathogenesis of relapsing polychondritis. Immunoglobulin and complement deposits are found at sites of inflammation. In addition, antibodies to type II collagen and to matrilin-1 and immune complexes are detected in the sera of some patients. The possibility that an immune response to type II collagen may be important in the pathogenesis is supported experimentally by the occurrence of auricular chondritis in rats immunized with type II collagen. Antibodies to type II collagen are found in the sera of these animals, and immune deposits are detected at sites of ear inflammation. Humoral immune responses to type IX and type XI collagen, matrilin-1, and cartilage oligomeric matrix protein have been demonstrated in some patients. In a study, rats immunized with matrilin-1 were found to develop severe inspiratory stridor and swelling of the nasal septum. The rats had severe inflammation with erosions of the involved cartilage, which was characterized by increased numbers of CD4+ and CD8+ T cells in the lesions. The cartilage of the joints and ear pinna was not involved. All had IgG antibodies to matrilin-1. Matrilin-1 is a noncollagenous protein present in the extracellular matrix in cartilage. It is present in high concentrations in the trachea and is also present in the nasal septum but not in articular cartilage. A subsequent study demonstrated serum anti-matrilin-1 antibodies in approximately 13% of patients with relapsing polychondritis; approximately 70% of these patients had respiratory symptoms. Cell-mediated immunity may also be operative in causing tissue injury, since lymphocyte transformation can be demonstrated when lymphocytes of patients are exposed to cartilage extracts. T cells specific for type II collagen have been found in some patients, and CD4+ T cells have been observed at sites of cartilage inflammation. The accumulating data strongly suggest that both humoral and cell-mediated immunity play an important role in the pathogenesis of relapsing polychondritis.

Dissolution of cartilage matrix can be induced by the intravenous injection of crude papain, a proteolytic enzyme, into young rabbits, which results in collapse of their normally rigid ears within 4 h. Reconstitution of the matrix occurs in about 7 days. In relapsing polychondritis, loss of cartilage matrix also most likely results from action of proteolytic enzymes released from chondrocytes, polymorphonuclear white cells, and monocytes that have been activated by inflammatory mediators.

CLINICAL MANIFESTATIONS

The onset of relapsing polychondritis is frequently abrupt with the appearance of one or two sites of cartilaginous inflammation. Fever, fatigue, and weight loss occur and may precede the clinical signs of relapsing polychondritis by several weeks. Relapsing polychondritis may go unrecognized for several months or even years in patients who only initially manifest intermittent joint pain and/or swelling, or who have unexplained eye inflammation, hearing loss, valvular heart disease, or pulmonary symptoms. The pattern of cartilaginous involvement and the frequency of episodes vary widely among patients.

Auricular chondritis is the most frequent presenting manifestation of relapsing polychondritis in 40% of patients and eventually affects about 85% of patients (Table 12-2). One or both ears are involved, either sequentially or simultaneously. Patients experience the sudden onset of pain, tenderness, and swelling of the

TABLE 12-2

CLINICAL MANIFESTATIONS OF RELAPSING POLYCHONDRITIS

CLINICAL FEATURE	FREQUENCY, %	
	PRESENTING	CUMULATIVE
Auricular chondritis	43	89
Arthritis	32	72
Nasal chondritis	21	61
Ocular inflammation	18	59
Laryngotracheal symptoms	23	55
Reduced hearing	7	40
Saddle nose deformity	11	25
Cutaneous	4	25
Laryngotracheal stricture	15	23
Vasculitis	2	14
Elevated creatinine	7	13
Aortic or mitral regurgitation	0	12

Source: Modified from Kent et al.

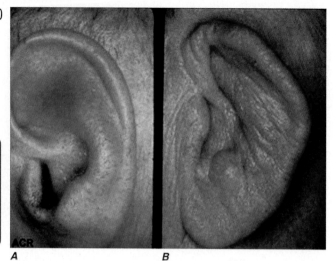

FIGURE 12-1

A. The pinna is erythematous, swollen, and tender. Not shown is the ear lobule that is spared as there is no underlying cartilage. **B.** The pinna is thickened and deformed. The destruction of the underlying cartilage results in a floppy ear. *(Reprinted from the Clinical Slide Collection on the Rheumatic Diseases, © 1991, 1995, 1997, 1998, 1999. Used by permission of the American College of Rheumatology.)*

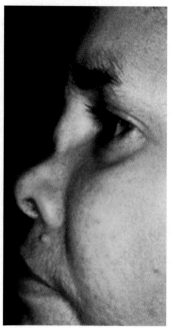

FIGURE 12-2

Saddle nose results from destruction and collapse of the nasal cartilage. *(Reprinted from the Clinical Slide Collection on the Rheumatic Diseases, © 1991, 1995, 1997, 1998, 1999. Used by permission of the American College of Rheumatology.)*

cartilaginous portion of the ear (**Fig. 12–1**). Earlobes are spared because they do not contain cartilage. The overlying skin has a beefy red or violaceous color. Prolonged or recurrent episodes result in a flabby or droopy ear as a sequela of cartilage destruction. Swelling may close off the eustachian tube (causing otitis media) or the external auditory meatus, either of which can impair hearing. Inflammation of the internal auditory artery or its cochlear branch produces hearing loss, vertigo, ataxia, nausea, and vomiting. Vertigo is almost always accompanied by hearing loss. The cartilage of the nose becomes inflamed during the first or subsequent attacks. Approximately 50% of patients will eventually have nose involvement. Patients may experience nasal stuffiness, rhinorrhea, and epistaxis. The bridge of the nose becomes red, swollen, and tender and may collapse, producing a saddle deformity (**Fig. 12–2**). In some patients, the saddle deformity develops insidiously without overt inflammation. Saddle nose is observed more frequently in younger patients, especially in women.

Arthritis is the presenting manifestation in relapsing polychondritis in approximately one-third of patients and may be present for several months before other features appear. Eventually, more than half the patients will have arthritis. The arthritis is usually asymmetric and oligo- or polyarticular, and it involves both large and small peripheral joints. An episode of arthritis lasts from a few days to several weeks and resolves spontaneously without residual joint deformity. Attacks of arthritis may not be temporally related to other manifestations of relapsing polychondritis. The joints are warm, tender, and swollen. Joint fluid has been reported to be noninflammatory. In addition to

peripheral joints, inflammation may involve the costochondral, sternomanubrial, and sternoclavicular cartilages. Destruction of these cartilages may result in a pectus excavatum deformity or even a flail anterior chest wall. Relapsing polychondritis may occur in patients with preexisting rheumatoid arthritis, Reiter's syndrome, psoriatic arthritis, or ankylosing spondylitis.

Eye manifestations occur in more than half of patients and include conjunctivitis, episcleritis, scleritis, iritis, and keratitis. Eye involvement is seldom the presenting feature. Ulceration and perforation of the cornea may occur and cause blindness. Other manifestations include eyelid and periorbital edema, proptosis, cataracts, optic neuritis, extraocular muscle palsies, retinal vasculitis, and renal vein occlusion.

Laryngotracheobronchial involvement occurs in ~50% of patients. Symptoms include hoarseness, a nonproductive cough, and tenderness over the larynx and proximal trachea. Mucosal edema, strictures, and/or collapse of laryngeal or tracheal cartilage may cause stridor and life-threatening airway obstruction necessitating tracheostomy. Collapse of cartilage in bronchi leads to pneumonia and, when extensive, to respiratory insufficiency.

Aortic regurgitation occurs in about 5% of patients and is due to progressive dilation of the aortic ring or to destruction of the valve cusps. Mitral and other heart valves are affected less often. Other cardiac manifestations include pericarditis, myocarditis, and conduction abnormalities. Aneurysms of the proximal, thoracic, or abdominal aorta may occur even in the absence of active chondritis and occasionally rupture.

Systemic vasculitis may occur in association with relapsing polychondritis. Vasculitides include isolated cutaneous vasculitis, polyarteritis nodosa, giant cell arteritis, and Takayasu's arteritis (Chap. 10). Neurologic abnormalities usually occur as a result of underlying vasculitis, manifesting as seizures, strokes, ataxia, and peripheral and cranial nerve neuropathies. Cranial nerves II, III, VI, and VII are most often involved. Approximately 25% of patients have skin lesions, none of which is characteristic for relapsing polychondritis but can reflect an associated vasculitis. These include purpura, erythema nodosum, erythema multiforme, angioedema/urticaria, livedo reticularis, and panniculitis. Segmental necrotizing glomerulonephritis with crescent formation has been noted in some patients, usually in association with microscopic polyangiitis, but may occur in the absence of systemic vasculitis.

The course of disease is highly variable, with episodes lasting from a few days to several weeks and then subsiding spontaneously. Attacks may recur at intervals varying from weeks to months. In other patients, the disease has a chronic, smoldering course. In a few patients, the disease may be limited to one or two episodes of cartilage inflammation. In one study, the 5-year estimated survival rate was 74% and the 10-year survival rate 55%. In contrast to earlier series, only about half the deaths could be attributed to relapsing polychondritis or complications of treatment. Pulmonary complications accounted for only 10% of all fatalities. In general, patients with more widespread disease have a worse prognosis.

LABORATORY FINDINGS

Mild leukocytosis and normocytic, normochromic anemia are often present. Eosinophilia is observed in 10% of patients. The erythrocyte sedimentation rate and C-reactive protein are usually elevated. Rheumatoid factor and antinuclear antibody tests are occasionally positive in low titers. Antibodies to type II collagen are present in fewer than half the patients and are not specific. Circulating immune complexes may be detected, especially in patients with early active disease. Elevated levels of γ globulin may be present. Antineutrophil cytoplasmic antibodies (ANCA), either cytoplasmic (cANCA) or perinuclear (pANCA), are found in some patients with active disease. The upper and lower airways can be evaluated by imaging techniques such as linear tomography, laryngotracheography, and CT, and by bronchoscopy. MRI is helpful in evaluation of the larynx and trachea. Bronchography is performed to demonstrate bronchial narrowing. Intrathoracic airway obstruction can also be evaluated by inspiratory-expiratory flow studies. The chest film may show narrowing of the trachea and/or the main bronchi, widening of the ascending or

descending aorta due to an aneurysm, and cardiomegaly when aortic insufficiency is present. MRI can be used in assessing aortic aneurysmal dilatation. Radiographs may show calcification at previous sites of cartilage damage involving ear, nose, larynx, or trachea.

DIAGNOSIS

Diagnosis is based on recognition of the typical clinical features. Biopsies of the involved cartilage from the ear, nose, or respiratory tract will confirm the diagnosis but are only necessary when clinical features are not typical. Patients with Wegener's granulomatosis may have a saddle nose and pulmonary involvement but can be distinguished by the absence of auricular involvement and the presence of granulomatous lesions in the tracheobronchial tree. Patients with Cogan's syndrome have interstitial keratitis and vestibular and auditory abnormalities, but this syndrome does not involve the respiratory tract or ears. Reiter's syndrome may initially resemble relapsing polychondritis because of oligoarticular arthritis and eye involvement, but it is distinguished in time by the appearance of urethritis and typical mucocutaneous lesions and the absence of nose or ear cartilage involvement. Rheumatoid arthritis may initially suggest relapsing polychondritis because of arthritis and eye inflammation. The arthritis in rheumatoid arthritis, however, is erosive and symmetric. In addition, rheumatoid factor titers are usually high compared with those in relapsing polychondritis. Bacterial infection of the pinna may be mistaken for relapsing polychondritis but differs by usually involving only one ear, including the earlobe. Auricular cartilage may also be damaged by trauma or frostbite.

Relapsing polychondritis may develop in patients with a variety of autoimmune disorders, including SLE, rheumatoid arthritis, Sjögren's syndrome, and vasculitis. In most cases, these disorders antedate the appearance of polychondritis, usually by months or years. It is likely that these patients have an immunologic abnormality that predisposes them to development of this group of autoimmune disorders.

℞ **Treatment:**
RELAPSING POLYCHONDRITIS

In patients with active chondritis, prednisone, 40–60 mg/d, is often effective in suppressing disease activity; it is tapered gradually once disease is controlled. In some patients, prednisone can be stopped, while in others low doses in the range of 10–15 mg/d are required for continued suppression of disease. Dapsone instead of prednisone has been effective in suppressing inflammation in some patients. Immunosuppressive drugs such as methotrexate, cyclophosphamide, azathioprine, or cyclosporine should be reserved for patients who fail to respond to prednisone or who require high doses for control of disease activity. Patients with significant ocular inflammation often require intraocular steroids as well as high doses of prednisone. A small retrospective series of nine patients did not find anti-CD20 (rituximab) to provide benefit, although this experience remains too small to draw firm conclusions. Heart valve replacement or repair of an aortic aneurysm may be necessary. When obstruction is severe, tracheostomy is required. Stents may be necessary in patients with tracheobronchial collapse.

FURTHER READINGS

BUCKNER JH et al: Identification of type II collagen peptide 261-273–specific T cell clones in a patient with relapsing polychondritis. Arthritis Rheum 46:238, 2002

DAMIANI JM, LEVINE HL: Relapsing polychondritis—Report of ten cases. Laryngoscope 89:929, 1979

ERNST A et al: Relapsing polychondritis and airway involvement. Chest 135:1024, 2009

FRANCES C et al: Dermatologic manifestations of relapsing polychondritis. A study of 200 cases at a single center. Medicine (Baltimore) 80:173, 2001

HANSSON AS et al: A new animal model for relapsing polychondritis, induced by cartilage matrix protein (matrilin-1). J Clin Invest 104:589, 1999

——— et al: The occurrence of autoantibodies to matrilin 1 reflects a tissue-specific response to cartilage of the respiratory tract in patients with relapsing polychondritis. Arthritis Rheum 44:2402, 2001

ISAAK BL et al: Ocular and systemic findings in relapsing polychondritis. Ophthalmology 93:681, 1986

KENT PD et al: Relapsing polychondritis. Curr Opin Rheumatol 16:56, 2004

LANG B et al: Susceptibility to relapsing polychondritis is associated with HLA-DR4. Arthritis Rheum 36:660, 1993

LEROUX G et al: Treatment of relapsing polychondritis with rituximab: A retrospective study of nine patients. Arthritis Rheum 61:577, 2009

LETKO E et al: Relapsing polychondritis: A clinical review. Semin Arthritis Rheum 31:384, 2002

MCADAM LP et al: Relapsing polychondritis. Medicine (Baltimore) 55:193, 1976

MICHET CJ et al: Relapsing polychondritis. Survival and predictive role of early disease manifestations. Ann Intern Med 104:74, 1986

STAATS BA et al: Relapsing polychondritis. Semin Respir Crit Care Med 23:145, 2002

TILLIE-LEBLOND I et al: Respiratory involvement in relapsing polychondritis: Clinical, functional, endoscopic, and radiographic evaluations. Medicine (Baltimore) 77:168, 1998

TRENTHAM DE, LE CH: Relapsing polychondritis. Ann Intern Med 129:114, 1998

ZEUNER M et al: Relapsing polychondritis: Clinical and immunogenic analysis of 62 patients. J Rheumatol 24:96, 1997

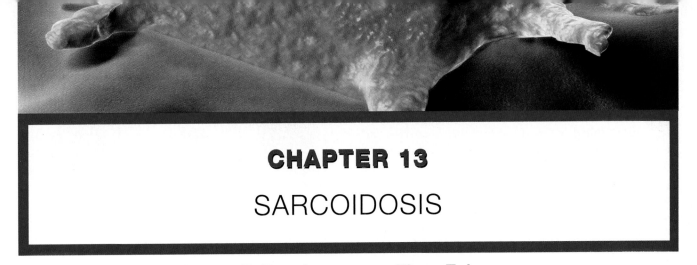

CHAPTER 13

SARCOIDOSIS

Robert P. Baughman ■ Elyse E. Lower

DEFINITION

Sarcoidosis is an inflammatory disease characterized by the presence of noncaseating granulomas. The disease is often multisystem and requires the presence of involvement in two or more organs for a specific diagnosis. The finding of granulomas is not specific for sarcoidosis, and other conditions known to cause granulomas must be ruled out. These conditions include mycobacterial and fungal infections, malignancy, and environmental agents such as beryllium. While sarcoidosis can affect virtually every organ of the body, the lung is most commonly affected. Other organs commonly affected are the liver, skin, and eye. The clinical outcome of sarcoidosis varies, with remission occurring in over half the patients within a few years of diagnosis; however, the remaining patients develop a chronic disease that lasts for decades.

ETIOLOGY

Despite multiple investigations, the cause of sarcoidosis remains unknown. Currently, the most likely etiology is an infectious or noninfectious environmental agent that triggers an inflammatory response in a genetically susceptible host. Among the possible infectious agents, careful studies have shown a much higher incidence of *Propionibacter acnes* in the lymph nodes of sarcoidosis patients compared to controls. An animal model has shown that *P. acnes* can induce a granulomatous response in mice similar to sarcoidosis. Other studies support the possibility of an atypical mycobacterium, although these have yet to be confirmed by blinded studies with adequate controls. Recent studies have demonstrated the presence of a mycobacterial protein [*Mycobacterium tuberculosis* catalase-peroxidase (mKatG)] in the granulomas of some sarcoidosis patients. This protein is very resistant to degradation and may represent the persistent antigen in sarcoidosis. Environmental exposures to insecticides and mold have been associated with an increased risk for disease. In addition, health care workers appear to have an increased risk. Some authors have suggested that sarcoidosis is not due to a single agent but represents a particular host response to multiple agents. An interesting approach to finding the etiology of sarcoidosis is to correlate the environmental exposures to genetic markers. These studies have supported the hypothesis that a genetically susceptible host is a key factor in the disease.

INCIDENCE AND PREVALENCE

Sarcoidosis is seen worldwide, with the highest prevalence reported in the Nordic population. In the United States, the disease has been reported more commonly in blacks than whites, with the ratio of blacks to whites ranging from 3:1 to 17:0. Women appear to be slightly more susceptible than men. The lower estimate is the result of a recent study from a large health maintenance organization in Detroit. The earlier American studies finding the higher incidence in blacks may have been influenced by the fact that blacks seem to develop more extensive and chronic pulmonary disease. Since most sarcoidosis clinics are run by pulmonologists, a selection bias may have occurred. Worldwide, the prevalence of the disease varies from 20–60 per 100,000 for many groups such as Japanese, Italians, and American whites. Higher rate occurs in Ireland and Nordic countries. In one closely observed community in Sweden, the lifetime risk for developing sarcoidosis was 3%.

Sarcoidosis often occurs in young, otherwise healthy adults. It is uncommon to diagnose the disease in someone under age 18. However, it has become clear that a second peak in incidence develops around age 60. In a study of >700 newly diagnosed sarcoidosis patients in the United States, half the patients were ≥40 years at the time of diagnosis.

Although most cases of sarcoidosis are sporadic, a familial form of the disease exists. At least 5% of patients with sarcoidosis will have a family member with sarcoidosis. Sarcoidosis patients who are Irish or American blacks seem to have a two to three times higher rate of familial disease.

PATHOPHYSIOLOGY AND IMMUNOPATHOGENESIS

The granuloma is the pathologic hallmark of sarcoidosis. A distinct feature of sarcoidosis is the local accumulation of inflammatory cells. Extensive studies in the lung using bronchoalveolar lavage (BAL) have demonstrated that the initial inflammatory response is an influx of T helper cells. In addition, there is an accumulation of activated monocytes. **Figure 13-1** is a proposed model for sarcoidosis. Using the HLA-CD4 complex, antigen-presenting cells present an unknown antigen to the helper T cell. Studies have clarified that specific HLA haplotypes such as HLA-DRB1*1101 are associated with an increased risk for developing sarcoidosis. In addition, different HLA haplotypes are associated with different clinical outcomes.

The macrophage/helper T cell cluster leads to activation with the increased release of several cytokines. These include interleukin (IL) 2 released from the T cell and interferon γ and tumor necrosis factor (TNF) released by the macrophage. The T cell is a necessary part of the initial inflammatory response. In advanced,

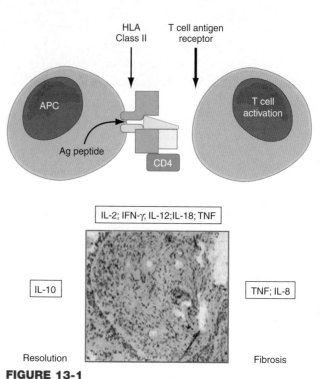

FIGURE 13-1

Schematic representation of initial events of sarcoidosis. The antigen-presenting cell and helper T cell complex leads to the release of multiple cytokines. This forms a granuloma. Over time, the granuloma may resolve or lead to chronic disease, including fibrosis.

untreated HIV infection, patients who lack helper T cells rarely develop sarcoidosis. In contrast, several reports confirm that sarcoidosis becomes unmasked as HIV-infected individuals receive antiretroviral therapy, with subsequent restoration of their immune system. In contrast, treatment of established pulmonary sarcoidosis with cyclosporine, a drug that downregulates helper T cell responses, seems to have little impact on sarcoidosis.

The granulomatous response of sarcoidosis can resolve with or without therapy. However, in at least 20% of patients with sarcoidosis, a chronic form of the disease develops. This persistent form of the disease is associated with the secretion of high levels of IL-8. Also, studies have reported that in patients with this chronic form of disease, excessive amounts of TNF are released in the areas of inflammation.

It is sometimes difficult to determine early on the ultimate clinical outcome of sarcoidosis. One form of the disease, *Löfgren's syndrome*, consists of erythema nodosum, hilar adenopathy on chest roentgenogram, and uveitis. Löfgren's syndrome is associated with a good prognosis, with >90% of patients experiencing disease resolution within 2 years. Recent studies have demonstrated that the HLA-DQB1*0201 is highly associated with Löfgren's syndrome. In contrast, patients with the disfiguring skin condition lupus pernio or cardiac or neurologic involvement rarely experience disease remission.

CLINICAL MANIFESTATIONS

The presentation of sarcoidosis ranges from patients who are asymptomatic to those with organ failure. It is unclear how often sarcoidosis is asymptomatic. In countries where routine chest roentgenogram screening is performed, 20–30% of pulmonary cases are detected in asymptomatic individuals. The inability to screen for other asymptomatic forms of the disease would suggest that as many as a third of sarcoidosis patients are asymptomatic.

Respiratory complaints including cough and dyspnea are the most common presenting symptoms. In many cases, the patient presents with a 2–4 week history of these symptoms. Unfortunately, due to the nonspecific nature of pulmonary symptoms, the patient may see physicians for up to a year before a diagnosis is confirmed. The diagnosis of sarcoidosis is usually only suggested when a chest roentgenogram is performed.

Symptoms related to cutaneous and ocular disease are the next two most common complaints. Skin lesions are often nonspecific. However, since these lesions are readily observed, the patient and treating physician are often led to a diagnosis. In contrast to patients with pulmonary disease, patients with cutaneous lesions are more likely to be diagnosed within 6 months of symptoms.

Nonspecific constitutional symptoms include fatigue, fever, night sweats, and weight loss. Fatigue is perhaps the most common constitutional symptom that affects these patients. Given its insidious nature, patients are usually not aware of the association with their sarcoidosis until their disease resolves.

The overall incidence of sarcoidosis at the time of diagnosis and eventual common organ involvement are summarized in Table 13-1. Over time, skin, eye, and neurologic involvement seem more apparent. In the United States, the frequency of specific organ involvement appears to be affected by age, race, and gender. For example, eye disease is more common among blacks. Under the age of 40, it occurs more frequently in women. However, in those diagnosed over the age of 40, eye disease is more common in men.

LUNG

Lung involvement occurs in >90% of sarcoidosis patients. The most commonly used method for detecting lung disease is still the chest roentgenogram. **Figure 13-2** illustrates the chest roentgenogram from a sarcoidosis patient with bilateral hilar adenopathy. Although the CT scan has changed the diagnostic approach to interstitial lung disease, the CT scan is not usually considered a monitoring tool for patients with sarcoidosis. **Figure 13-3** demonstrates some of the characteristic CT features, including peribronchial thickening and reticular nodular changes, which are predominantly subpleural. The peribronchial thickening seen on CT scan seems to explain the high yield of granulomas from bronchial biopsies performed for diagnosis.

While the CT scan is more sensitive, the standard scoring system described by Scadding in 1961 for chest roentgenograms remains the preferred method of characterizing the chest involvement. Stage 1 is hilar adenopathy alone (Fig. 13-2), often with right paratracheal involvement. Stage 2 is a combination of adenopathy plus infiltrates, whereas stage 3 reveals infiltrates alone. Stage 4 consists of fibrosis. Usually the infiltrates in sarcoidosis are predominantly an upper lobe process. Only in a few noninfectious diseases is an upper lobe predominance noted. In addition to sarcoidosis, the differential diagnosis of upper lobe disease includes hypersensitivity pneumonitis, silicosis, and Langerhans cell histiocytosis. For infectious

TABLE 13-1

FREQUENCY OF COMMON ORGAN INVOLVEMENT AND LIFETIME RISK[a]

	PRESENTATION, %[b]	FOLLOW-UP, %[c]
Lung	95	94
Skin	24	43
Eye	12	29
Extrathoracic lymph node	15	16
Liver	12	14
Spleen	7	8
Neurologic	5	16
Cardiac	2	3

[a]Patients could have more than one organ involved.
[b]From ACCESS study of 736 patients evaluated within 6 months of diagnosis.
[c]From follow-up of 1024 sarcoidosis patients seen at the University of Cincinnati Interstitial Lung Disease and Sarcoidosis Clinic from 2002–2006.

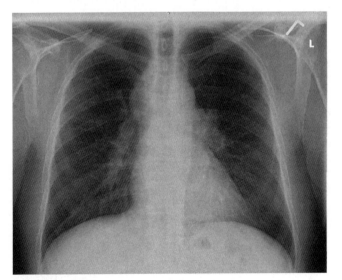

FIGURE 13-2
Posterior-anterior chest roentgenogram demonstrating bilateral hilar adenopathy, stage 1 disease.

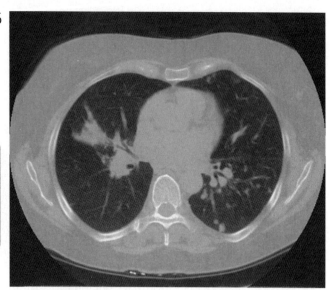

FIGURE 13-3

High-resolution CT scan of chest demonstrating patchy reticular nodularity, including areas of confluence.

diseases, tuberculosis and *Pneumocystis* pneumonia can often present as upper lobe diseases.

Lung volumes, mechanics, and diffusion all are useful in evaluating interstitial lung diseases such as sarcoidosis. The diffusion of carbon monoxide (DL_{CO}) is the most sensitive test for an interstitial lung disease. Reduced lung volumes are a reflection of the restrictive lung disease seen in sarcoidosis. However, a third of the patients presenting with sarcoidosis still have lung volumes within the normal range, despite abnormal chest roentgenograms and dyspnea.

Approximately half of sarcoidosis patients present with obstructive disease, reflected by a reduced ratio of forced vital capacity expired in time interval t (FEV_t/FVC). Cough is a very common symptom. Airway involvement causing varying degrees of obstruction underlies the cough in most sarcoidosis patients. However, airway hyperreactivity as determined by methacholine challenge will be positive in some of these patients. A few patients with cough will respond to traditional bronchodilators as the only form of treatment. In some cases, high-dose inhaled glucocorticoids alone are useful.

Pulmonary arterial hypertension is reported in at least 5% of sarcoidosis patients. Either direct vascular involvement or the consequence of fibrotic changes in the lung can lead to pulmonary arterial hypertension. In sarcoidosis patients with end-stage fibrosis awaiting lung transplant, 70% will have pulmonary arterial hypertension. This is a much higher incidence than that reported for other fibrotic lung diseases. In less advanced, but still symptomatic patients pulmonary arterial hypertension has been noted in up to 50% of the cases. Because sarcoidosis-associated pulmonary arterial hypertension

may respond to therapy, evaluation for this should be considered in persistently symptomatic patients.

SKIN

Skin involvement is eventually identified in over a third of patients with sarcoidosis. The classic cutaneous lesions include erythema nodosum, maculopapular lesions, hyper- and hypopigmentation, keloid formation, and sub-cutaneous nodules. A specific complex of involvement of the bridge of the nose, the area beneath the eyes, and the cheeks is referred to as *lupus pernio* (**Fig. 13-4**) and is diagnostic for a chronic form of sarcoidosis.

In contrast, erythema nodosum is a transient rash that can be seen in association with hilar adenopathy and uveitis (Löfgren's syndrome). Erythema nodosum is more common in women and in certain self-described demographic groups including Caucasians and Puerto Ricans. In the United States, the other manifestations of skin sarcoidosis, especially lupus pernio, are more common in blacks than whites.

The maculopapular lesions from sarcoidosis are the most common chronic form of the disease (**Fig. 13-5**). These are often overlooked by the patient and physician, since they are chronic and not painful. Initially, these lesions are usually purplish papules elevated up to 1 cm and <3 cm in diameter. They can become confluent and infiltrate large areas of the skin. With treatment, the color and induration may fade. Because these lesions are caused by noncaseating granulomas, the diagnosis of sarcoidosis can be readily made by a skin biopsy.

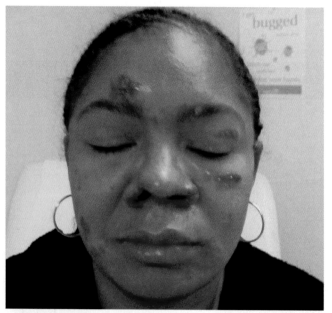

FIGURE 13-4

Chronic inflammatory lesions around nose, eyes, and cheeks, referred to as lupus pernio.

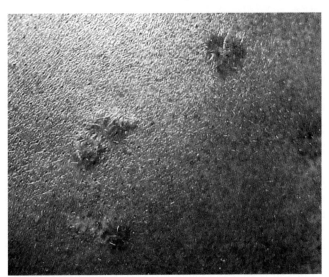

FIGURE 13-5
Maculopapular lesions on the trunk of a sarcoidosis patient.

EYE

The frequency of ocular manifestations for sarcoidosis varies depending on race. In Japan, >70% of sarcoidosis patients develop ocular disease, while in the United States only 30% have eye disease, with problems more common in blacks than whites. Although the most common manifestation is an anterior uveitis, over a quarter of patients will have inflammation at the posterior of the eye, including retinitis and pars planitis. While symptoms such as photophobia, blurred vision, and increased tearing can occur, some asymptomatic patients still have active inflammation. Initially asymptomatic patients with ocular sarcoidosis can eventually develop blindness. Therefore, it is recommended that all patients with sarcoidosis receive a dedicated ophthalmologic examination. Sicca is seen in over half of the chronic sarcoidosis patients. Dry eyes appear to be a reflection of prior lacrimal gland disease. Although the patient may no longer have active inflammation, the dry eyes may require natural tears or other lubricants.

LIVER

Using biopsies to detect granulomatous disease, liver involvement can be identified in over half of sarcoidosis patients. However, using liver function studies, only 20–30% of patients will have evidence of liver involvement. The most common abnormality of liver function is an elevation of the alkaline phosphatase level, consistent with an obstructive pattern. In addition, elevated transaminase levels can occur. An elevated bilirubin level is a marker for more advanced liver disease. Overall, only 5% of sarcoidosis patients have sufficient

symptoms from their liver disease to require specific therapy. Although symptoms can be due to hepatomegaly, more frequently symptoms result from extensive intrahepatic cholestasis leading to portal hypertension. In this case, ascites and esophageal varices can occur. It is rare that a sarcoidosis patient will require a liver transplant, because even the patient with cirrhosis due to sarcoidosis can respond to systemic therapy. On a cautionary note, patients with both sarcoidosis and hepatitis C should avoid therapy with interferon α because of its association with the development or worsening of granulomatous disease.

BONE MARROW AND SPLEEN

One or more bone marrow manifestations can be identified in many sarcoidosis patients. The most common hematologic problem is lymphopenia, which is a reflection of sequestration of the lymphocytes into the areas of inflammation. Anemia occurs in 20% of patients and leukopenia is less common. Bone marrow examination will reveal granulomas in about a third of patients. Splenomegaly can be detected in 5–10% of patients, but splenic biopsy reveals granulomas in 60% of patients. The CT scan can be relatively specific for sarcoidosis involvement of the spleen (Fig. 13-6). Both bone marrow and spleen involvement are more common in blacks than whites. These manifestations alone are rarely an indication for therapy. On occasion, splenectomy may be indicated for massive symptomatic splenomegaly or profound pancytopenia.

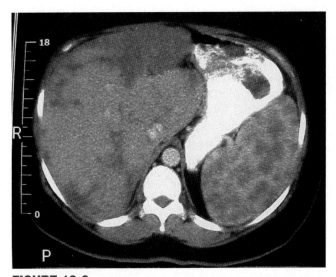

FIGURE 13-6
CT scan of the abdomen after oral and intravenous contrast. The stomach is compressed by the enlarged spleen. Within the spleen, areas of hypo- and hyperdensity are identified.

CALCIUM METABOLISM

Hypercalcemia and/or hypercalciuria occurs in about 10% of sarcoidosis patients. It is more common in whites than blacks and in men. The mechanism of abnormal calcium metabolism is increased production of 1,25-dihydroxyvitamin D by the granuloma itself. The 1,25-dihydroxyvitamin D causes increased intestinal absorption of calcium, leading to hypercalcemia with a suppressed parathyroid hormone (PTH) level. Increased exogenous vitamin D from diet or sunlight exposure may exacerbate this problem. Serum calcium should be determined as part of the initial evaluation of all sarcoidosis patients, and a repeat determination may be useful during the summer months with increased sun exposure. In patients with a history of renal calculi, a 24-h urine calcium measurement should be obtained. If a sarcoidosis patient with a history of renal calculi is to be placed on calcium supplements, a follow-up 24-h urine calcium level should be measured.

RENAL DISEASE

Direct kidney involvement occurs in <5% of sarcoidosis patients. It is associated with granulomas in the kidney itself and can lead to nephritis. However, hypercalcemia is the most likely cause of sarcoidosis-associated renal disease. In 1–2% of sarcoidosis patients, acute renal failure has been encountered as a result of hypercalcemia. Treatment of the hypercalcemia with glucocorticoids and other therapies often improves, but does not totally resolve, the renal dysfunction.

NERVOUS SYSTEM

Neurologic disease is reported in 5–10% of sarcoidosis patients and appears to be of equal frequency across all ethnic groups. Any part of the central or peripheral nervous system can be affected. The presence of granulomatous inflammation is often visible on MRI studies. The MRI with gadolinium enhancement may demonstrate space-occupying lesions, but the MRI can be negative due to small lesions or the effect of systemic therapy in reducing the inflammation. The cerebral spinal fluid (CSF) findings include a lymphocytic meningitis with a mild increase in protein. The CSF glucose is usually normal but can be low. Certain areas of the nervous system are more commonly affected in neurosarcoidosis. These include cranial nerve involvement, basilar meningitis, myelopathy, and anterior hypothalamic disease with associated diabetes insipidus. Seizures and cognitive changes also occur. Of the cranial nerves, seventh nerve paralysis can be transient and can be mistaken for Bell's palsy (idiopathic seventh nerve paralysis). Since this form of neurosarcoidosis often resolves within weeks and does not recur, it may have occurred prior to a definitive

diagnosis of sarcoidosis. Optic neuritis is another cranial nerve manifestation of sarcoidosis. This manifestation is more chronic and usually requires long-term systemic therapy. It can be associated with both anterior and posterior uveitis. Differentiating between neurosarcoidosis and multiple sclerosis can be difficult at times. Optic neuritis can occur in both diseases. In some patients with sarcoidosis, multiple enhancing white matter abnormalities may be detected by MRI, suggesting multiple sclerosis. In such cases, the presence of meningeal enhancement or hypothalamic involvement suggests neurosarcoidosis, as does evidence of extraneurologic disease such as pulmonary or skin involvement, which also suggests sarcoidosis. Since the response of neurosarcoidosis to glucocorticoids and cytotoxic therapy is different from that of multiple sclerosis, differentiating between these disease entities is important.

CARDIAC

The presence of cardiac involvement is influenced by race. Over a quarter of Japanese sarcoidosis patients develop cardiac disease, whereas only 5% of sarcoidosis patients in the United States and Europe develop cardiac disease. However, there is no apparent difference between whites and blacks. Cardiac disease usually presents as either congestive heart failure or cardiac arrhythmias. Both manifestations result from infiltration of the heart muscle by granulomas. Diffuse granulomatous involvement of the heart muscle can lead to ejection fractions below 10%. Even in this situation, improvement in the ejection fraction can occur with systemic therapy. Arrhythmias can also occur with diffuse infiltration or with more patchy cardiac involvement. If the AV node is infiltrated, heart block can occur. This can be detected by routine electrocardiography. Ventricular arrhythmias and sudden death due to ventricular tachycardia are common causes of death. Arrhythmias are best detected using 24-h ambulatory monitoring. Because ventricular arrhythmias are usually multifocal due to patchy multiple granulomas in the heart, ablation therapy is not useful. Patients with significant ventricular arrhythmias should be considered for an implanted defibrillator, which appears to have reduced the rate of death in cardiac sarcoidosis. While systemic therapy can be useful in treating the arrhythmias, patients may still have malignant arrhythmias up to 6 months after starting successful treatment, and the risk for recurrent arrhythmias occurs whenever medications are tapered.

MUSCULOSKELETAL SYSTEM

Direct granulomatous bone and muscle involvement as documented by x-ray, MRI (**Fig. 13-7**), gallium scan, or biopsy can be seen in about 10% of sarcoidosis patients.

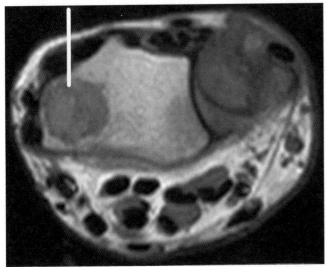

FIGURE 13-7
MRI of wrist demonstrating large cyst in a sarcoidosis patient (*line*).

However, a larger percentage of sarcoidosis patients complain of myalgias and arthralgias. These complaints are similar to those reported by patients with other inflammatory diseases, including chronic infections such as mononucleosis. Fatigue associated with sarcoidosis may be overwhelming for many patients. Recent studies have demonstrated a link between fatigue and small peripheral nerve fiber disease in sarcoidosis.

OTHER ORGAN INVOLVEMENT

Although sarcoidosis can affect any organ of the body, rarely does it involve the breast, testes, ovary, or stomach. Because of the rarity of involvement, a mass in one of these areas requires a biopsy to rule out other diseases including cancer. For example, in a study of breast problems in female sarcoidosis patients, a breast lesion was more likely to be granulomas from sarcoidosis than from breast cancer. However, findings on the physical examination or mammogram cannot reliably differentiate between these lesions. More importantly, as women with sarcoidosis age, breast cancer becomes more common. Therefore, it is recommended that routine screening including mammography be performed along with other imaging studies (ultrasound, MRI) or biopsy as clinically indicated.

COMPLICATIONS

Sarcoidosis is usually a self-limited, non–life-threatening disease. However, organ-threatening disease can occur. These complications can include blindness, paraplegia, or renal failure. Death from sarcoidosis occurs in about 5% of patients seen in sarcoidosis referral clinics. The usual causes of death related to sarcoidosis are from

lung, cardiac, neurologic, or liver involvement. In respiratory failure, an elevation of the right atrial pressure is a poor prognostic finding. Lung complications can also include infections such as mycetoma, which can subsequently lead to massive bleeding. In addition, the use of immunosuppressive agents can increase the incidence of serious infections.

LABORATORY FINDINGS

The chest roentgenogram remains the most commonly used tool to assess lung involvement in sarcoidosis. As noted above, the chest roentgenogram classifies involvement into four stages, with stages 1 and 2 having hilar and paratracheal adenopathy. The CT scan has been used increasingly in evaluating interstitial lung disease. In sarcoidosis, the presence of adenopathy and a nodular infiltrate is not specific for sarcoidosis. Adenopathy up to 2 cm can be seen in other inflammatory lung diseases such as idiopathic pulmonary fibrosis. However, adenopathy >2 cm in the short axis supports the diagnosis of sarcoidosis over other interstitial lung diseases.

Gallium 67 scanning has been used over the years to detect inflammatory activity in various parts of the body. A negative scan can be easily misinterpreted as the scan will quickly revert to normal during glucocorticoid therapy. In addition, the test requires that the patient return 2–4 days later. More recently, the positron emission tomography (PET) scan, using radiolabeled fluorodeoxy glucose as the marker, has provided information similar to that of the gallium scan. While the sensitivity of PET scanning has not been fully evaluated in sarcoidosis, it is important to recognize that a positive PET scan may be due to the granulomas from sarcoidosis and not to disseminated malignancy.

Serum levels of angiotensin-converting enzyme (ACE) can be helpful in the diagnosis of sarcoidosis. However, the test has somewhat low sensitivity and specificity. Elevated levels of ACE are reported in 60% of patients with acute disease and only 20% of patients with chronic disease. Although there are several causes for mild elevation of ACE, including diabetes, elevations of >50% of the upper limit of normal are seen in only a few conditions including sarcoidosis, leprosy, Gaucher's disease, hyperthyroidism, and disseminated granulomatous infections such as miliary tuberculosis. The ACE level in lymphoma is usually lower than normal, which may provide a useful distinction from sarcoidosis. There is an insertion/deletion (I/D) polymorphism of the *ACE* gene on what is felt to be in the noncritical part of the gene. There is a phenotypic difference for ACE levels, with II polymorphism having the lowest and DD polymorphism the highest levels of ACE for both sarcoidosis patients and healthy controls. There is no clear-cut association between ACE phenotype and clinical manifestation of disease. Because the

ACE level is determined by a biologic assay, the concurrent use of an ACE inhibitor such as lisinopril will lead to a very low ACE level.

DIAGNOSIS

The diagnosis of sarcoidosis requires both compatible clinical features and pathologic findings. Since the cause of sarcoidosis remains elusive, the diagnosis cannot be made with 100% certainty. Nevertheless, the diagnosis can be made with reasonable certainty based on history and physical features along with laboratory and pathologic findings.

Patients are usually evaluated for possible sarcoidosis based on two scenarios (**Fig. 13-8**). In the first scenario, a patient may undergo a biopsy revealing a noncaseating granuloma in either a pulmonary or an extrapulmonary organ. If the clinical presentation is consistent with sarcoidosis and there is no alternative cause for the granulomas identified, then the patient is felt to have sarcoidosis.

In the second scenario, signs or symptoms suggesting sarcoidosis such as the presence of bilateral adenopathy may be present in an otherwise asymptomatic patient or a patient with uveitis or a rash consistent with sarcoidosis. At this point, a diagnostic procedure should be performed. For the patient with a compatible skin lesion, a skin biopsy should be considered. Other biopsies to consider could include liver, extrathoracic lymph node, or muscle. In some cases, a biopsy of the affected organ may not be easy to perform (such as a brain or spinal cord lesion). In other cases, such as an endomyocardial biopsy, the likelihood of a positive biopsy is low. Because of the high rate of pulmonary involvement in these cases, the lung may be easier to approach by bronchoscopy. During the bronchoscopy, a transbronchial biopsy, bronchial biopsy, or transbronchial needle aspirate of an enlarged mediastinal lymph node can be performed.

If the biopsy reveals granulomas, an alternative diagnosis such as infection or malignancy must be excluded. Bronchoscopic washings can be sent for cultures for fungi and tuberculosis. For the pathologist, the more tissue that is provided, the more comfortable is the diagnosis of sarcoidosis. A needle aspirate may be adequate in an otherwise classic case of sarcoidosis, but may be insufficient in a patient in whom lymphoma or fungal infection is a likely alternative diagnosis. Since granulomas can be seen on the edge of a lymphoma, the presence of a few granulomas from a needle aspirate may not be sufficient to clarify the diagnosis. Mediastinoscopy remains the procedure of choice to confirm the presence or absence of lymphoma in the mediastinum. Alternatively, for most patients, evidence of extrathoracic disease (e.g., eye involvement) may further support the diagnosis of sarcoidosis.

For patients with negative pathology, positive supportive tests may increase the likelihood of the diagnosis of sarcoidosis. These tests include an elevated ACE level, which can also be elevated in other granulomatous diseases but not in malignancy. A positive gallium scan can support the diagnosis if increased activity is noted in the parotids and lacrimal glands (*Panda sign*) or in the right paratracheal and

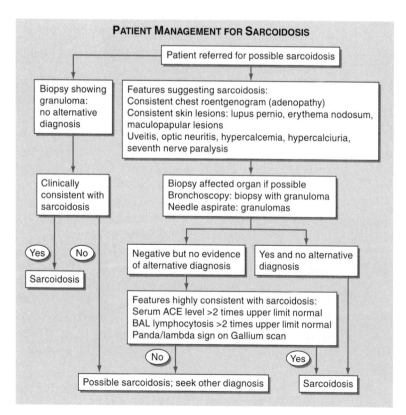

FIGURE 13-8

Proposed approach to management of patient with possible sarcoidosis. Presence of one or more of these features supports the diagnosis of sarcoidosis: uveitis, optic neuritis, hypercalcemia, hypercalciuria, seventh cranial nerve paralysis, diabetes insipidus.

left hilar area (*lambda sign*). A BAL is often performed during the bronchoscopy. An increase in the percentage of lymphocytes supports the diagnosis of sarcoidosis. The use of the lymphocyte markers CD4 and CD8 can be used to determine the CD4/CD8 ratio of these increased lymphocytes in the BAL fluid. A ratio of >3.5 is strongly supportive of sarcoidosis but is less sensitive than an increase in lymphocytes alone. Although in general, an increase in BAL lymphocytes is supportive of the diagnosis, other conditions must be considered.

These supportive tests when combined with commonly associated clinical features of the disease, which are not diagnostic of sarcoidosis, can enhance the diagnostic probability. These nondiagnostic features include uveitis, renal stones, hypercalcemia, seventh cranial nerve paralysis, or erythema nodosum.

The *Kviem-Siltzbach procedure* is a specific diagnostic test for sarcoidosis. An intradermal injection of specially prepared tissue derived from the spleen of a known sarcoidosis patient is biopsied 4–6 weeks after injection. If noncaseating granulomas are seen, this is highly specific for the diagnosis of sarcoidosis. Unfortunately, there is no commercially available Kviem-Siltzbach reagent, and some locally prepared batches have lower specificity. Thus, this test is of historic interest and is rarely used in current clinical practice.

Because the diagnosis of sarcoidosis can never be certain, over time other features may arise that lead to an alternative diagnosis. On the other hand, evidence for new organ involvement may eventually confirm the diagnosis of sarcoidosis.

PROGNOSIS

The risk of death or loss of organ function remains low in sarcoidosis. Poor outcomes usually occur in patients who present with advanced disease in whom treatment

seems to have little impact. In these cases, irreversible fibrotic changes have frequently occurred.

For the majority of patients, initial presentation occurs during the granulomatous phase of the disease as depicted in Fig. 13-1. It is clear that many patients resolve their disease within 2–5 years. These patients are felt to have acute, self-limiting sarcoidosis. On the other hand, there is a form of the disease that does not resolve within the first 2–5 years. These chronic patients can be identified at presentation by certain risk factors at presentation such as fibrosis on chest roentgenogram, presence of lupus pernio, bone cysts, cardiac or neurologic disease (except isolated seventh nerve paralysis), and presence of renal calculi due to hypercalciuria. Recent studies also indicate that patients who require glucocorticoids for any manifestation of their disease in the first 6 months of presentation have a >50% chance of having chronic disease. In contrast, <10% of patients who require systemic therapy in the first 6 months will require chronic therapy.

℞ **Treatment:**
SARCOIDOSIS

The indications for therapy should be based on symptoms. The patient with elevated liver function tests or an abnormal chest roentgenogram probably does not benefit from treatment. However, these patients should be monitored for evidence of progressive, symptomatic disease.

One approach to therapy is summarized in **Figs. 13-9** and **13-10**. We have divided the approach into treating acute versus chronic disease. For acute disease, no therapy remains a viable option for patients with no or mild symptoms. For symptoms confined to only one organ, topical therapy is preferable. For multiorgan disease or disease too extensive for topical therapy, an approach

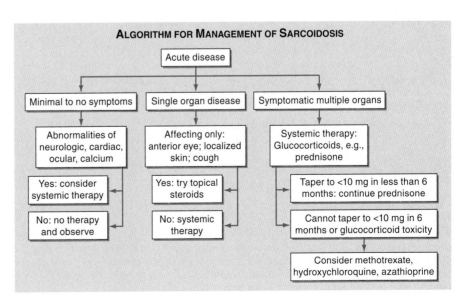

FIGURE 13-9

The management of acute sarcoidosis is based on level of symptoms and extent of organ involvement. In patients with mild symptoms, no therapy may be needed unless specified manifestations are noted.

ALGORITHM FOR MANAGEMENT OF SARCOIDOSIS

Acute disease

Minimal to no symptoms | Single organ disease | Symptomatic multiple organs

Abnormalities of neurologic, cardiac, ocular, calcium | Affecting only: anterior eye; localized skin; cough | Systemic therapy: Glucocorticoids, e.g., prednisone

Yes: consider systemic therapy | Yes: try topical steroids | Taper to <10 mg in less than 6 months: continue prednisone

No: no therapy and observe | No: systemic therapy | Cannot taper to <10 mg in 6 months or glucocorticoid toxicity

Consider methotrexate, hydroxychloroquine, azathioprine

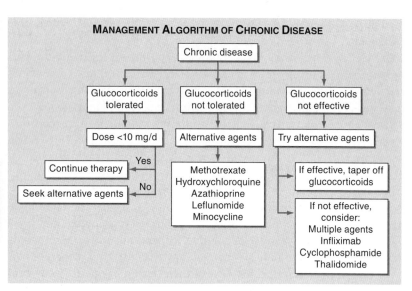

FIGURE 13-10

Approach to chronic disease is based on whether glucocorticoid therapy is tolerated or not.

to systemic therapy is outlined. Glucocorticoids remain the drugs of choice for this disease. However, the decision to continue to treat with glucocorticoids or to add steroid-sparing agents depends on the tolerability, duration, and dosage of glucocorticoids. Table 13-2 summarizes the dosage and monitoring of several commonly used drugs. According to the available trials, evidence-based recommendations are made. Most of

these recommendations are for pulmonary disease because most of the trials were performed only in pulmonary disease. Treatment recommendations for extrapulmonary disease are usually similar with a few modifications. For example, the dosage of glucocorticoids is usually higher for neurosarcoidosis and lower for cutaneous disease. There was some suggestion that higher doses would be beneficial for cardiac sarcoidosis, but

TABLE 13-2

COMMONLY USED DRUGS TO TREAT SARCOIDOSIS

DRUG	INITIAL DOSE	MAINTENANCE DOSE	MONITORING	TOXICITY	SUPPORT THERAPY[a]	SUPPORT MONITORING[a]
Prednisone	20–40 mg qd	Taper to 5–10 mg	Glucose, blood pressure, bone density	Diabetes, osteoporosis	A: Acute pulmonary D: Extrapulmonary	
Hydroxychloroquine	200–400 mg qd	400 mg qd	Eye exam q6–12 mo	Ocular	B: Some forms of disease	D: Routine eye exam
Methotrexate	10 mg qw	2.5–15 mg qw	CBC, renal, hepatic q2mo	Hematologic, nausea, hepatic, pulmonary	B: Steroid sparing C: Some forms chronic disease	D: Routine hematologic, renal, and hepatic monitoring
Azathioprine	50–150 mg qd	50–200 mg qd	CBC, renal q2mo	Hematologic, nausea	C: Some forms chronic disease	D: Routine hematologic monitoring
Infliximab	3–5 mg/kg q2wk for 2 doses	3–10 mg/kg q4–8 wk	Initial PPD	Infections, allergic reaction, carcinogen	B: Chronic pulmonary disease	C: Caution in patients with latent tuberculosis or advanced congestive heart failure

[a]Grade A: supported by at least two double-blind randomized control trials; grade B: supported by prospective cohort studies; grade C: supported primarily by two or more retrospective studies; grade D: only one retrospective study or based on experience in other diseases.
Note: CBC, complete blood count; PPD, purified protein derivative test for tuberculosis.
Source: Adapted from Baughman and Selroos.

one study found that initial doses >40 mg/d prednisone were associated with a worse outcome.

While most patients receive glucocorticoids as their initial systemic therapy, toxicity associated with prolonged therapy often leads to steroid-sparing alternatives. The antimalarial drugs such as hydroxychloroquine are more effective for skin than pulmonary disease. Minocycline may also be useful for cutaneous sarcoidosis. For pulmonary and other extrapulmonary disease, cytotoxic agents are often employed. These include methotrexate, azathioprine, chlorambucil, and cyclophosphamide. The most widely studied cytotoxic agent has been methotrexate. This agent works in approximately two-thirds of sarcoidosis patients, regardless of the disease manifestation. As noted in Table 13-2, specific guidelines for monitoring therapy have been recommended. Cytokine modulators such as thalidomide and pentoxifylline have also been used in a limited number of cases.

The anti-TNF agents have recently been studied in sarcoidosis, with prospective randomized trials of both etanercept and infliximab completed. Etanercept has a limited role as a steroid-sparing agent. On the other hand, infliximab significantly improves lung function when given to patients with chronic disease already on glucocorticoids and cytotoxic agents. The difference in response for these two agents is similar to that observed in Crohn's disease, where infliximab is effective and etanercept is not. In addition, increased risks for reactivation of tuberculosis are reported for infliximab compared to etanercept. The differential response rate could be explained by differences in mechanism of action since etanercept is a TNF receptor antagonist and infliximab is a monoclonal antibody against TNF. The peak dosage of the drug may also be different, since etanercept is given SC whereas infliximab is given IV. A higher peak dose may lead to better intracellular penetration and therefore affect the transmembrane TNF. In contrast to etanercept, infliximab binds to TNF on the surface of some cells that are releasing TNF and this can lead to cell lysis. This effect has been documented in Crohn's disease.

The role of the newer therapeutic agents for sarcoidosis is still evolving. However, these targeted therapies confirm that TNF may be an important target, especially in the treatment of chronic disease. However, the majority of cases either do not require therapy or can be controlled with glucocorticoids and cytotoxic agents.

FURTHER READINGS

Baughman RP, Selroos O: Evidence-based approach to treatment of sarcoidosis, in *Evidence-Based Respiratory Medicine*, PG Gibson et al (eds). Oxford, BMJ Books Blackwell, 2005, pp 491–508

——— et al: Clinical characteristics of patients in a case control study of sarcoidosis. Am J Respir Crit Care Med 164:1885, 2001

——— et al: Treatment of sarcoidosis. Clin Chest Med 29:533, 2008

Hunninghake GW et al: ATS/ERS/WASOG statement on sarcoidosis. American Thoracic Society/European Respiratory Society/World Association of Sarcoidosis and Other Granulomatous Disorders. Sarcoidosis Vasc Diffuse Lung Dis 16:149, 1999

Iannuzzi MC et al: Sarcoidosis. N Engl J Med 357:2153, 2007

Judson MA and the ACCESS Research Group: Defining organ involvement in sarcoidosis: The ACCESS proposed instrument. Sarcoidosis Vasc Diffuse Lung Dis 16:75, 1999

——— et al: Comparison of sarcoidosis phenotypes among affected African-American siblings. Chest 130:855, 2006

Mehta D et al: Cardiac involvement in patients with sarcoidosis: Diagnostic and prognostic value of outpatient testing. Chest 133:1426, 2008

Newman LS et al: A case control etiologic study of sarcoidosis: Environmental and occupational risk factors. Am J Respir Crit Care Med 170:1324, 2004

Rossman MD et al: HLA-DRB1*1101: A significant risk factor for sarcoidosis in blacks and whites. Am J Hum Genet 73:720, 2003

Sato H et al: HLA-DQB1*0201: A marker for good prognosis in British and Dutch patients with sarcoidosis. Am J Respir Cell Mol Biol 27:406, 2002

Song Z et al: Mycobacterial catalase-peroxidase is a tissue antigen and target of the adaptive immune response in systemic sarcoidosis. J Exp Med 201:755, 2005

Torralba KD, Quismorio FP Jr: Sarcoidosis and the rheumatologist. Curr Opin Rheumatol 21:62, 2009

Yeager H et al: Pulmonary and psychosocial findings at enrollment in the ACCESS study. Sarcoidosis Vasc Diffuse Lung Dis 22:147, 2005

Ziegenhagen MW et al: Exaggerated TNF-alpha release of alveolar macrophages in corticosteroid resistant sarcoidosis. Sarcoidosis Vasc Diffuse Lung Dis 19:185, 2002

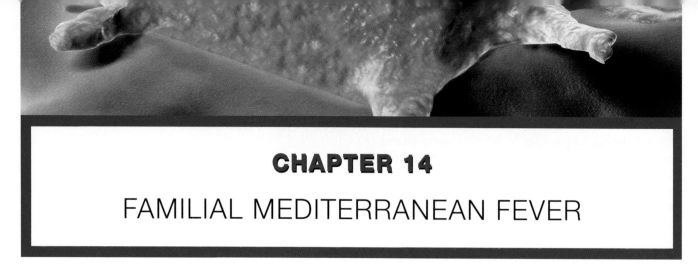

CHAPTER 14

FAMILIAL MEDITERRANEAN FEVER

Daniel L. Kastner

Familial Mediterranean fever (FMF) is the prototype of a group of inherited diseases (Table 14-1) that are characterized by recurrent episodes of fever with serosal, synovial, or cutaneous inflammation and, in some individuals, the eventual development of systemic AA amyloidosis (Chap. 15). Because of the relative infrequency of high-titer autoantibodies or antigen-specific T cells, the term *autoinflammatory* has been proposed to describe these disorders, rather than autoimmune.

BACKGROUND AND PATHOPHYSIOLOGY

FMF was first recognized among Armenians, Arabs, Turks, and non-Ashkenazi (primarily North African and Iraqi) Jews. With the advent of genetic testing, FMF has been documented with increasing frequency among Ashkenazi Jews and Italians, and occasional cases have been confirmed even in the absence of known Mediterranean ancestry. FMF is recessively inherited, but, particularly in countries where families are small, a positive family history can only be elicited in ~50% of cases. DNA testing demonstrates carrier frequencies as high as 1:3 among affected populations, suggesting a heterozygote advantage.

The FMF gene encodes a 781-amino acid, ~95 kDa protein denoted *pyrin* (or *marenostrin*) that is expressed in granulocytes, eosinophils, monocytes, dendritic cells, and synovial and peritoneal fibroblasts. The N-terminal 92 amino acids of pyrin define a motif, the PYRIN domain, which is similar in structure to death domains, death

effector domains, and caspase recruitment domains. PYRIN domains mediate homotypic protein-protein interactions and have been found in several other proteins, including cryopyrin, which is mutated in three other recurrent fever syndromes. Through a number of mechanisms, including the interaction of the PYRIN domain with an intermediary adaptor protein, pyrin regulates caspase-1 [interleukin (IL) 1β-converting enzyme], and thereby IL-1β secretion. Pyrin-deficient mice exhibit heightened sensitivity to endotoxin, excessive IL-1β production, and impaired monocyte apoptosis.

ACUTE ATTACKS

Febrile episodes in FMF may begin even in early infancy; 90% of patients have had their first attack by age 20. Typical FMF episodes generally last 24–72 h, with arthritic attacks tending to last somewhat longer. In some patients the episodes occur with great regularity, but more often the frequency of attacks varies over time, ranging from as often as once every few days to remissions lasting several years. Attacks are often unpredictable, although some patients relate them to physical exertion, emotional stress, or menses; pregnancy may be associated with remission.

If measured, fever is nearly always present throughout FMF attacks. Severe hyperpyrexia and even febrile seizures may be seen in infants, and fever is sometimes the only manifestation of FMF in young children.

TABLE 14-1

THE HEREDITARY PERIODIC FEVER SYNDROMES

	FMF	TRAPS	HIDS	MWS	FCAS	NOMID
Ethnicity	Jewish, Arab, Turkish, Armenian, Italian	Any ethnic group	Predominantly Dutch, northern European	Any ethnic group	Any ethnic group	Any ethnic group
Inheritance	Recessive	Dominant	Recessive	Dominant	Dominant	Usually de novo mutations
Gene/chromosome	MEFV/16p13.3	TNFRSF1A/12p13	MVK/12q24	CIAS1/1q44	CIAS1/1q44	CIAS1/1q44
Protein	Pyrin	p55 TNF receptor	Mevalonate kinase	Cryopyrin	Cryopyrin	Cryopyrin
Attack length	1–3 days	Often >7 days	3–7 days	1–2 days	Minutes–3 days	Continuous, with flares
Serosa	Pleurisy, peritonitis; asymptomatic pericardial effusions	Pleurisy, peritonitis, pericarditis	Abd pain, but seldom peritonitis; pleurisy, pericarditis uncommon	Abd pain common; pleurisy, pericarditis rare	Rare	Rare
Skin	Erysipeloid erythema	Centrifugally migrating erythema	Diffuse maculopapular rash; oral ulcers	Diffuse urticaria-like rash	Cold-induced urticaria-like rash	Diffuse urticaria-like rash
Joints	Acute monoarthritis; chronic hip arthritis (rare)	Acute monoarthritis, arthralgia	Arthralgia, oligoarthritis	Arthralgia, large joint oligoarthritis	Polyarthralgia	Epiphyseal, patellar overgrowth, clubbing
Muscle	Exercise-induced myalgia common; protracted febrile myalgia rare	Migratory myalgia	Uncommon	Myalgia common	Sometimes myalgia	Sometimes myalgia
Eyes, ears	Uncommon	Periorbital edema, conjunctivitis, rarely uveitis		Conjunctivitis, episcleritis, optic disc edema; sensorineural hearing loss	Conjunctivitis	Conjunctivitis, uveitis, optic disc edema, blindness, sensorineural hearing loss
CNS	Aseptic meningitis rare	Headache	Headache	Headache	Headache	Aseptic meningitis, seizures
Amyloidosis	Most common in M694V homozygotes	~15% of cases	Not described	~25% of cases	Uncommon	Late complication
Treatment	Oral colchicine prophylaxis	Glucocorticoids, etanercept	NSAIDs for fever; IL-1β and TNF inhibitors investigational	Anakinra (IL-1 receptor antagonist)	Anakinra	Anakinra

Note: FMF, familial Mediterranean fever; TNF, tumor necrosis factor; TRAPS, TNF receptor–associated periodic syndrome; HIDS, hyperimmunoglobulin D with periodic fever syndrome; MWS, Muckle-Wells syndrome; FACS, familial cold autoinflammatory syndrome; NOMID, neonatal-onset multisystem inflammatory disease; Abd, abdominal; CNS, central nervous system; NSAIDs, nonsteroidal anti-inflammatory drugs.

Over 90% of FMF patients experience abdominal attacks at some time. Episodes range in severity from dull, aching pain and distention with mild tenderness on direct palpation to severe generalized pain with absent bowel sounds, rigidity, rebound tenderness, and air-fluid levels on upright radiographs. CT scanning may demonstrate a small amount of fluid in the abdominal cavity. If such patients undergo exploratory laparotomy, a sterile, neutrophil-rich peritoneal exudate is present, sometimes with adhesions from previous episodes. Ascites is rare.

Pleural attacks are usually manifested by unilateral, sharp, stabbing chest pain. Radiographs may show atelectasis and sometimes an effusion. If performed, thoracentesis demonstrates an exudative fluid rich in neutrophils. After repeated attacks, pleural thickening may develop.

FMF arthritis is most frequent among individuals homozygous for the M694V mutation, which is especially common in the non-Ashkenazi Jewish population. Acute arthritis in FMF is usually monoarticular, affecting the knee, ankle, or hip, although other patterns can be seen, particularly in children. Large sterile effusions rich in neutrophils are frequent, without commensurate erythema or warmth. Even after repeated arthritic attacks, radiographic changes are rare. Before the advent of colchicine prophylaxis, chronic arthritis of the knee or hip were seen in ~5% of FMF patients with arthritis. Chronic sacroiliitis can occur in FMF irrespective of the HLA-B27 antigen, even in the face of colchicine therapy. In the United States, FMF patients are much more likely to have arthralgia than arthritis.

The most characteristic cutaneous manifestation of FMF is erysipelas-like erythema, a raised erythematous rash that most commonly occurs on the dorsum of the foot, ankle, or lower leg, alone or in combination with abdominal pain, pleurisy, or arthritis. Biopsy demonstrates perivascular infiltrates of granulocytes and monocytes. This rash is seen most often in M694V homozygotes and is relatively rare in the United States.

Exercise-induced (nonfebrile) myalgia is common in FMF, and a small percentage of patients develop a protracted febrile myalgia that can last several weeks. Symptomatic pericardial disease is rare, although some patients have small pericardial effusions as an incidental echocardiographic finding. Unilateral acute scrotal inflammation may occur in prepubertal boys. Aseptic meningitis has been reported in FMF but the causal connection is controversial. Vasculitis, including Henoch-Schönlein purpura and polyarteritis nodosa (Chap. 10) may be seen at increased frequency in FMF.

Laboratory features of FMF attacks are consistent with acute inflammation and include an elevated erythrocyte sedimentation rate, leukocytosis, thrombocytosis (in children), and elevations in C-reactive protein, fibrinogen, haptoglobin, and serum immunoglobulins. Transient albuminuria and hematuria may also be seen.

AMYLOIDOSIS

Before the advent of colchicine prophylaxis, systemic amyloidosis was a common complication of FMF. It is caused by deposition of a fragment of serum amyloid A, an acute-phase reactant, in the kidneys, adrenals, intestine, spleen, lung, and testes (Chap. 15). Amyloidosis should be suspected in patients who have proteinuria between attacks; renal or rectal biopsy is used most often to establish the diagnosis. Risk factors include the M694V homozygous genotype, positive family history (independent of FMF mutational status), the SAA 1 genotype, male gender, noncompliance with colchicine therapy, and having grown up in the Middle East.

DIAGNOSIS

For typical cases, physicians experienced with FMF can often make the diagnosis on clinical grounds alone. Clinical criteria sets for FMF have been shown to have high sensitivity and specificity in parts of the world where the pretest probability of FMF is high. Genetic testing can provide a useful adjunct in ambiguous cases or for physicians not experienced in FMF. Most of the disease-associated FMF mutations are in exon 10 of the gene, with a smaller group of mutations in exon 2. An updated list of mutations for FMF and other hereditary periodic fevers can be found online at *http://fmf.igh.cnrs.fr/infevers/*.

Genetic testing has permitted a broadening of the clinical spectrum and geographic distribution of FMF and may be of prognostic value. Most studies indicate that M694V homozygotes have an earlier age of onset and a higher frequency of arthritis, rash, and amyloidosis. In contrast, the E148Q mutation is usually associated with milder disease. E148Q is sometimes found in *cis* with exon 10 mutations, which complicates the interpretation of genetic test results. Only ~70% of patients with clinically typical FMF have two identifiable mutations in *trans*, suggesting either that current screening methods do not detect all of the relevant mutations or that one mutation may be sufficient to cause disease under some circumstances. In these cases clinical judgment is very important, and sometimes a therapeutic trial of colchicine may help to confirm the diagnosis. Genetic testing of unaffected individuals is usually inadvisable, because of the possibility of nonpenetrance and the potential impact of a positive test on future insurability.

If a patient is seen during his or her first attack, the differential diagnosis may be broad, although delimited by the specific organ involvement. After several attacks the differential diagnosis may include the other hereditary periodic fever syndromes (Table 14-1); the syndrome of periodic fever with aphthous ulcers, pharyngitis, and cervical adenopathy (PFAPA); systemic-onset juvenile rheumatoid arthritis or adult Still's disease; porphyria; hereditary angioedema; inflammatory bowel disease; and, in women, gynecologic disorders.

℞ Treatment: FAMILIAL MEDITERRANEAN FEVER

The treatment of choice for FMF is daily oral colchicine, which decreases the frequency and intensity of attacks and prevents the development of amyloidosis in compliant patients. Intermittent dosing at the onset of attacks is not as effective as daily prophylaxis and is of unproven value in preventing amyloidosis. The usual adult dose of colchicine is 1.2–1.8 mg/d, which causes substantial reduction in symptoms in two-thirds of patients and some improvement in >90%. Children may require lower doses, although not proportionately to body weight.

Common side effects of colchicine include bloating, abdominal cramps, lactose intolerance, and diarrhea. They can be minimized by starting at a low dose and gradually advancing as tolerated, splitting the dose, use of simethecone for flatulence, and avoidance of dairy products. If taken by either parent at the time of conception, colchicine may cause a small increase in the risk of trisomy 21 (Down syndrome). In elderly patients with renal insufficiency, colchicine can cause a myoneuropathy characterized by proximal muscle weakness and elevation of the creatine kinase. Cyclosporine inhibits hepatic excretion of colchicine by its effects on the MDR-1 transport system, sometimes leading to colchicine toxicity in patients who have undergone renal transplantation for amyloidosis. Intravenous colchicine should generally not be administered to patients already taking oral colchicine, because severe, sometimes fatal, toxicity can occur in this setting.

There are no established alternatives for the small number of patients who do not respond to colchicine or cannot tolerate therapeutic dosages, although the IL-1 receptor antagonist and inhibitors of interferon-α and tumor necrosis factor (TNF) are investigational. Bone marrow transplantation has been suggested for refractory FMF, but the risk-benefit ratio is currently regarded as unacceptable.

OTHER HEREDITARY RECURRENT FEVERS

Within 5 years of the discovery of the FMF gene, three additional genes causing five other hereditary periodic fever syndromes were identified, catalyzing a paradigm shift in diagnosis and treatment of these disorders.

■ TNF Receptor–Associated Periodic Syndrome (TRAPS)

TRAPS is caused by dominantly inherited mutations in the extracellular domains of the 55-kDa TNF receptor (TNFRSF1A, p55). Although originally described in a large Irish family (and hence the name *familial Hibernian fever*), TRAPS has a broad ethnic distribution. TRAPS episodes often begin in childhood. The duration of attacks ranges from 1–2 days to as long as several weeks, and in severe cases symptoms may be nearly continuous. In addition to peritoneal, pleural, and synovial attacks similar to FMF, TRAPS patients frequently have ocular inflammation (most often conjunctivitis and/or periorbital edema), and a distinctive migratory myalgia with overlying painful erythema may be present. TRAPS patients generally respond better to glucocorticoids than to prophylactic colchicine. About 15% develop amyloidosis. The diagnosis of TRAPS is based on the demonstration of *TNFRSF1A* mutations in the presence of characteristic symptoms. Leukocytes from patients with certain TRAPS mutations exhibit a defect in TNF receptor-shedding, possibly impairing normal homeostasis. However, a more complex picture is emerging, with a number of functional abnormalities, some of which are ligand independent, contributing to the autoinflammatory phenotype. Etanercept, a TNF inhibitor, ameliorates TRAPS attacks, although its effect on amyloidosis is unproven.

Hyperimmunoglobulinemia D with Periodic Fever Syndrome (HIDS)

HIDS is a recessively inherited recurrent fever syndrome found primarily in individuals of northern European ancestry. It is caused by mutations in mevalonate kinase (*MVK*), encoding an enzyme involved in the synthesis of cholesterol and nonsterol isoprenoids. Attacks usually begin in infancy, and last 3–5 days. Clinically distinctive features include painful cervical adenopathy, a diffuse maculopapular rash sometimes affecting the palms and soles, and aphthous ulcers; pleurisy is rare, as is amyloidosis. Although originally defined by the persistent elevation of serum IgD, disease activity is not related to IgD levels, and some patients with FMF or TRAPS may have modestly increased serum IgD. Moreover, occasional patients with *MVK* mutations and periodic fever have normal IgD levels. All patients with mutations have markedly elevated urinary mevalonate levels during their febrile attacks, although the inflammatory manifestations are likely to be due to a deficiency of isoprenoids rather than an excess of mevalonate. There is currently no established treatment for HIDS.

The Cryopyrinopathies

Three hereditary febrile syndromes, familial cold autoinflammatory syndrome (FCAS), Muckle-Wells syndrome (MWS), and neonatal-onset multisystem inflammatory disease (NOMID), are all caused by mutations in *CIAS1*, the gene encoding cryopyrin (or NALP3), and represent a clinical spectrum of disease. FCAS patients develop chills, fever, headache, arthralgia, conjunctivitis, and an urticaria-like rash in response to generalized cold exposure. In

MWS, an urticarial rash is noted, but it is not usually induced by cold; MWS patients also develop fevers, abdominal pain, limb pain, arthritis, conjunctivitis, and, over time, sensorineural hearing loss. NOMID is the most severe of the three disorders, with chronic aseptic meningitis, a characteristic arthropathy, and rash. Like the FMF protein, pyrin, cryopyrin has an N-terminal PYRIN domain. Cryopyrin regulates IL-1β production through the formation of a macromolecular complex termed the *inflammasome*. Macrophages from cryopyrin-deficient mice exhibit decreased IL-1β production in response to certain gram-positive bacteria, bacterial RNA, and monosodium urate crystals. Patients with all three cryopyrinopathies show a dramatic response to daily injections of anakinra, the IL-1 receptor antagonist.

FURTHER READINGS

AKSENTIJEVICH I et al: An autoinflammatory disease with deficiency of the interleukin-1-receptor antagonist. N Engl J Med 360:2426, 2009

BOOTY MG et al: Familial Mediterranean fever with a single MEFV mutation: Where is the second hit? Arthritis Rheum 60:1851, 2009

DRENTH JPH, VAN DER MEER JWM: Hereditary periodic fever. N Engl J Med 345:1748, 2001

GOLDBACH-MANSKY R et al: Neonatal onset multisystem inflammatory disease responsive to IL-1β inhibition. N Engl J Med 355:581, 2006

HOFFMAN HM et al: Prevention of cold-associated acute inflammation in familial cold autoinflammatory syndrome by interleukin-1 receptor antagonist. Lancet 364:1779, 2004

——— et al: Recurrent febrile syndromes: What a rheumatologist needs to know. Nat Rev Rheumatol 5:249, 2009

HULL KM et al: The TNF receptor–associated periodic syndrome (TRAPS). Emerging concepts of an autoinflammatory disorder. Medicine (Baltimore) 81:349, 2002

LOBITO AA et al: Abnormal disulfide-linked oligomerization results in ER retention and altered signaling by TNFR1 mutants in TNFR1-associated periodic fever syndrome (TRAPS). Blood 108:1320, 2006

MANDEY SH et al: A role for geranylgeranylation in interleukin-1β secretion. Arthritis Rheum 54:3690, 2006

MARIATHASAN S, MONACK DM: Inflammasome adaptors and sensors: Intracellular regulators of infection and inflammation. Nat Rev Immunol 7:31, 2007

MASTERS SL et al: Recent advances in the molecular pathogenesis of hereditary recurrent fevers. Curr Opin Allergy Clin Immunol 6:428, 2006

——— et al: Horror autoinflammaticus: The molecular pathophysiology of autoinflammatory disease (*). Annu Rev Immunol 27:621, 2009

RYAN JG, GOLDBACH-MANSKY R: The spectrum of autoinflammatory diseases: Recent bench to bedside observations. Curr Opin Rheumatol 20:66, 2008

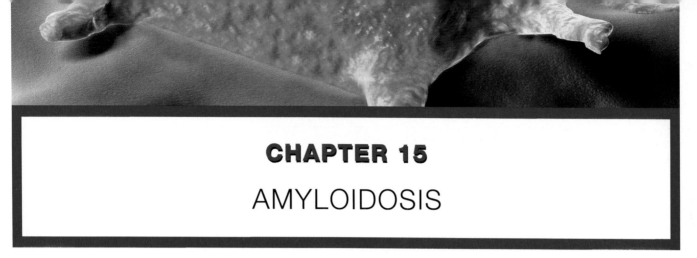

CHAPTER 15

AMYLOIDOSIS

David C. Seldin ■ Martha Skinner

GENERAL PRINCIPLES

Amyloidosis is a term for diseases that are due to the extracellular deposition of insoluble polymeric protein fibrils in tissues and organs. These diseases are a subset of a growing group of disorders caused by misfolding of proteins. Among these are Alzheimer's disease and other neurodegenerative diseases, transmissible prion diseases, and some genetic diseases caused by mutations that lead to misfolding and protein loss of function, such as certain of the cystic fibrosis mutations. Amyloid fibrils share a common β-pleated sheet structural conformation that confers unique staining properties. The name *amyloid* is attributed to the pathologist Virchow, who in 1854 thought such deposits were cellulose-like.

Amyloid diseases are defined by the biochemical nature of the protein in the fibril deposits and are classified according to whether they are systemic or localized, acquired or inherited, and by their clinical patterns (Table 15–1). The accepted nomenclature is *AX*, where *A* indicates amyloidosis and *X* represents the protein in the fibril. *AL* is amyloid composed of immunoglobulin (Ig) light chains (LCs), and is called *primary systemic amyloidosis*; it arises from a clonal B cell disorder, usually myeloma. *AF* groups the familial amyloidoses, most commonly due to transthyretin, the transport protein for thyroid hormone and retinol binding protein. *AA* amyloid is composed of the acute phase reactant serum amyloid A protein and occurs in the setting of chronic

inflammatory or infectious diseases. The disease associated with AA amyloid is called *secondary amyloidosis*. *Aβ₂M* is amyloid composed of β₂-microglobulin and occurs in individuals with end-stage renal disease (ESRD) of long duration. *Aβ* is the most common form of localized amyloidosis. *Aβ* is in the brain in Alzheimer's disease and is derived from abnormal proteolytic processing of the amyloid precursor protein (APP).

Diagnosis and treatment of the amyloidoses rests upon the pathologic diagnosis of amyloid deposits and immunohistochemical or biochemical identification of amyloid type (Fig. 15–1). In the systemic amyloidoses, the involved organs can be biopsied, but amyloid deposits may be found in any tissue of the body. Historically, blood vessels of the gingiva or rectal mucosa were examined, but the most easily accessible tissue, positive in more than 80% of patients with systemic amyloid, is fat. After local anesthesia, needle aspiration of fat from the abdominal wall can be expelled onto a slide and stained, avoiding even a minor surgical procedure. If this material is negative, kidney biopsy, endomyocardial biopsy, liver biopsy, or an endoscopic biopsy can be considered. The regular β sheet structure of amyloid deposits exhibits a unique green birefringence by polarized light microscopy when stained with Congo red dye; the 10-nm diameter fibrils can be seen by electron microscopy. Once amyloid is found, the protein type must be determined, usually by immunohistochemistry or immunoelectron microscopy. Careful evaluation of

TABLE 15-1

AMYLOID FIBRIL PROTEINS AND THEIR PRECURSORS

AMYLOID PROTEIN	PRECURSOR	SYSTEMIC (S) OR LOCALIZED (L)	SYNDROME OR INVOLVED TISSUES
AL	Immunoglobulin light chain	S, L	Primary Myeloma-associated
AH	Immunoglobulin heavy chain	S, L	Primary Myeloma-associated
ATTR	Transthyretin	S	Familial Senile systemic
		L?	Tenosynovium
Aβ_2M	β_2-microglobulin	S	Hemodialysis
		L?	Joints
AA	(Apo)serum AA	S	Secondary, reactive
AApoAI	Apolipoprotein AI	S	Familial
		L	Aortic
AApoAII	Apolipoprotein AII	S	Familial
AGel	Gelsolin	S	Familial
ALys	Lysozyme	S	Familial
AFib	Fibrinogen α-chain	S	Familial
ACys	Cystatin C	S	Familial
ABri[a]	ABriPP	L, S?	Familial dementia, British
ADan[a]	*ADanPP*	*L*	*Familial dementia, Danish*
Aβ	Aβ protein precursor (AβPP)	L	Alzheimer's disease, aging
APrP	Prion protein	L	Spongiform encephalopathies
ACal	(Pro)calcitonin	L	C-cell thyroid tumors
AIAPP	Islet amyloid polypeptide	L	Islets of Langerhans Insulinomas
AANF	Atrial natriuretic factor	L	Cardiac atria
APro	Prolactin	L	Aging pituitary Prolactinomas
AIns	Insulin	L	Iatrogenic
AMed	Lactadherin	L	Senile aortic, media
AKer	Kerato-epithelin	L	Cornea; familial
A(tbn)[b]	*tbn[b]*	*L*	*Pindborg tumors*
ALac	*Lactoferrin*	*L*	*Cornea; familial*

[a] ADan is coming from the same gene as ABri and has identical N-terminal sequence. It will be a matter of further discussion whether ADan should be included in the nomenclature as a separate protein (see text).
[b] To be named.
Note: Proteins in italics are preliminary.
Source: Reprinted from P Westermark et al: A primer of amyloid nomenclature. Amyloid 14(3):179–183, 2007. With permission from Taylor & Francis Ltd. (http://www.tandf.co.uk/journals).

the patient profile and clinical presentation, including age and ethnic origin, organ system involvement, underlying diseases, and family history should provide a clue to the type of amyloid.

The mechanisms of fibril formation and tissue toxicity remain controversial. A common underlying mechanism involves formation of intermolecular dimers by trans β sheet interactions of partially unfolded APP, leading to the formation of multimers and higher-order polymers. Factors that contribute to fibrillogenesis include variant or unstable protein structure; extensive β-sheet conformation of the precursor protein; proteolytic processing of the precursor protein; association with components of the serum or extracellular matrix (e.g., amyloid P-component, "amyloid enhancing factor" in spleen extracts, apolipoprotein E, or glycosaminoglycans), and local physical properties, including pH of the tissue. Once the fibrils reach a critical size, they become insoluble and deposit in extracellular tissue sites. These macromolecular deposits interfere with organ function, at least in part due to cellular uptake of oligomeric amyloid precursors producing toxicity to target cells.

The clinical syndromes of the amyloidoses are associated with relatively nonspecific alterations in routine laboratory tests. Blood counts are usually normal, although the erythrocyte sedimentation rate is frequently

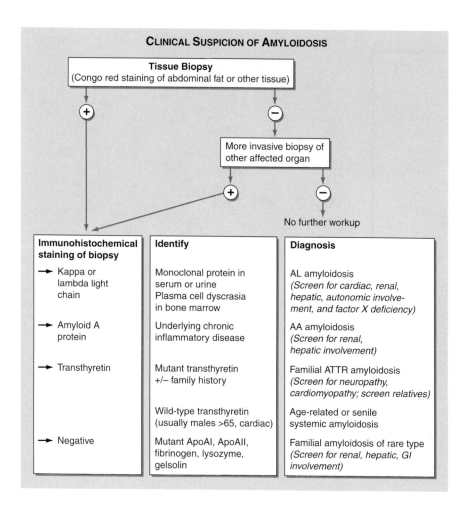

CLINICAL SUSPICION OF AMYLOIDOSIS

Tissue Biopsy
(Congo red staining of abdominal fat or other tissue)

(+)

(−) More invasive biopsy of other affected organ

(+)

(−) No further workup

Immunohistochemical staining of biopsy	Identify	Diagnosis
→ Kappa or lambda light chain	Monoclonal protein in serum or urine Plasma cell dyscrasia in bone marrow	AL amyloidosis *(Screen for cardiac, renal, hepatic, autonomic involvement, and factor X deficiency)*
→ Amyloid A protein	Underlying chronic inflammatory disease	AA amyloidosis *(Screen for renal, hepatic involvement)*
→ Transthyretin	Mutant transthyretin +/− family history	Familial ATTR amyloidosis *(Screen for neuropathy, cardiomyopathy; screen relatives)*
	Wild-type transthyretin (usually males >65, cardiac)	Age-related or senile systemic amyloidosis
→ Negative	Mutant ApoAI, ApoAII, fibrinogen, lysozyme, gelsolin	Familial amyloidosis of rare type *(Screen for renal, hepatic, GI involvement)*

FIGURE 15-1

Algorithm for the diagnosis of amyloidosis and determination of type: Clinical suspicion: unexplained nephropathy, cardiomyopathy, neuropathy, enteropathy, arthropathy, and macroglossia. ApoAI, apolipoprotein AI; ApoAII, apolipoprotein AII; GI, gastrointestinal.

elevated. Patients with renal involvement will usually have proteinuria, which can be as much as 30 g/d, producing hypoalbuminemia lower than 1 g/dL. Patients with cardiac involvement will often have elevation of brain naturietic peptide (BNP), pro–BNP, and troponin. These can be useful for monitoring disease activity and have been proposed as prognostic factors; they can be falsely elevated in the presence of renal insufficiency. Patients with liver involvement, even when it is advanced, usually develop cholestasis with an elevated alkaline phosphatase but minimal elevation of the transaminases and preservation of synthetic function. In AL amyloidosis, endocrinopathies can occur, with laboratory testing demonstrating hypothyroidism, hypoadrenalism, or even hypopituitarism. These findings are not specific for amyloidosis. Diagnosis of amyloidosis rests upon two pillars: the identification of fibrillar deposits in tissues and the typing of the amyloid.

AL AMYLOIDOSIS

ETIOLOGY AND INCIDENCE

AL amyloidosis is most frequently caused by a clonal expansion of plasma cells in the bone marrow that secrete a clonal Ig LC that deposits as amyloid fibrils in tissues. It may be purely serendipitous whether the clonal plasma cells produce an LC that misfolds and produces AL amyloidosis, or folds properly, allowing the cells to inexorably expand over time and develop into multiple myeloma. It is also possible that the two processes have differing molecular etiologies. AL amyloidosis can occur in multiple myeloma and other B lymphoproliferative diseases, including non-Hodgkin's lymphoma and Waldenstrom's macroglobulinemia. AL amyloidosis is the most common type of systemic amyloidosis in North America. Its incidence has been estimated at 4.5 per 100,000; however, ascertainment continues to be inadequate, and the true incidence may be much higher. AL amyloidosis, like other plasma cell diseases, usually occurs after age 40 and is often rapidly progressive and fatal if untreated. It occurs in about 15% of myelomas. About 20% of all patients with AL amyloidosis have myeloma; the rest have other B cell disorders.

DIAGNOSIS

Identification of a clonal plasma cell dyscrasia distinguishes AL from other types of amyloidosis. More than 90% of patients have a serum or urine monoclonal Ig protein that can be detected by immunofixation

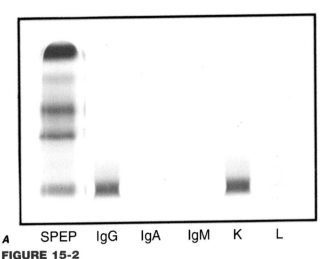

A | SPEP | IgG | IgA | IgM | K | L

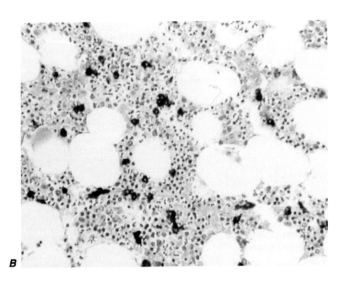

B

FIGURE 15-2

Laboratory features of AL amyloidosis. A. Serum immunofixation electrophoresis reveals an IgGκ monoclonal protein; the serum protein electrophoresis is often normal. **B.** Bone marrow biopsy specimen in another patient, stained with antibody to

λ light chain and developed with horseradish peroxidase, exhibits clonotypic λ-positive plasma cells (400×); antibody staining for κ would reveal few or no κ-positive cells. *(Photomicrograph courtesy of C. O'Hara; with permission.)*

electrophoresis (Fig. 15-2*A*) or free light chain assay. The standard serum protein electrophoresis (SPEP) and urine protein electrophoresis (UPEP) are not useful screening tests because the clonal Ig in AL amyloidosis, unlike in multiple myeloma, is often not present in sufficient quantity in the serum to produce a monoclonal "M-spike" by these tests. A commercially available nephelometric assay accurately quantifies abnormal LCs that circulate free of heavy chains in both multiple myeloma and AL amyloidosis. In AL, elevated levels of free LCs with a shift in the normal ratio of free kappa to lambda is seen in 75% of patients. Lambda LCs are more common than kappa LCs in AL amyloidosis. Examining the ratio is essential because in renal failure free light chain clearance is reduced, and both types of LCs will be elevated. In addition, an increased percentage of plasma cells in the bone marrow is noted in about 90% of patients; those cells are monoclonal by immunohistochemical staining for kappa and lambda (Fig. 15-2*B*), or by fluorescence-activated cell sorter. However, a monoclonal serum protein by itself is not diagnostic of amyloidosis, since monoclonal gammopathy of uncertain significance (MGUS) is common in older patients. However, when MGUS is present in a patient with biopsy-proven amyloidosis, the AL type is strongly suspected. Immunohistochemical staining of the amyloid deposits is useful if they bind one light chain antibody in preference to the other; some AL deposits bind many antisera nonspecifically. Immunoelectron microscopy can be more reliable but is not widely available. Mass spectrometry–based microsequencing of small amounts of protein extracted from fibril deposits may ultimately be the most reliable way to identify the components of

the fibrils. In ambiguous cases, other forms of amyloidosis should be thoroughly excluded.

PATHOLOGY AND CLINICAL FEATURES

Amyloid deposits are usually widespread in AL amyloidosis and can be present in the interstitium of any organ except the central nervous system. The amyloid fibril deposits are composed of intact 23 kDa monoclonal Ig LCs or smaller fragments, 11–18 kDa in size, representing the variable (V) region alone, or the V region and a portion of the constant (C) region. Although all kappa and lambda LC subtypes have been identified in AL amyloid fibrils, lambda subtypes predominate, and the lambda VI subtype appears to have unique structural properties that predispose it to fibril formation, often in the kidney.

AL amyloidosis is usually a rapidly progressive disease that presents with characteristic clinical syndromes, recognition of which is key to making the diagnosis. Initial symptoms of fatigue and weight loss are common, but the diagnosis is rarely made until symptoms referable to a specific organ appear. The kidneys are the most frequently affected organ (80%). Renal amyloidosis is usually manifested by proteinuria, which is often in the nephrotic range and associated with significant hypoalbuminemia and edema or anasarca; rarely, tubular rather than glomerular deposition of amyloid can produce azotemia without significant proteinuria. Cardiac symptoms are the second most common presentation (40%), but cardiac dysfunction is associated with death in 75% of patients. The electrocardiogram may show low voltage with a pseudo-infarct pattern. With significant cardiac

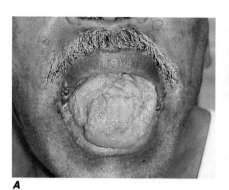

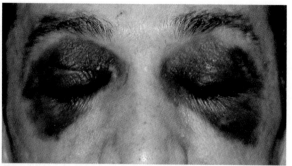

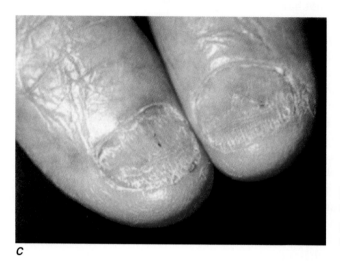

193

CHAPTER 15

Amyloidosis

FIGURE 15-3
Clinical signs of AL amyloidosis. A. Macroglossia. **B.** Periorbital ecchymoses. **C.** Fingernail dystrophy.

involvement, the echocardiogram will display concentrically thickened ventricles (the interventricular septal thickness is a useful parameter to monitor) and diastolic dysfunction; however, systolic function is preserved until late in the disease. Nervous system features include a peripheral sensory neuropathy (18%), carpal tunnel syndrome (25%), and/or autonomic dysfunction with gastrointestinal motility disturbances (early satiety, diarrhea, constipation) and orthostatic hypotension (16%). Macroglossia, with an enlarged, indented, or immobile tongue, is pathognomonic of AL amyloidosis and is seen in 10% of patients. Hepatomegaly, seen in 34% of patients, may be massive with cholestatic liver function abnormalities, although liver failure is uncommon. The spleen is frequently involved, and there may be functional hyposplenism in the absence of significant splenomegaly. Many patients report "easy bruising" due to amyloid deposits in capillaries and deficiency of clotting factor X; cutaneous ecchymoses appear, particularly around the eyes, giving the "raccoon-eyes" sign. Other findings include nail dystrophy, alopecia, and amyloid arthropathy with thickening of synovial membranes (**Fig. 15-3**).

Rx Treatment:
AL AMYLOIDOSIS

Extensive multisystem involvement typifies AL amyloidosis, and median survival with no treatment is usually about one year from the time of diagnosis. Current therapies target the clonal bone marrow plasma cells using approaches employed for multiple myeloma. Treatment with cyclic oral melphalan and prednisone can decrease the plasma cell burden but produces complete hematologic remission in only a few percent of patients and minimal organ responses and improvement in survival (median 2 years). The substitution of pulses of high-dose dexamethasone for prednisone produces a higher response rate and more durable remissions, although dexamethasone is not always well tolerated by patients with significant edema or cardiac disease. High-dose intravenous melphalan followed by autologous stem cell transplantation is far more effective than oral melphalan and prednisone. Complete hematologic response rates are about 40%, as measured by complete loss of clonal plasma cells in the bone marrow and disappearance of the monoclonal LC by immunofixation electrophoresis. In patients without a complete hematologic response, a significant improvement is often seen in hematologic parameters. Similar rates of improvement are seen in organ function and quality of life, with an extended survival exceeding that previously seen in this disease. The complete hematologic responses appear to be more durable than those seen in multiple myeloma and may even signal cure, as remissions of more than 10 years are documented. Unfortunately, only about half of AL amyloidosis patients are eligible for such aggressive treatment, and even at specialized treatment centers, peritransplant mortality is higher than for other hematologic diseases because of impaired organ function. Amyloid cardiomyopathy, poor nutritional status, impaired performance status, and multiple-organ disease contribute to excess morbidity and mortality. The bleeding diathesis due to adsorption of clotting factor X to amyloid fibrils also confers high mortality during myelosuppressive therapy; however, this syndrome occurs in only a few percent of patients. Age alone, or renal insufficiency, does not have a major impact on morbidity or outcome, and these factors alone should not exclude patients from such treatment. In selected patients, tandem transplantation may offer an even higher rate of hematologic response.

For patients with impaired cardiac function or arrhythmias due to amyloid involvement of the myocardium, median survival is only about 6 months without treatment, and stem cell mobilization and high-dose chemotherapy are dangerous. In these patients, cardiac transplantation can be performed, followed by treatment with high-dose melphalan and stem cell rescue to prevent amyloid deposition in the transplanted heart or other organs. Thalidomide and lenalidomide have activity; lenalidomide is reasonably well tolerated and, particularly in combination with dexamethasone, produces complete hematologic remissions and improvement in organ function. Novel agents such as the proteasome inhibitor bortezomib are also under investigation for AL amyloidosis.

Supportive care is important for patients with any type of amyloidosis. For nephrotic syndrome, diuretics and supportive stockings can ameliorate edema; angiotensin-converting enzyme inhibitors should be used with caution and have not been shown to slow renal disease progression. Congestive heart failure due to amyloid cardiomyopathy is also best treated with diuretics; it is important to note that digitalis, calcium channel blockers, and beta blockers are relatively contraindicated as they can interact with amyloid fibrils and produce heart block and worsening heart failure. Amiodarone has been used for atrial and ventricular arrhythmias. Automatic implantable defibrillators have reduced effectiveness due to the thickened myocardium. Atrial ablation is another effective approach for atrial fibrillation. For conduction abnormalities, ventricular pacing may be indicated. Atrial contractile dysfunction is common in amyloid cardiomyopathy, and is an indication for anticoagulation. Autonomic neuropathy can be treated with α agonists such as midodrine to support the blood pressure; gastrointestinal dysfunction may respond to motility or bulk agents. Nutritional supplementation, either orally or parenterally, is also important.

In localized AL, amyloid deposits can be produced by clonal plasma cells infiltrating local sites in the airways, bladder, skin, or lymph nodes (Table 15-1). Deposits may respond to surgical intervention or radiation therapy; systemic treatment is generally not appropriate. Patients should be referred to a center familiar with management of these rare manifestations of amyloidosis.

AA AMYLOIDOSIS

ETIOLOGY AND INCIDENCE

AA amyloidosis can occur in association with almost any of the chronic inflammatory states (e.g., rheumatoid arthritis, lupus, Crohn's disease) or chronic infections such as tuberculosis or subacute bacterial endocarditis. In the United States and Europe, AA amyloidosis has become uncommon, occurring in <1% of patients with these diseases, perhaps because of advances in anti-inflammatory and antimicrobial therapies. Nonetheless, in Finland AA amyloidosis was reported to be the most common cause of nephrotic syndrome in patients with rheumatoid arthritis. AA amyloidosis is more common in Turkey and the Middle East, where it occurs in association with familial Mediterranean fever. It is the only type of systemic amyloidosis that occurs in children.

PATHOLOGY AND CLINICAL FEATURES

Deposits are more limited in AA amyloidosis than in AL amyloidosis; they usually begin in the kidneys. Hepatomegaly, splenomegaly, and autonomic neuropathy can occur as the disease progresses; cardiomyopathy occurs rarely. The symptoms and signs are similar to those described for AL amyloidosis. The AA amyloid fibrils are usually composed of an 8-kDa, 76 amino acid N-terminal portion of a 12-kDa precursor protein, serum amyloid A (SAA). SAA is an acute-phase apoprotein synthesized in the liver and transported by high-density lipoprotein, HDL3, in the plasma. Several years of an underlying inflammatory disease causing chronic elevation of SAA usually precedes fibril formation, although infections can produce AA deposition more quickly. In mouse models and perhaps in people, AA fibril formation can be accelerated by an amyloid enhancing factor present in high concentration in the spleen (which may be early SAA aggregates or deposits), by basement membrane heparan sulfate proteoglycan, or by seeding with AA or heterologous fibrils.

℞ **Treatment:**
AA AMYLOIDOSIS

The primary therapy in AA amyloidosis is treatment of the underlying inflammatory or infectious disease. Treatment that suppresses or eliminates the inflammation or infection also decreases the SAA protein concentration. For familial Mediterranean fever, colchicine in a dose of 1.2–1.8 mg/d is the appropriate treatment. Colchicine has not been helpful for AA amyloidosis of other causes or for other amyloidoses. A multicenter randomized phase III trial has recently been completed using eprodisate, designed to interfere with the interaction of AA amyloid protein with glycosaminoglycans in tissues and thus prevent or disrupt fibril formation. This drug is well tolerated and appears to markedly delay progression of AA renal disease, regardless of the underlying inflammatory process. Eprodisate is the first targeted inhibitor for diseases of protein misfolding and deposition to become available to patients.

AF AMYLOIDOSIS

The inherited AF amyloidoses are autosomal dominant diseases in which a variant plasma protein forms amyloid deposits, beginning in midlife. These diseases are rare, with an estimated incidence of <1 per 100,000. The most common form of AF is caused by mutation of the abundant plasma protein transthyretin (TTR, also known as *prealbumin*). More than 100 TTR mutations are known, and most are associated with ATTR amyloidosis. One variant, Ile122, has a carrier frequency that may be as high as 4% in the African-American population and is associated with late-onset cardiac amyloidosis. The actual incidence of disease in the African-American population is the subject of ongoing clinical research, but it would be wise to consider this in the differential diagnosis of African-American patients who present with concentric cardiac hypertrophy and evidence of diastolic dysfunction, whether or not they have a history of hypertension. Even wild-type TTR can form fibrils, leading to so-called senile systemic amyloidosis (SSA) in older patients. It can be found in up to 25% of autopsies in patients over age 80, and it can produce a clinical syndrome of amyloid cardiomyopathy that is similar to that occurring in younger patients with mutant TTR. Other familial amyloidoses, caused by variant apolipoproteins AI or AII, gelsolin, fibrinogen Aα, or lysozyme, are reported in only a few families worldwide.

In ATTR and in other forms of familial amyloidosis, the variant structure of the precursor protein is the key factor in fibril formation. The role of aging is intriguing, since patients born with the variant proteins do not have clinically apparent disease until middle age, despite the lifelong presence of the abnormal protein. Further evidence of an age-related "trigger" is the occurrence of SSA in the elderly, caused by the deposition of fibrils derived from normal TTR.

AF amyloidosis has a variable presentation but is usually consistent within affected kindreds with the same mutant protein. A family history makes AF more likely, but many patients present sporadically with new mutations. ATTR usually presents as a syndrome of familial amyloidotic polyneuropathy or familial amyloidotic cardiomyopathy; within a family, the age of disease onset is usually consistent. Peripheral neuropathy begins as a lower-extremity sensory and motor neuropathy and progresses to the upper extremities. Autonomic neuropathy is manifest by gastrointestinal symptoms of diarrhea with weight loss and orthostatic hypotension. Patients with TTR Met-30, the most common mutation, have normal echocardiograms but may have conduction defects and require a pacemaker. Patients with TTR Ala-60 and several other mutations have myocardial thickening similar to that caused by AL amyloidosis, although heart failure is less common and the prognosis is better. Vitreous opacities caused by amyloid deposits are pathognomonic of ATTR amyloidosis.

Other AF syndromes include those associated with inherited mutations in apolipoprotein AI (AApoAI), apolipoprotein AII (AApoAII), fibrinogen (AFib), lysozyme (ALys), and gelsolin (AGel) that cause amyloid fibril deposition. These are very rare disorders with slowly progressing dysfunction of kidneys, liver, gastrointestinal tract, and, in the case of gelsolin, abnormalities of the cranial nerves and cornea.

Patients with AF amyloidosis can present with clinical syndromes that mimic those of patients with AL. Patients who do not have a plasma cell disorder should be screened for AF. This is particularly important in ethnic populations with a high carrier frequency of AF alleles (e.g., patients of Portuguese decent, African Americans). Variant TTR proteins can usually be detected by isoelectric focusing, but DNA sequencing is the gold standard for diagnosis for ATTR and the other AF mutations.

℞ **Treatment:**
ATTR AMYLOIDOSIS

Without intervention, survival after ATTR disease onset is 5–15 years. Orthotopic liver transplantation removes the major source of variant TTR production and replaces it with a source of normal TTR; it also arrests disease progression and leads to improvement in autonomic and peripheral neuropathy in some patients. Cardiomyopathy often does not improve, and in some patients it can worsen after liver transplantation, perhaps due to deposition of wild-type TTR as seen in SSA. Compounds have been identified that stabilize TTR in a nonpathogenic tetrameric conformation. The first of these, diflunisal, is being studied in a multicenter phase III trial, and screens for other agents are ongoing.

Aβ₂M AMYLOIDOSIS

Aβ₂M amyloidosis is composed of β₂-microglobulin, the invariant chain of class I human leukocyte antigens, and produces rheumatologic manifestations in patients on long-term hemodialysis. β₂-microglobulin is excreted by the kidney, and levels become elevated in ESRD. The molecular mass of β₂M is 11.8 kDa, above the molecular mass cutoff of some dialysis membranes. The incidence of this disease appears to be declining with newer dialysis techniques.

Aβ₂M amyloidosis usually presents with carpal tunnel syndrome, persistent joint effusions, spondyloarthropathy, and cystic bone lesions. Carpal tunnel syndrome is often the first symptom of disease. In the past, persistent joint effusions accompanied by mild discomfort had been seen in up to 50% of patients on dialysis for more than 12 years. Involvement is bilateral, and large joints (shoulders, knees, wrists, and hips) are more frequently affected. The synovial fluid is non-inflammatory, and β₂M amyloid deposits can be found if the sediment is stained with Congo red. Although less common, visceral β₂M amyloid deposits do occasionally occur in the gastrointestinal tract, heart, tendons, and subcutaneous tissues of the buttocks. There is no specific therapy for Aβ₂M amyloidosis, but cessation of dialysis after renal allograft may lead to symptomatic improvement.

SUMMARY

A diagnosis of amyloidosis should be considered in patients with unexplained nephropathy, cardiomyopathy (particularly with diastolic dysfunction), neuropathy (either peripheral or autonomic), enteropathy, or the pathognomonic soft tissue findings of macroglossia and periorbital ecchymoses. Pathologic identification of amyloid fibrils can be made; Congo red staining of aspirated abdominal fat is the initial test of choice in most cases. Accurate typing using a combination of immunologic, biochemical, and genetic testing is essential to choosing the appropriate therapy (see algorithm for workup, Fig. 15-1). For difficult cases, referral centers can provide specialized diagnostic techniques and access to clinical trials.

FURTHER READINGS

AKAR H et al: Quantitative serum free light-chain assay in the diagnostic evaluation of AL amyloidosis. Amyloid J Protein Folding Disorders 12:210, 2005

BENSON M: AMYLOIDOSIS, in *The Metabolic and Molecular Bases of Inherited Disease*, 8th ed, CR Scriver et al (eds). New York, McGraw- Hill, 2001, pp 5345–5378

DEMBER LM et al: Effect of intravenous melphalan and autologous blood stem cell transplant on AL amyloidosis–associated renal disease. Ann Intern Med 134:746, 2001

——— et al: Eprodisate for the treatment of renal disease in AA amyloidosis. N Engl J Med 356:2349, 2007

———: Modern treatment of amyloidosis: Unresolved questions. J Am Soc Nephrol 20:469, 2009

MERLINI G, BELLOTTI V: Molecular mechanisms of amyloidosis. N Engl J Med 349:583, 2003

RAJKUMAR SV, GERTZ MA: Advances in the treatment of amyloidosis. N Engl J Med 356:2413, 2007

SELDIN DC et al: Improvement in quality of life of patients with AL amyloidosis treated with high-dose melphalan and autologous stem cell transplantation. Blood 104:1888, 2004

——— et al: Successful treatment of AL amyloidosis with high-dose melphalan and autologous stem cell transplantation in patients over age 65. Blood 108:3945, 2006

SKINNER M et al: High-dose melphalan and autologous stem-cell transplantation in patients with AL amyloidosis: An 8-year study. Ann Intern Med 140:85, 2004

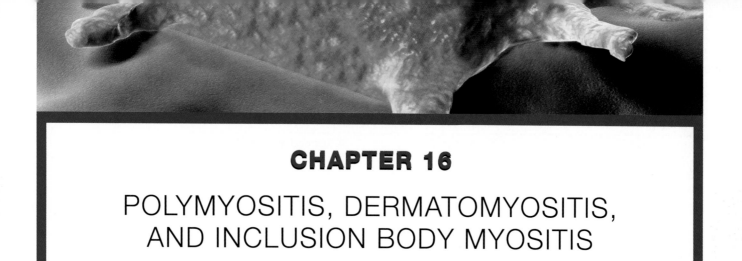

CHAPTER 16

POLYMYOSITIS, DERMATOMYOSITIS, AND INCLUSION BODY MYOSITIS

Marinos C. Dalakas

The inflammatory myopathies represent the largest group of acquired and potentially treatable causes of skeletal muscle weakness. They are classified into three major groups: polymyositis (PM), dermatomyositis (DM), and inclusion body myositis (IBM).

CLINICAL FEATURES

The prevalence of the inflammatory myopathies is estimated at 1 in 100,000. PM as a stand-alone entity is a rare disease affecting adults. DM affects both children and adults and women more often than men. IBM is three times more frequent in men than in women, more common in Caucasians than blacks, and is most likely to affect persons >50 years of age.

These disorders present as progressive and symmetric muscle weakness except for IBM, which can have an asymmetric pattern. Patients usually report increasing difficulty with everyday tasks requiring the use of proximal muscles, such as getting up from a chair, climbing steps, stepping onto a curb, lifting objects, or combing hair. Fine-motor movements that depend on the strength of distal muscles, such as buttoning a shirt, sewing, knitting, or writing, are affected only late in the course of PM and DM, but fairly early in IBM. Falling is common in IBM because of early involvement of the quadriceps muscle with buckling of the knees. Ocular muscles are spared, even in advanced, untreated cases; if these muscles are affected, the diagnosis of inflammatory

myopathy should be questioned. Facial muscles are unaffected in PM and DM, but mild facial muscle weakness is common in patients with IBM. In all forms of inflammatory myopathy, pharyngeal and neck-flexor muscles are often involved, causing dysphagia or difficulty in holding up the head (*head drop*). In advanced and rarely in acute cases, respiratory muscles may also be affected. Severe weakness, if untreated, is almost always associated with muscle wasting. Sensation remains normal. The tendon reflexes are preserved but may be absent in severely weakened or atrophied muscles, especially in IBM where atrophy of the quadriceps and the distal muscles is common. Myalgia and muscle tenderness may occur in a small number of patients, usually early in the disease, and particularly in DM associated with connective tissue disorders. Weakness in PM and DM progresses subacutely over a period of weeks or months and rarely acutely; by contrast, IBM progresses very slowly, over years, simulating a late-life muscular dystrophy or slowly progressive motor neuron disorder.

SPECIFIC FEATURES

(Table 16-1)

Polymyositis

The actual onset of PM is often not easily determined, and patients typically delay seeking medical advice for

TABLE 16-1

FEATURES ASSOCIATED WITH INFLAMMATORY MYOPATHIES

CHARACTERISTIC	POLYMYOSITIS	DERMATOMYOSITIS	INCLUSION BODY MYOSITIS
Age at onset	>18 yr	Adulthood and childhood	>50 yr
Familial association	No	No	Yes, in some cases
Extramuscular manifestations	Yes	Yes	Yes
Associated conditions			
Connective tissue diseases	Yes[a]	Scleroderma and mixed connective tissue disease (overlap syndromes)	Yes, in up to 20% of cases[a]
Systemic autoimmune diseases[b]	Frequent	Infrequent	Infrequent
Malignancy	No	Yes, in up to 15% of cases	No
Viruses	Yes[c]	Unproven	Yes[c]
Drugs[d]	Yes	Yes, rarely	No
Parasites and bacteria[e]	Yes	No	No

[a]Systemic lupus erythematosus, rheumatoid arthritis, Sjögren's syndrome, systemic sclerosis, mixed connective tissue disease.

[b]Crohn's disease, vasculitis, sarcoidosis, primary biliary cirrhosis, adult celiac disease, chronic graft-versus-host disease, discoid lupus, ankylosing spondylitis, Behçet's syndrome, myasthenia gravis, acne fulminans, dermatitis herpetiformis, psoriasis, Hashimoto's disease, granulomatous diseases, agammaglobulinemia, monoclonal gammopathy, hypereosinophilic syndrome, Lyme disease, Kawasaki disease, autoimmune thrombocytopenia, hypergammaglobulinemic purpura, hereditary complement deficiency, IgA deficiency.

[c]HIV (human immunodeficiency virus) and HTLV-I (human T cell lymphotropic virus type I).

[d]Drugs include penicillamine (dermatomyositis and polymyositis), zidovudine (polymyositis), and contaminated tryptophan (dermatomyositis-like illness). Other myotoxic drugs may cause myopathy but not an inflammatory myopathy (see text for details).

[e]Parasites (protozoa, cestodes, nematodes), tropical and bacterial myositis (pyomyositis).

several months. This is in contrast to DM, in which the rash facilitates early recognition (see below). PM mimics many other myopathies and is a diagnosis of exclusion. It is a subacute inflammatory myopathy affecting adults, and rarely children, who *do not have* any of the following: rash, involvement of the extraocular and facial muscles, family history of a neuromuscular disease, history of exposure to myotoxic drugs or toxins, endocrinopathy, neurogenic disease, muscular dystrophy, biochemical muscle disorder (deficiency of a muscle enzyme), or IBM as excluded by muscle biopsy analysis (see below). As an isolated entity, PM is a rare (and overdiagnosed) disorder; more commonly, PM occurs in association with a systemic autoimmune or connective tissue disease, or with a known viral or bacterial infection. Drugs, especially D-penicillamine or zidovudine (AZT), may also produce an inflammatory myopathy similar to PM.

Dermatomyositis

DM is a distinctive entity identified by a characteristic rash accompanying, or more often preceding, muscle weakness. The rash may consist of a blue–purple discoloration on the upper eyelids with edema (heliotrope rash), a flat red rash on the face and upper trunk, and erythema of the knuckles with a raised violaceous scaly eruption (*Gottron's sign*). The erythematous rash can also occur on other body surfaces, including the knees, elbows, malleoli, neck and anterior chest (often in a *V sign*), or back and shoulders (*shawl sign*), and may worsen after sun exposure. In some patients the rash is pruritic, especially on the scalp, chest, and back. Dilated capillary loops at the base of the fingernails are also characteristic. The cuticles may be irregular, thickened, and distorted, and the lateral and palmar areas of the fingers may become rough and cracked, with irregular, "dirty" horizontal lines, resembling *mechanic's hands*. The weakness can be mild, moderate, or severe enough to lead to quadriparesis. At times, the muscle strength appears normal, hence the term *dermatomyositis sine myositis*. When muscle biopsy is performed in such cases, however, significant perivascular and perimysial inflammation is often seen.

DM usually occurs alone but may overlap with scleroderma and mixed connective tissue disease. Fasciitis and thickening of the skin, similar to that seen in chronic cases of DM, have occurred in patients with the *eosinophilia-myalgia syndrome* associated with the ingestion of contaminated L-tryptophan.

Inclusion Body Myositis

In patients ≥50 years of age, IBM is the most common of the inflammatory myopathies. It is often misdiagnosed as PM and is suspected only later when a patient with presumed PM does not respond to therapy. Weakness and atrophy of the distal muscles, especially foot extensors and deep finger flexors, occur in almost all cases of IBM and may be a clue to early diagnosis. Some patients present with falls because their knees collapse due to early quadriceps weakness. Others present with weakness in the small muscles of the hands, especially finger flexors, and complain of inability to hold objects such as golf clubs or perform tasks such as turning keys or tying knots. On occasion, the weakness and accompanying atrophy can be asymmetric and selectively involve the quadriceps, iliopsoas, triceps, biceps, and finger flexors, resembling a lower motor neuron disease. Dysphagia is common, occurring in up to 60% of IBM patients, and may lead to episodes of choking. Sensory examination is generally normal; some patients have mildly diminished vibratory sensation at the ankles that presumably is age related. The pattern of distal weakness, which superficially resembles motor neuron or peripheral nerve disease, results from the myopathic process affecting distal muscles selectively. Disease progression is slow but steady, and most patients require an assistive device such as a cane, walker, or wheelchair within several years of onset.

In at least 20% of cases, IBM is associated with systemic autoimmune or connective tissue diseases. Familial aggregation of typical IBM may occur; such cases have been designated as *familial inflammatory IBM*. This disorder is distinct from *hereditary inclusion body myopathy* (h-IBM), which describes a heterogeneous group of recessive, and less frequently dominant, inherited syndromes; the h-IBMs are noninflammatory myopathies. A subset of h-IBM that spares the quadriceps muscles has emerged as a distinct entity. This disorder, originally described in Iranian Jews and now seen in many ethnic groups, is linked to chromosome 9p1 and results from mutations in the UDP-*N*-acetylglucosamine 2-epimerase/*N*-acetylmannosamine kinase (*GNE*) gene.

ASSOCIATED CLINICAL FINDINGS

Extramuscular Manifestations

These may be present to a varying degree in patients with PM or DM, and include:

1. *Systemic symptoms,* such as fever, malaise, weight loss, arthralgia, and Raynaud's phenomenon, especially when inflammatory myopathy is associated with a connective tissue disorder.
2. *Joint contractures,* mostly in DM and especially in children.
3. *Dysphagia and gastrointestinal symptoms,* due to involvement of oropharyngeal striated muscles and upper esophagus, especially in DM and IBM.
4. *Cardiac disturbances,* including atrioventricular conduction defects, tachyarrhythmias, dilated cardiomyopathy, a low ejection fraction, and congestive heart failure, which may rarely occur, either from the disease itself or from hypertension associated with long-term use of glucocorticoids.

5. *Pulmonary dysfunction,* due to weakness of the thoracic muscles, interstitial lung disease, or drug-induced pneumonitis (e.g., from methotrexate), which may cause dyspnea, nonproductive cough, and aspiration pneumonia. Interstitial lung disease may precede myopathy or occur early in the disease and develops in up to 10% of patients with PM or DM, most of whom have antibodies to t-RNA synthetases, as described below.
6. *Subcutaneous calcifications,* in DM, sometimes extruding on the skin and causing ulcerations and infections.
7. *Arthralgias,* synovitis, or deforming arthropathy with subluxation in the interphalangeal joints can occur in some patients with DM and PM who have Jo-1 antibodies (see below).

Association with Malignancies

Although all the inflammatory myopathies can have a chance association with malignant lesions, especially in older age groups, the incidence of malignant conditions appears to be specifically increased only in patients with DM and not in those with PM or IBM. The most common tumors associated with DM are ovarian cancer, breast cancer, melanoma, colon cancer, and non-Hodgkin's lymphoma. The extent of the search that should be conducted for an occult neoplasm in adults with DM depends on the clinical circumstances. Tumors in these patients are usually uncovered by abnormal findings in the medical history and physical examination and not through an extensive blind search. The weight of evidence argues against performing expensive, invasive, and nondirected tumor searches. A complete annual physical examination with pelvic, breast (mammogram, if indicated), and rectal examinations (with colonoscopy according to age and family history); urinalysis; complete blood count; blood chemistry tests; and a chest film should suffice in most cases. In Asians, nasopharyngeal cancer is common, and a careful examination of ears, nose, and throat is indicated.

Overlap Syndromes

These describe the association of inflammatory myopathies with connective tissue diseases. A well-characterized overlap syndrome occurs in patients with DM who also have manifestations of systemic sclerosis or mixed connective tissue disease, such as sclerotic thickening of the dermis, contractures, esophageal hypomotility, microangiopathy, and calcium deposits (Table 16-1). By contrast, signs of rheumatoid arthritis, systemic lupus erythematosus, or Sjögren's syndrome are very rare in patients with DM. Patients with the overlap syndrome of DM and systemic sclerosis may have a specific antinuclear antibody, the anti-PM/Scl, directed against a nucleolar-protein complex.

An autoimmune etiology of the inflammatory myopathies is indirectly supported by an association with other autoimmune or connective tissue diseases; the presence of various autoantibodies; an association with specific major histocompatibility complex (MHC) genes; demonstration of T cell–mediated myocytotoxicity or complement-mediated microangiopathy; and a response to immunotherapy.

Autoantibodies and Immunogenetics

Various autoantibodies against nuclear antigens (antinuclear antibodies) and cytoplasmic antigens are found in up to 20% of patients with inflammatory myopathies. The antibodies to cytoplasmic antigens are directed against ribonucleoproteins involved in protein synthesis (anti-synthetases) or translational transport (anti–signal-recognition particles). The antibody directed against the histidyl-transfer RNA synthetase, called *anti–Jo-1*, accounts for 75% of all the anti-synthetases and is clinically useful because up to 80% of patients with anti–Jo-1 antibodies have interstitial lung disease. Some patients with the anti–Jo-1 antibody also have Raynaud's phenomenon, nonerosive arthritis, and the MHC molecules DR3 and DRw52. DR3 haplotypes (molecular designation DRB1*0301, DQB1*0201) occur in up to 75% of patients with PM and IBM, whereas in juvenile DM there is an increased frequency of DQA1*0501 (Chap. 2).

Immunopathologic Mechanisms

In DM, humoral immune mechanisms are implicated, resulting in a microangiopathy and muscle ischemia (**Fig. 16-1**). Endomysial inflammatory infiltrates are composed of B cells located in proximity to CD4 T cells,

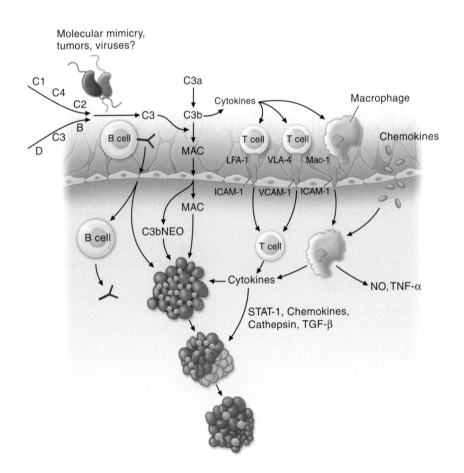

FIGURE 16-1

Immunopathogenesis of dermatomyositis. Activation of complement, possibly by autoantibodies (Y), against endothelial cells and formation of C3 via the classic or alternative pathway. Activated C3 leads to formation of C3b, C3bNEO, and membrane attack complexes (MAC), which are deposited in and around the endothelial cell wall of the endomysial capillaries. Deposition of MAC leads to destruction of capillaries, ischemia, or microinfarcts most prominent in the periphery of the fascicles, and perifascicular atrophy. B cells, CD4 T cells, and macrophages traffic from the circulation to the muscle. Endothelial expression of vascular cell adhesion molecule (VCAM) and intercellular adhesion molecule (ICAM) is induced by cytokines released by the mononuclear cells. Integrins, specifically very late activation antigen (VLA)-4 and leukocyte function-associated antigen (LFA)-1, bind VCAM and ICAM and promote T-cell and macrophage infiltration of muscle through the endothelial cell wall.

dendritic cells, and macrophages; there is a relative absence of lymphocytic invasion of nonnecrotic muscle fibers. Activation of the complement C5b-9 membranolytic attack complex is thought to be a critical early event that triggers release of proinflammatory cytokines and chemokines, induces expression of vascular cell adhesion molecule (VCAM) 1 and intracellular adhesion molecule (ICAM) 1 on endothelial cells, and facilitates migration of activated lymphoid cells to the perimysial and endomysial spaces. Necrosis of the endothelial cells, reduced numbers of endomysial capillaries, ischemia, and muscle-fiber destruction resembling microinfarcts occur. The remaining capillaries often have dilated lumens in response to the ischemic process. Larger intramuscular blood vessels may also be affected in the same pattern. Residual perifascicular atrophy reflects the endofascicular hypoperfusion that is prominent in the periphery of the muscle fascicles.

By contrast, in PM and IBM a mechanism of T cell–mediated cytotoxicity is likely. CD8 T cells, along with macrophages, initially surround and eventually invade and destroy healthy, nonnecrotic muscle fibers

that aberrantly express class I MHC molecules. MHC-I expression, absent from the sarcolemma of normal muscle fibers, is probably induced by cytokines secreted by activated T cells and macrophages. The CD8/MHC-I complex is characteristic of PM and IBM; its detection can aid in confirming the histologic diagnosis of PM, as discussed below. The cytotoxic CD8 T cells contain perforin and granzyme granules directed towards the surface of the muscle fibers and capable of inducing myonecrosis. Analysis of T-cell receptor molecules expressed by the infiltrating CD8 cells have revealed clonal expansion and conserved sequences in the antigen-binding region, both suggesting an antigen-driven T-cell response. Whether the putative antigens are endogenous (e.g., muscle) or exogenous (e.g., viral) sequences is unknown. Viruses have not been identified within the muscle fibers. Co-stimulatory molecules and their counterreceptors, which are fundamental for T-cell activation and antigen recognition, are strongly upregulated in PM and IBM. Key molecules involved in T cell–mediated cytotoxicity are depicted in **Fig. 16-2**.

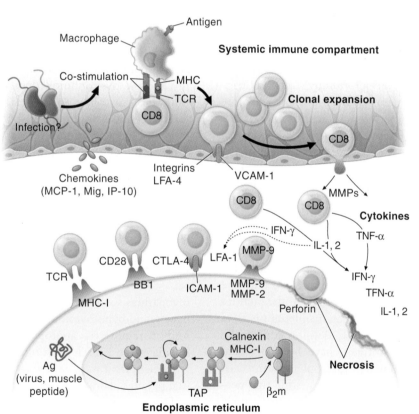

FIGURE 16-2

Cell-mediated mechanisms of muscle damage in polymyositis (PM) and inclusion body myositis (IBM). Antigen-specific CD8 cells are expanded in the periphery, cross the endothelial barrier, and bind directly to muscle fibers via T-cell receptor (TCR) molecules that recognize aberrantly expressed MHC-I. Engagement of co-stimulatory molecules (BB1 and ICOSL) with their ligands (CD28, CTLA-4, and ICOS) along with ICAM-1/LFA-1, stabilize the CD8–muscle fiber interaction. Metalloproteinases (MMP) facilitate the migration of T cells and their attachment to the muscle surface. Muscle fiber necrosis occurs via perforin granules released by the autoaggressive T cells. A direct myocytotoxic effect exerted by the cytokines interferon (IFN) γ, interleukin (IL) 1, or tumor necrosis factor (TNF) α may also play a role. Death of the muscle fiber is mediated by necrosis. MHC class I molecules consist of a heavy chain and a light chain [β_2 microglobulin (β_2m)] complexed with an antigenic peptide that is transported into the endoplasmic reticulum by TAP proteins (Chap. 2).

The Role of Nonimmune Factors in IBM

In IBM, the presence of β-amyloid deposits within vacuolated muscle fibers and abnormal mitochondria with cytochrome oxidase–negative fibers suggest that, in addition to the autoimmune component, there is also a degenerative process. Similar to Alzheimer's disease, the amyloid deposits in IBM are immunoreactive against amyloid precursor protein (APP), chymotrypsin, apolipoprotein E, and phosphorylated tau, but it is unclear whether these deposits are directly pathogenic or represent secondary phenomena. The same is true for the mitochondrial abnormalities, which may also be secondary to the effects of aging or a bystander effect of upregulated cytokines. Expression of cytokines and upregulation of MHC class I by the muscle fibers may cause an endoplasmic reticulum stress response resulting in intracellular accumulation of misfolded glycoproteins and activation of nuclear factor κB (NFκB), leading to further cytokine activation.

Association with Viral Infections and the Role of Retroviruses

Several viruses, including coxsackieviruses, influenza, paramyxoviruses, mumps, cytomegalovirus, and Epstein-Barr virus, have been indirectly associated with myositis. For the coxsackieviruses, an autoimmune myositis triggered by molecular mimicry has been proposed because of structural homology between histidyl-transfer RNA synthetase, which is the target of the Jo-1 antibody (see above), and genomic RNA of an animal picornavirus, the encephalomyocarditis virus. Sensitive polymerase chain reaction (PCR) studies, however, have repeatedly failed to confirm the presence of such viruses in muscle biopsies.

The best evidence of a viral connection in PM and IBM is with the retroviruses. Some individuals infected with HIV or with human T cell lymphotropic virus I (HTLV-I) develop PM or IBM; a similar disorder has been described in nonhuman primates infected with the simian immunodeficiency virus. The inflammatory myopathy may occur as the initial manifestation of a retroviral infection, or myositis may develop later in the disease course. Retroviral antigens have been detected only in occasional endomysial macrophages and not within the muscle fibers themselves, suggesting that persistent infection and viral replication within the muscle do not occur. Histologic findings are identical to retroviral-negative PM or IBM. The infiltrating T cells in the muscle are clonally driven and a number of them are retroviral specific. This disorder should be distinguished from a toxic myopathy related to long-term therapy with AZT, characterized by fatigue, myalgia, mild muscle weakness, and mild elevation of creatine kinase (CK). AZT-induced myopathy, which generally improves when the drug is discontinued, is a mitochondrial disorder characterized histologically by "ragged-red"

fibers. AZT inhibits γ-DNA polymerase, an enzyme found solely in the mitochondrial matrix.

DIFFERENTIAL DIAGNOSIS

The clinical picture of the typical skin rash and proximal or diffuse muscle weakness has few causes other than DM. However, proximal muscle weakness without skin involvement can be due to many conditions other than PM or IBM.

Subacute or Chronic Progressive Muscle Weakness

This may be due to denervating conditions such as the spinal muscular atrophies or amyotrophic lateral sclerosis. In addition to the muscle weakness, upper motor neuron signs in the latter and signs of denervation detected by electromyography (EMG) aid in the diagnosis. The muscular dystrophies may be additional considerations; however, these disorders usually develop over years rather than weeks or months and rarely present after the age of 30. It may be difficult, even with a muscle biopsy, to distinguish chronic PM from a rapidly advancing muscular dystrophy. This is particularly true of facioscapulohumeral muscular dystrophy, dysferlin myopathy, and the dystrophinopathies where inflammatory cell infiltration is often found early in the disease. Such doubtful cases should always be given an adequate trial of glucocorticoid therapy and undergo genetic testing to exclude muscular dystrophy. Identification of the MHC/CD8 lesion by muscle biopsy is helpful to identify cases of PM. Some metabolic myopathies, including glycogen storage disease due to myophosphorylase or acid maltase deficiency, lipid storage myopathies due to carnitine deficiency, and mitochondrial diseases produce weakness that is often associated with other characteristic clinical signs; diagnosis rests upon histochemical and biochemical studies of the muscle biopsy. The endocrine myopathies such as those due to hypercorticosteroidism, hyper- and hypothyroidism, and hyper- and hypoparathyroidism require the appropriate laboratory investigations for diagnosis. Muscle wasting in patients with an underlying neoplasm may be due to disuse, cachexia, or rarely to a paraneoplastic neuromyopathy.

Diseases of the neuromuscular junction, including myasthenia gravis or the Lambert-Eaton myasthenic syndrome, cause fatiguing weakness that also affects ocular and other cranial muscles. Repetitive nerve stimulation and single-fiber EMG studies aid in diagnosis.

Acute Muscle Weakness

This may be caused by an acute neuropathy such as Guillain-Barré syndrome, transverse myelitis, a neurotoxin, or a neurotropic viral infection such as poliomyelitis or

West Nile virus. When acute weakness is associated with painful muscle cramps, rhabdomyolysis, and myoglobinuria, it may be due to a viral infection or a metabolic disorder such as myophosphorylase deficiency or carnitine palmitoyltransferase deficiency. Several animal parasites, including protozoa (*toxoplasma, trypanosoma*), cestodes (*cysticerci*), and nematodes (*trichinae*), may produce a focal or diffuse inflammatory myopathy known as *parasitic polymyositis*. *Staphylococcus aureus*, *Yersinia*, *Streptococcus*, or anaerobic bacteria may produce a suppurative myositis, known as *tropical polymyositis*, or *pyomyositis*. Pyomyositis, previously rare in the West, is now occasionally seen in AIDS patients. Other bacteria, such as *Borrelia burgdorferi* (Lyme disease) and *Legionella pneumophila* (Legionnaire's disease) may infrequently cause myositis.

Patients with periodic paralysis experience recurrent episodes of acute muscle weakness without pain, always beginning in childhood. Chronic alcoholics may develop painful myopathy with myoglobinuria after a bout of heavy drinking. Acute painless muscle weakness with myoglobinuria may occur with prolonged hypokalemia, or hypophosphatemia and hypomagnesemia, usually in chronic alcoholics or in patients on nasogastric suction receiving parenteral hyperalimentation.

Myofasciitis

This distinctive inflammatory disorder affecting muscle and fascia presents as diffuse myalgias, skin induration, fatigue, and mild muscle weakness; mild elevations of serum CK are usually present. The most common form is eosinophilic myofasciitis characterized by peripheral blood eosinophilia and eosinophilic infiltrates in the endomysial tissue. In some patients, the eosinophilic myositis/fasciitis occurs in the context of parasitic infections, vasculitis, mixed connective tissue disease, hypereosinophilic syndrome, or toxic exposures (e.g., toxic oil syndrome, contaminated L-tryptophan) or with mutations in the calpain gene. A distinct subset of myofasciitis is characterized by pronounced infiltration of the connective tissue around the muscle by sheets of periodic acid–Schiff-positive macrophages and occasional CD8 T cells (macrophagic myofasciitis). Such histologic involvement is focal and limited to sites of previous vaccinations, which may have been administered months or years earlier. This disorder, which to date has not been observed outside of France, has been linked to an aluminum-containing substrate in vaccines. Most patients respond to glucocorticoid therapy, and the overall prognosis seems favorable.

Necrotizing Myositis

This is an increasingly recognized entity that has distinct features, even though it is often labeled as PM. It presents often in the fall or winter as an acute or subacute onset of symmetric muscle weakness; CK is typically extremely high. The weakness can be severe. Coexisting interstitial lung disease and cardiomyopathy may be present. The disorder may develop after a viral infection or in association with cancer. Some patients have antibodies against signal recognition particle (SRP). The muscle biopsy demonstrates necrotic fibers infiltrated by macrophages but only rare, if any, T-cell infiltrates. Muscle MHC-I expression is only slightly and focally upregulated. The capillaries may be swollen with hyalinization, thickening of the capillary wall, and deposition of complement. Some patients respond to immunotherapy, but others are resistant.

Drug-Induced Myopathies

D-Penicillamine and procainamide may produce a true myositis resembling PM, and a DM-like illness had been associated with the contaminated preparations of L-tryptophan. As noted above, AZT causes a mitochondrial myopathy. Other drugs may elicit a toxic noninflammatory myopathy that is histologically different from DM, PM, or IBM. These include cholesterol-lowering agents such as clofibrate, lovastatin, simvastatin, or pravastatin, especially when combined with cyclosporine or gemfibrozil. Rhabdomyolysis and myoglobinuria have been rarely associated with amphotericin B, ε-aminocaproic acid, fenfluramine, heroin, and phencyclidine. The use of amiodarone, chloroquine, colchicine, carbimazole, emetine, etretinate, ipecac syrup, chronic laxative or licorice use resulting in hypokalemia, and glucocorticoids or growth hormone administration have also been associated with myopathic muscle weakness. Some neuromuscular blocking agents such as pancuronium, in combination with glucocorticoids, may cause an acute critical illness myopathy. A careful drug history is essential for diagnosis of these drug-induced myopathies, which do not require immunosuppressive therapy.

"Weakness" Due to Muscle Pain and Muscle Tenderness

A number of conditions including *polymyalgia rheumatica* (Chap. 10) and arthritic disorders of adjacent joints may enter into the differential diagnosis of inflammatory myopathy, even though they do not cause myositis. The muscle biopsy is either normal or discloses type II muscle fiber atrophy. Patients with *fibromyalgia* (Chap. 21) complain of focal or diffuse muscle tenderness, fatigue, and aching, which is sometimes poorly differentiated from joint pain. Some patients, however, have muscle tenderness, painful muscles on movement, and signs suggestive of a collagen vascular disorder, such as an increased erythrocyte sedimentation rate, C-reactive protein, antinuclear antibody, or rheumatoid factor, along with modest elevation of the serum CK and aldolase. They demonstrate a "give-way" pattern of weakness with difficulty sustaining effort but not true muscle weakness. The muscle biopsy is usually normal or nonspecific. Many such patients show some response to nonsteroidal anti-inflammatory agents or glucocorticoids, though most continue to have indolent complaints. An indolent fasciitis in the setting of an ill-defined connective tissue disorder may be present, and these patients should not be labeled as having a psychosomatic disorder. *Chronic fatigue syndrome*, which may follow a viral infection, can present with debilitating fatigue, fever, sore throat, painful lymphadenopathy, myalgia, arthralgia, sleep disorder, and headache. These patients do not have muscle weakness, and the muscle biopsy is normal.

DIAGNOSIS

The clinically suspected diagnosis of PM, DM, or IBM is confirmed by examining the serum muscle enzymes, EMG findings, and muscle biopsy (Table 16-2).

The most sensitive enzyme is CK, which in active disease can be elevated as much as 50-fold. Although the

CK level usually parallels disease activity, it can be normal in some patients with active IBM or DM, especially when associated with a connective tissue disease. The CK is always elevated in patients with active PM. Along with the CK, the serum glutamic-oxaloacetic and glutamate pyruvate transaminases, lactate dehydrogenase, and aldolase may be elevated.

Needle EMG shows myopathic potentials characterized by short-duration, low-amplitude polyphasic units on voluntary activation and increased spontaneous activity with fibrillations, complex repetitive discharges, and positive sharp waves. Mixed potentials (polyphasic units of short and long duration) indicating a chronic process and muscle fiber regeneration are often present in IBM. These EMG findings are not diagnostic of an inflammatory myopathy but are useful to identify the presence of active or chronic myopathy and to exclude neurogenic disorders.

MRI is not routinely used for the diagnosis of PM, DM, or IBM. However, it may guide the location of the muscle biopsy in certain clinical settings.

Muscle biopsy is the definitive test for establishing the diagnosis of inflammatory myopathy and for excluding other neuromuscular diseases. Inflammation is the

TABLE 16-2

CRITERIA FOR DIAGNOSIS OF INFLAMMATORY MYOPATHIES

CRITERION	POLYMYOSITIS DEFINITE	POLYMYOSITIS PROBABLE	DERMATOMYOSITIS	INCLUSION BODY MYOSITIS
Myopathic muscle weakness[a]	Yes	Yes	Yes[b]	Yes; slow onset, early involvement of distal muscles, frequent falls
Electromyographic findings	Myopathic	Myopathic	Myopathic	Myopathic with mixed potentials
Muscle enzymes	Elevated (up to 50-fold)	Elevated (up to 50-fold)	Elevated (up to 50-fold) or normal	Elevated (up to 10-fold) or normal
Muscle biopsy findings[c]	"Primary" inflammation with the CD8/MHC-I complex and no vacuoles	Ubiquitous MCH-I expression but minimal inflammation and no vacuoles[d]	Perifascicular, perimysial, or perivascular infiltrates, perifascicular atrophy	Primary inflammation with CD8/MHC-I complex; vacuolated fibers with β-amyloid deposits; cytochrome oxygenase–negative fibers; signs of chronic myopathy[e]
Rash or calcinosis	Absent	Absent	Present[f]	Absent

[a]Myopathic muscle weakness, affecting proximal muscles more than distal ones and sparing eye and facial muscles, is characterized by a subacute onset (weeks to months) and rapid progression in patients who have no family history of neuromuscular disease, no endocrinopathy, no exposure to myotoxic drugs or toxins, and no biochemical muscle disease (excluded on the basis of muscle-biopsy findings).
[b]In some cases with the typical rash, the muscle strength is seemingly normal (dermatomyositis sine myositis); these patients often have new onset of easy fatigue and reduced endurance. Careful muscle testing may reveal mild muscle weakness.
[c]See text for details.
[d]An adequate trial of prednisone or other immunosuppressive drugs is warranted in probable cases. If, in retrospect, the disease is unresponsive to therapy, another muscle biopsy should be considered to exclude other diseases or possible evolution in inclusion body myositis.
[e]If the muscle biopsy does not contain vacuolated fibers but shows chronic myopathy with hypertrophic fibers, primary inflammation with the CD8/MHC-I complex and cytochrome oxygenase–negative fibers, the diagnosis is probable inclusion body myositis.
[f]If rash is absent but muscle biopsy findings are characteristic of dermatomyositis, the diagnosis is probable DM.

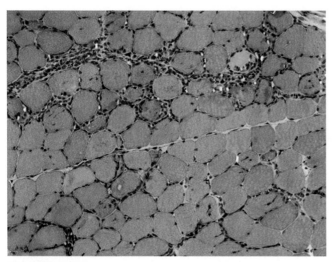

FIGURE 16-3

Cross section of a muscle biopsy from a patient with polymyositis demonstrates scattered inflammatory foci with lymphocytes invading or surrounding muscle fibers. Note lack of chronic myopathic features (increased connective tissue, atrophic or hypertrophic fibers) as seen in inclusion body myositis.

histologic hallmark for these diseases; however, additional features are characteristic of each subtype (**Figs. 16-3, 16-4,** and **16-5**).

In PM the inflammation is *primary*, a term used to indicate that T-cell infiltrates, located primarily within the muscle fascicles (endomysially), surround individual, healthy muscle fibers and result in phagocytosis and necrosis (Fig. 16-3). The MHC-I molecule is ubiquitously expressed on the sarcolemma, even in fibers not invaded by CD8+ cells. The CD8/MHC-I lesion is now fundamental for confirming or establishing the diagnosis and to exclude disorders with secondary, nonspecific,

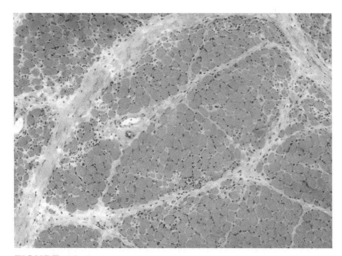

FIGURE 16-4

Cross section of a muscle biopsy from a patient with dermatomyositis demonstrates atrophy of the fibers at the periphery of the fascicle (perifascicular atrophy).

inflammation. When the disease is chronic, connective tissue is increased and may react positively with alkaline phosphatase.

In DM the endomysial inflammation is predominantly perivascular or in the interfascicular septae and around, rather than within, the muscle fascicles (Fig. 16-4). The intramuscular blood vessels show endothelial hyperplasia with tuboreticular profiles, fibrin thrombi, and obliteration of capillaries. The muscle fibers undergo necrosis, degeneration, and phagocytosis, often in groups involving a portion of a muscle fasciculus in a wedgelike shape or at the periphery of the fascicle, due to microinfarcts within the muscle. This results in perifascicular atrophy, characterized by 2–10 layers of atrophic fibers at the periphery of the fascicles. The presence of perifascicular atrophy is diagnostic of DM, *even in the absence of inflammation.*

In IBM (Fig. 16-5), there is endomysial inflammation with T cells invading MHC-I–expressing nonvacuolated muscle fibers; basophilic granular deposits distributed around the edge of slitlike vacuoles (rimmed vacuoles); loss of fibers, replaced by fat and connective tissue, hypertrophic fibers, and angulated or round fibers; eosinophilic cytoplasmic inclusions; abnormal mitochondria characterized by the presence of ragged-red fibers or cytochrome oxidase–negative fibers; amyloid deposits within or next to the vacuoles; and filamentous inclusions seen by electron microscopy in the vicinity of the rimmed vacuoles.

℞ **Treatment:**
INFLAMMATORY MYOPATHIES

The goal of therapy is to improve muscle strength, thereby improving function in activities of daily living, and ameliorate the extramuscular manifestations (rash, dysphagia, dyspnea, fever). When strength improves, the serum CK falls concurrently; however, the reverse is not always true. Unfortunately, there is a common tendency to "chase" or treat the CK level instead of the muscle weakness, a practice that has led to prolonged and unnecessary use of immunosuppressive drugs and erroneous assessment of their efficacy. It is prudent to discontinue these drugs if, after an adequate trial, there is no objective improvement in muscle strength whether or not CK levels are reduced. Agents used in the treatment of PM and DM include:

1. *Glucocorticoids.* Oral prednisone is the initial treatment of choice; the effectiveness and side effects of this therapy determine the future need for stronger immunosuppressive drugs. High-dose prednisone, at least 1 mg/kg per d, is initiated as early in the disease as possible. After 3–4 weeks, prednisone is tapered slowly over a period of 10 weeks to 1 mg/kg every

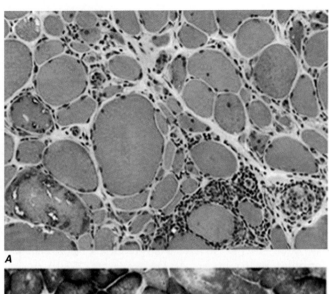

A

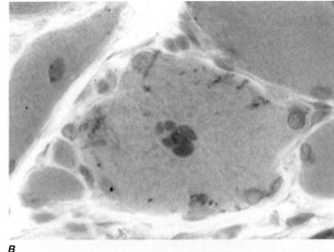

B

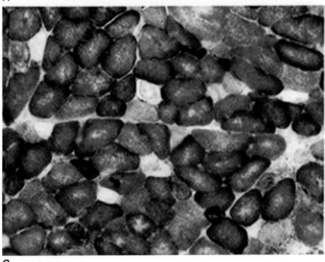

C

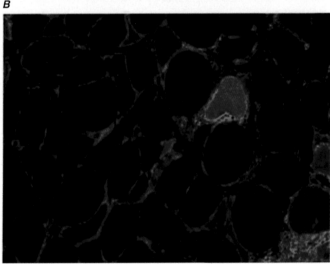

D

FIGURE 16-5

Cross sections of a muscle biopsy from a patient with inclusion body myositis demonstrate the typical features of vacuoles with lymphocytic infiltrates surrounding nonvacuolated or necrotic fibers *(A)*, tiny endomysial deposits of amyloid visualized with crystal violet *(B)*, cytochrome oxidase-negative fibers, indicative of mitochondrial dysfunction *(C)*, and ubiquitous MHC-I expression at the periphery of all fibers *(D)*.

other day. If there is evidence of efficacy and no serious side effects, the dosage is then further reduced by 5 or 10 mg every 3–4 weeks until the lowest possible dose that controls the disease is reached. The efficacy of prednisone is determined by an objective increase in muscle strength and activities of daily living, which almost always occurs by the third month of therapy. A feeling of increased energy or a reduction of the CK level without a concomitant increase in muscle strength is not a reliable sign of improvement. If prednisone provides no objective benefit after ~3 months of high-dose therapy, the disease is probably unresponsive to the drug and tapering should be accelerated while the next-in-line immunosuppressive drug is started. Although controlled trials have not been performed, almost all patients with true PM or DM respond to glucocorticoids to *some degree and for some period of time*; in general, DM responds better than PM.

The long-term use of prednisone may cause increased weakness associated with a normal or unchanged CK level; this effect is referred to as *steroid myopathy*. In a patient who previously responded to high doses of prednisone, the development of new weakness may be related to steroid myopathy or to disease activity that either will respond to a higher dose of glucocorticoids or has become glucocorticoid resistant. In uncertain cases, the prednisone dosage can be steadily increased or decreased as desired: the cause of the weakness is usually evident in 2–8 weeks.

2. *Other immunosuppressive drugs.* Approximately 75% of patients ultimately require additional treatment. This occurs when a patient fails to respond adequately to glucocorticoids after a 3-month trial, the patient

becomes glucocorticoid resistant, glucocorticoid-related side effects appear, attempts to lower the prednisone dose repeatedly result in a new relapse, or rapidly progressive disease with evolving severe weakness and respiratory failure develops.

The following drugs are commonly used but have never been tested in controlled studies: (1) *Azathioprine* is well tolerated, has few side effects, and appears to be as effective for long-term therapy as other drugs. The dose is up to 3 mg/kg daily. (2) *Methotrexate* has a faster onset of action than azathioprine. It is given orally starting at 7.5 mg weekly for the first 3 weeks (2.5 mg every 12 h for 3 doses), with gradual dose escalation by 2.5 mg per week to a total of 25 mg weekly. A rare side effect is methotrexate pneumonitis, which can be difficult to distinguish from the interstitial lung disease of the primary myopathy associated with Jo-1 antibodies (described above). (3) *Mycophenolate mofetil* also has a faster onset of action than azathioprine. At doses up to 2.5 mg/d, it is well tolerated and appears promising for long-term use. (4) Monoclonal anti-CD20 (rituximab) has been shown in a small uncontrolled series to benefit patients with DM. (5) *Cyclosporine* has inconsistent and mild benefit. (6) *Cyclophosphamide* (0.5–1 g IV monthly for 6 months) has limited success and significant toxicity. (7) Tacrolimus (formerly known as Fk506) has been effective in some difficult cases of PM.

3. *Immunomodulation*. In a controlled trial of patients with refractory DM, intravenous immunoglobulin (IVIg) improved not only strength and rash but also the underlying immunopathology. The benefit is often short-lived (≤8 weeks); repeated infusions every 6–8 weeks are generally required to maintain improvement. A dose of 2 g/kg divided over 2–5 days per course is recommended. Uncontrolled observations suggest that IVIg may also be beneficial for patients with PM. Neither plasmapheresis nor leukapheresis appears to be effective in PM and DM.

The following sequential empirical approach to the treatment of PM and DM is suggested: *Step 1*: high-dose prednisone; *Step 2*: azathioprine, mycophenolate, or methotrexate for steroid-sparing effect; *Step 3*: IVIg; *Step 4*: a trial, with guarded optimism, of one of the following agents, chosen according to the patient's age, degree of disability, tolerance, experience with the drug, and general health: rituximab, cyclosporine, cyclophosphamide, or tacrolimus. Patients with interstitial lung disease may benefit from aggressive treatment with cyclophosphamide or tacrolimus.

A patient with presumed PM who has not responded to any form of immunotherapy most likely has IBM or another disease, usually a metabolic myopathy, a muscular dystrophy, a drug-induced myopathy, or an endocrinopathy. In these cases, a repeat muscle biopsy and a renewed search for another cause of the myopathy is indicated.

Calcinosis, a manifestation of DM, is difficult to treat; however, new calcium deposits may be prevented if the primary disease responds to the available therapies. Bisphosphonates, aluminum hydroxide, probenecid, colchicine, low doses of warfarin, calcium blockers, and surgical excision have all been tried without success.

IBM is generally resistant to immunosuppressive therapies. Prednisone together with azathioprine or methotrexate is often tried for a few months in newly diagnosed patients, although results are generally disappointing. Because occasional patients may feel subjectively weaker after these drugs are discontinued, some clinicians prefer to maintain some patients on low-dose, every-other-day prednisone or weekly methotrexate in an effort to slow disease progression, even though there is no objective evidence or controlled study to support this practice. In two controlled studies of IVIg in IBM, minimal benefit in up to 30% of patients was found; the strength gains, however, were not of sufficient magnitude to justify its routine use. Another trial of IVIg combined with prednisone was ineffective. Nonetheless, many experts believe that a 2- to 3-month trial with IVIg may be reasonable for selected patients with IBM who experience rapid progression of muscle weakness or choking episodes due to worsening dysphagia.

PROGNOSIS

The 5-year survival rate for treated patients with PM and DM is ~95% and the 10-year survival is 84%; death is usually due to pulmonary, cardiac, or other systemic complications. Patients severely affected at presentation or treated after long delays, those with severe dysphagia or respiratory difficulties, older patients, and those with associated cancer have a worse prognosis. DM responds more favorably to therapy than PM and thus has a better prognosis. Most patients improve with therapy, and many make a full functional recovery, which is often sustained with maintenance therapy. Up to 30% may be left with some residual muscle weakness. Relapses may occur at any time.

IBM has the least favorable prognosis of the inflammatory myopathies. Most patients will require the use of an assistive device such as a cane, walker, or wheelchair within 5–10 years of onset. In general, the older the age of onset in IBM, the more rapidly progressive is the course.

FURTHER READINGS

AMATO AA et al: Inclusion body myositis: Clinical and pathological boundaries. Ann Neurol 40:581, 1996

ASKANAS V et al: Inclusion-body myositis: Clinical and pathologic aspects, and basic research potentially relevant to treatment. Neurology 24:66(Suppl 1), 2006

208 BRONNER IM et al: Necrotising myopathy, an unusual presentation of a steroid-responsive myopathy. J Neurol 250(4):480, 2003

CALLEN JP: Dermatomyositis. Lancet 355:53, 2000

DALAKAS MC: Polymyositis in patients with AIDS. JAMA 256:2381, 1986

————: Polymyositis, dermatomyositis, and inclusion-body myositis. N Engl J Med 325:1487, 1991

————: Muscle biopsy findings in inflammatory myopathies. Rheum Dis Clin North Am 28:779, 2002

————: Inflammatory disorders of muscle: Progress in polymyositis, dermatomyositis and inclusion body myositis. Curr Opin Neurol 17:561, 2004

————: Viral related muscle disease, in *Myology*, 3d ed, AG Engel, C Franzini-Armstrong (eds). New York, McGraw Hill, 2004, pp 1389–1417

————: Signaling pathways and immunobiology of inflammatory myopathies. Nat Clin Pract Rheumatol 2:219, 2006

————: Sporadic inclusion body myositis: Diagnosis, pathogenesis and therapeutic strategies. Nat Clin Pract Neurol 2:437, 2006

————: Therapeutic targets in patients with inflammatory myopathies: Present approaches and a look to the future. Neuromuscul Disord 16:223, 2006

————, HOHLFELD R: Polymyositis and dermatomyositis. Lancet 362:971, 2003

————, KARPATI G: The inflammatory myopathies, in *Disorders of Voluntary Muscle* 7th ed, G Karpati, D Hilton-Jones, RC Griggs (eds). Cambridge, Cambridge University Press, 2001, pp 636–659

———— et al: A controlled trial of high-dose intravenous immunoglobulin infusions as treatment for dermatomyositis. N Engl J Med 329:1993, 1993

———— et al: Inclusion body myositis with human immunodeficiency virus infection: Four cases with clonal expansion of viral-specific T cells. Ann Neurol 61:466, 2007

EISENBERG I et al: The UDP-*N*-acetylglucosamine 2-epimerase/*N*-acetylmannosamine kinase gene is mutated in recessive hereditary inclusion body myopathy. Nat Genet 29:83, 2001

ENGEL AG, HOHLFELD R: The polymyositis and dermatomyositis syndromes, in *Myology*, 3d ed, AG Engel, C Franzini-Armstrong (eds). New York, McGraw-Hill, 2004, pp 1321–1366

GERARDI RK et al: Macrophagic myofasciitis: An emerging entity. Lancet 352:347, 1998

GREENBERG SA et al: Interferon-alpha/beta-mediated innate immune mechanisms in dermatomyositis. Ann Neurol 57(5):664, 2005

GRIGGS RC et al: Inclusion body myositis and myopathies. Ann Neurol 38:705, 1995

GUNAWARDENA H et al: Myositis-specific autoantibodies: Their clinical and pathogenic significance in disease expression. Rheumatology 48:607, 2009

HENGSTMAN GJ et al: Myositis-specific autoantibodies: Overview and recent developments. Curr Opin Rheumatol 13(6):476, 2001

HILTON-JONES D: Inflammatory myopathies. Curr Opin Neurol 14:591, 2001

IOANNOU Y et al: Myositis overlap syndrome. Curr Opin Rheumatol 11:468, 1999

KARPATI G, CARPENTER S: Pathology of the inflammatory myopathies. Baillieres Clin Neurol 2:527, 1993

LEON-MONZON DM, DALAKAS MC: Absence of persistent infection with enteroviruses in muscles of patients with inflammatory myopathies. Ann Neurol 32:219, 1992

———— et al: Polymyositis in patients with HTLV-I: The role of the virus in the cause of the disease. Ann Neurol 36:643, 1994

LEVINE TD: Rituximab in the treatment of dermatomyositis: An open-label pilot study. Arthritis Rheum 52:601, 2005

MARIE I et al: Polymyositis and dermatomyositis: Short term and long term outcome and predictive factors of prognosis. J Rheumatol 28:2230, 2001

MASTAGLIA FL: Inflammatory myopathies: Clinical, diagnostic and therapeutic aspects. Muscle Nerve 27:407, 2003

MIKOL J, ENGEL AG: Inclusion body myositis, in *Myology*, 3d ed, AG Engel, C Franzini-Armstrong (eds). New York, McGraw-Hill, 2004, pp 1367–1388

MORGAN OSTC et al: HTLV-1 and polymyositis in Jamaica. Lancet 2:1184, 1989

NAGARAJU K et al: Activation of the endoplasmic reticulum stress response in autoimmune myositis: Potential role in muscle fiber damage and dysfunction. Arthritis Rheum 52:1824, 2005

ODDIS CV et al: Tacrolimus in refractory polymyositis with interstitial lung disease. Lancet 353:1762, 1999

SIVAKUMAR K et al: An inflammatory, familial, inclusion body myositis with autoimmune features and a phenotype identical to sporadic inclusion body myositis: Studies in three families. Brain 120:653, 1997

SONTHEIMER RD: Dermatomyositis: An overview of recent progress with emphasis on dermatologic aspects. Dermatol Clin 20:387, 2002

SULTAN SM et al: Outcome in patients with idiopathic inflammatory myositis: Morbidity and mortality. Rheumatology 41:22, 2002

TARGOFF IN et al: Update on myositis-specific and myositis-associated autoantibodies. Curr Opin Rheumatol 12(6):475, 2000

WALKER UA: Imaging tools for the clinical assessment of idiopathic inflammatory myositis. Curr Opin Rheumatol 20:656, 2008

WIENDL H et al: Immunobiology of muscle: Advances in understanding an immunological microenvironment. Trends Immunol 26:373, 2005

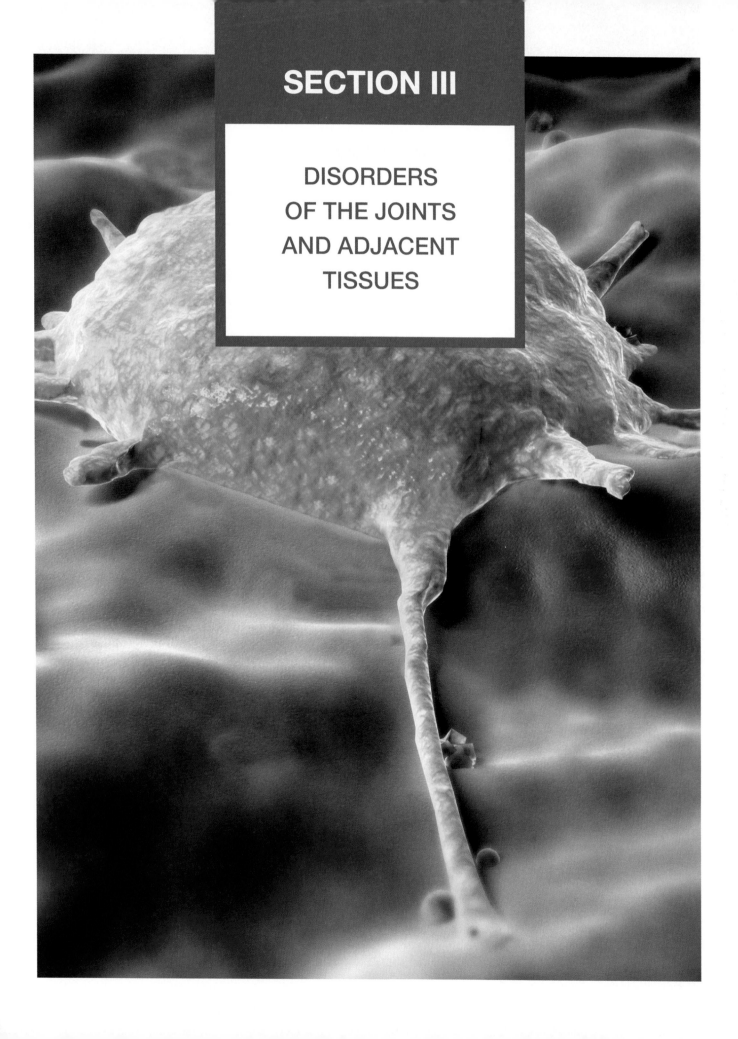

SECTION III

DISORDERS OF THE JOINTS AND ADJACENT TISSUES

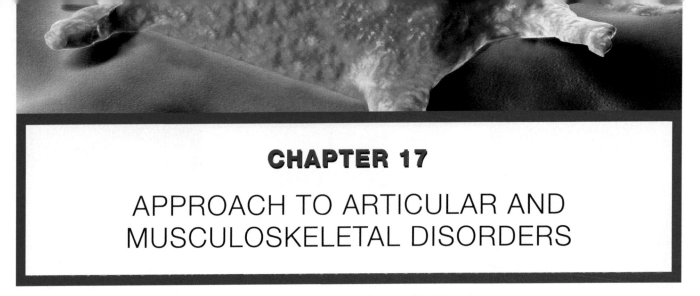

CHAPTER 17

APPROACH TO ARTICULAR AND MUSCULOSKELETAL DISORDERS

John J. Cush ■ Peter E. Lipsky

Musculoskeletal complaints account for >315 million outpatient visits per year. Recent surveys by the Centers for Disease Control and Prevention suggest that 33% (69.9 million) of the U.S. population is affected by arthritis or joint disorders. Many of these are self-limited conditions requiring minimal evaluation and only symptomatic therapy and reassurance. However, in some patients, specific musculoskeletal symptoms or their persistence may herald a more serious condition that requires further evaluation or laboratory testing to establish a diagnosis or document the extent and nature of the pathologic process. The goal of the musculoskeletal evaluation is to formulate a differential diagnosis that leads to an accurate diagnosis and timely therapy, while avoiding excessive diagnostic testing and unnecessary treatment (Table 17-1). There are several urgent conditions that must be diagnosed promptly to avoid significant morbid or mortal sequelae. These "red flag" diagnoses include septic arthritis, acute crystal-induced arthritis (e.g., gout), and fracture. Each may be suspected by its acute onset and monarticular or focal presentation (see below).

Individuals with musculoskeletal complaints should be evaluated with a thorough history, a comprehensive physical examination, and, if appropriate, laboratory testing. The initial encounter should determine whether the musculoskeletal complaint is (1) *articular* or *nonarticular* in origin, (2) *inflammatory* or *noninflammatory* in nature, (3) *acute* or *chronic* in duration, and (4) *localized* or *widespread* (*systemic*) in distribution.

With such an approach and an understanding of the pathophysiologic processes that underlie musculoskeletal complaints, a diagnosis can be made in the vast majority of individuals. However, some patients will not fit immediately into an established diagnostic category. Many musculoskeletal disorders resemble each other at the outset, and some may take weeks or months to evolve into a readily recognizable diagnostic entity. This consideration should temper the desire to establish a definitive diagnosis at the first encounter.

ARTICULAR VERSUS NONARTICULAR

The musculoskeletal evaluation must discriminate the anatomic origin(s) of the patient's complaint. For example, ankle pain can result from a variety of pathologic conditions involving disparate anatomic structures, including gonococcal arthritis, calcaneal fracture, Achilles tendinitis, cellulitis, and peripheral neuropathy. Distinguishing between articular and nonarticular conditions requires a careful and detailed examination.

TABLE 17-1

EVALUATION OF PATIENTS WITH MUSCULOSKELETAL COMPLAINTS

Goals
  Accurate diagnosis
  Timely provision of therapy
  Avoidance of unnecessary diagnostic testing
Approach
  Anatomic localization of complaint (articular vs nonarticular)
  Determination of the nature of the pathologic process (inflammatory vs. noninflammatory)
  Determination of the extent of involvement (monarticular, polyarticular, focal, widespread)
  Determination of chronology (acute vs chronic)
  Consider the most common disorders first
  Formulation of a differential diagnosis

Articular structures include the synovium, synovial fluid, articular cartilage, intraarticular ligaments, joint capsule, and juxtaarticular bone. Nonarticular (or periarticular) structures, such as supportive extraarticular ligaments, tendons, bursae, muscle, fascia, bone, nerve, and overlying skin, may be involved in the pathologic process. Although musculoskeletal complaints are often ascribed to the joints, nonarticular disorders (rather than articular) more frequently underlie such complaints. Distinguishing between these potential sources of pain may be challenging to the unskilled examiner. Articular disorders may be characterized by deep or diffuse pain, pain or limited range of motion on active and passive movement, and swelling (caused by synovial proliferation, effusion, or bony enlargement), crepitation, instability, "locking," or deformity. By contrast, nonarticular disorders tend to be painful on active, but not passive (or assisted), range of motion; demonstrate point or focal tenderness in regions adjacent to articular structures; and have physical findings remote from the joint capsule. Moreover, nonarticular disorders seldom demonstrate swelling, crepitus, instability, or deformity.

INFLAMMATORY VERSUS NONINFLAMMATORY DISORDERS

In the course of a musculoskeletal evaluation, the examiner should determine the nature of the underlying pathologic process and whether inflammatory or noninflammatory findings exist. Inflammatory disorders may be infectious (infection with *Neisseria gonorrhoeae* or *Mycobacterium tuberculosis*), crystal induced (gout, pseudogout), immune related [rheumatoid arthritis (RA), systemic lupus erythematosus (SLE)], reactive (rheumatic fever, Reiter's syndrome), or idiopathic. Inflammatory disorders may be identified by any of the four cardinal signs of inflammation (erythema, warmth, pain, or swelling), systemic symptoms (fatigue, fever, rash, weight loss), or laboratory evidence of inflammation [elevated erythrocyte sedimentation rate (ESR) or C-reactive protein (CRP), thrombocytosis, anemia of chronic disease, or hypoalbuminemia]. Articular stiffness commonly accompanies chronic musculoskeletal disorders. However, the severity and duration of stiffness may be diagnostically important. Morning stiffness related to inflammatory disorders (such as RA or polymyalgia rheumatica) is precipitated by prolonged rest, is described as severe, lasts for hours, and may improve with activity and anti-inflammatory medications. By contrast, intermittent stiffness (also known as gel phenomenon), associated with noninflammatory conditions [such as osteoarthritis (OA)], is precipitated by brief periods of rest, usually lasts <60 min, and is exacerbated by activity. Fatigue may accompany inflammation (as seen in RA and polymyalgia rheumatica) but may also be prominent in fibromyalgia (a noninflammatory disorder), anemia, cardiac failure, endocrinopathy, poor nutrition, poor sleep, or depression. Noninflammatory disorders may be related to trauma (rotator cuff tear), repetitive use (bursitis, tendonitis), degeneration or ineffective repair (OA), neoplasm (pigmented villonodular synovitis), or pain amplification (fibromyalgia). Noninflammatory disorders are often characterized by pain without synovial swelling or warmth, absence of inflammatory or systemic features, daytime gel phenomena rather than morning stiffness, and normal (for age) or negative laboratory investigations.

Identification of the nature of the underlying process and the site of the complaint will enable the examiner to narrow the diagnostic considerations and to assess the need for immediate diagnostic or therapeutic intervention, or for continued observation. **Figure 17-1** presents a logical approach to the evaluation of patients with musculoskeletal complaints.

In the formulation of a differential diagnosis, the examiner should be mindful of the most common causes of musculoskeletal complaints (**Fig. 17-2**). Thus, the prevalence of these disorders in the general population may facilitate an early diagnosis. As trauma, fracture, and fibromyalgia are among the most common causes of presentation, these should be considered during the initial encounter. The frequency of these disorders is best clarified by dividing patients according to their age. Hence, those >60 years are commonly affected by repetitive use/strain disorders, gout (men only), RA, spondyloarthritis, and infectious arthritis. Patients >60 years are frequently affected by

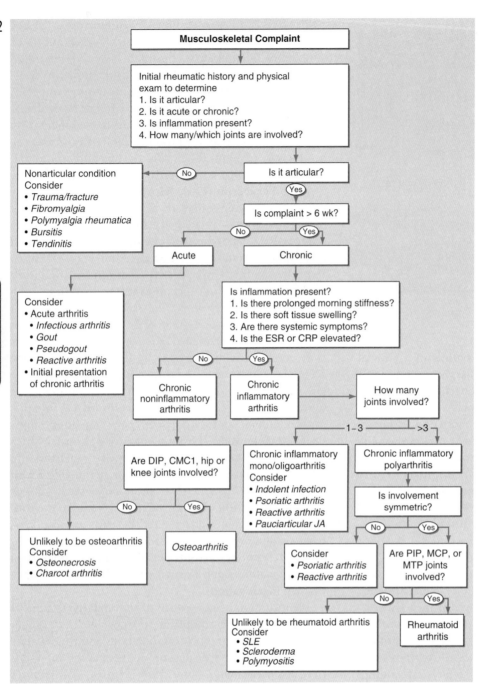

FIGURE 17-1

Algorithm for the diagnosis of musculoskeletal complaints. An approach to formulating a differential diagnosis (shown in italics). (ESR, erythrocyte sedimentation rate; CRP, C-reactive protein; DIP, distal interphalangeal; CMC, carpometacarpal; PIP, proximal interphalangeal; MCP, metacarpophalangeal; MTP, metatarsophalangeal; PMR, polymyalgia rheumatica; SLE, systemic lupus erythematosus; JA, juvenile arthritis.)

OA, crystal (gout and pseudogout) arthritis, polymyalgia rheumatica, osteoporotic fracture, and septic arthritis.

CLINICAL HISTORY

Additional historic features may reveal important clues to the diagnosis. Aspects of the patient profile, complaint chronology, extent of joint involvement, and precipitating factors can provide important information. Certain diagnoses are more frequent in different *age* groups (Fig. 17-2). SLE and reactive arthritis occur more frequently in the young, whereas fibromyalgia and

RA are frequent in middle age, and OA and polymyalgia rheumatica are more prevalent among the elderly. Diagnostic clustering is also evident when *sex* and *race* are considered. Gout and the spondyloarthropathies (e.g., ankylosing spondylitis) are more common in men, whereas RA, fibromyalgia, and lupus are more frequent in women. *Racial predilections* may be influential. Thus, polymyalgia rheumatica, giant cell arteritis, and Wegener's granulomatosis commonly affect whites, whereas sarcoidosis and SLE more commonly affect African Americans. *Familial aggregation* may be seen in disorders such as ankylosing spondylitis, gout, and Heberden's nodes of OA.

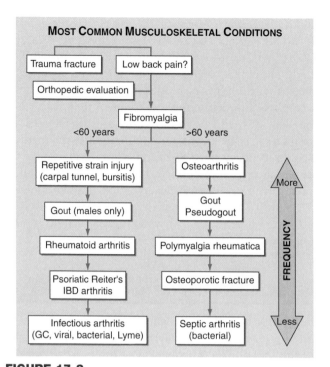

MOST COMMON MUSCULOSKELETAL CONDITIONS

FIGURE 17-2

Algorithm for consideration of the most common muscu-loskeletal conditions. (IBD, inflammatory bowel disease; GC, gonococcal.)

The chronology of the complaint is an important diagnostic feature and can be divided into *onset*, *evolution*, and *duration*. The onset of disorders such as septic arthritis or gout tends to be abrupt, whereas OA, RA, and fibromyalgia may have more indolent presentations. The patients' complaints may evolve differently and be classified as chronic (OA), intermittent (crystal or Lyme arthritis), migratory (rheumatic fever, gonococcal or viral arthritis), or additive (RA, psoriatic arthritis). Musculoskeletal disorders are typically classified as acute or chronic based upon a symptom duration that is either less than or greater than 6 weeks, respectively. Acute arthropathies tend to be infectious, crystal induced, or reactive. Chronic conditions include noninflammatory or immunologic arthritides (e.g., OA, RA) and nonarticular disorders (e.g., fibromyalgia).

The *extent* of articular involvement is often diagnostic. Articular disorders are classified based on the number of joints involved, as either *monarticular* (one joint), *oligoarticular* or *pauciarticular* (two or three joints), or *polyarticular* (more than three joints). Although crystal and infectious arthritides are often mono- or oligoarticular, OA and RA are polyarticular disorders. Nonarticular disorders may be classified as either focal or widespread. Complaints secondary to tendinitis or carpal tunnel syndrome are typically focal, whereas weakness and myalgia, due to polymyositis or fibromyalgia, are more diffuse in their presentation. Joint involvement in RA tends to be symmetric, whereas the spondyloarthropathies and

gout are often asymmetric and oligoarticular. The upper extremities are frequently involved in RA and OA, whereas lower extremity arthritis is characteristic of reactive arthritis and gout at their onset. Involvement of the axial skeleton is common in OA and ankylosing spondylitis but is infrequent in RA, with the notable exception of the cervical spine.

The clinical history should also identify *precipitating events*, such as trauma, drug administration (**Table 17-2**), or antecedent or intercurrent illnesses, that may have contributed to the patient's complaint. Certain comorbidities may predispose to musculoskeletal consequences. This is especially so for diabetes mellitus (carpal tunnel syndrome), renal insufficiency (gout), psoriasis (psoriatic arthritis), myeloma (low back pain), cancer (myositis), and osteoporosis (fracture) or when using certain drugs such as glucocorticoids (osteonecrosis, septic arthritis) and diuretics or chemotherapy (gout).

A thorough *rheumatic review of systems* may disclose useful diagnostic information. A variety of musculoskeletal

TABLE 17-2

DRUG-INDUCED MUSCULOSKELETAL CONDITIONS

Arthralgias
Quinidine, cimetidine, quinolones, chronic acyclovir, interferon, IL-2, nicardipine, vaccines, rifabutin, aromatase and HIV protease inhibitors

Myalgias/myopathy
Glucocorticoids, penicillamine, hydroxychloroquine, AZT, lovastatin, simvastatin, pravastatin, clofibrate, interferon, IL-2, alcohol, cocaine, taxol, docetaxel, colchicine, quinolones, cyclosporine

Tendon rupture
Quinolones, glucocorticoids

Gout
Diuretics, aspirin, cytotoxics, cyclosporine, alcohol, moonshine, ethambutol

Drug-induced lupus
Hydralazine, procainamide, quinidine, phenytoin, carbamazepine, methyldopa, isoniazid, chlorpromazine, lithium, penicillamine, tetracyclines, TNF inhibitors, ACE inhibitors, ticlopidine

Osteonecrosis
Glucocorticoids, alcohol, radiation, bisphosphonates

Osteopenia
Glucocorticoids, chronic heparin, phenytoin, methotrexate

Scleroderma
Vinyl chloride, bleomycin, pentazocine, organic solvents, carbidopa, tryptophan, rapeseed oil

Vasculitis
Allopurinol, amphetamines, cocaine, thiazides, penicillamine, propylthiouracil, montelukast, TNF inhibitors, hepatitis B vaccine, trimethoprim/sulfamethoxazole

Note: IL-2, interleukin 2; TNF, tumor necrosis factor; ACE, angiotensin-converting enzyme.

Modified Health Assessment Questionnaire				
Today are you able to (check box)	No difficulty	Some difficulty	Much difficulty	Cannot do
Dress yourself; including laces & buttons?				
Get in and out of bed?				
Lift a full cup or glass to your mouth?				
Walk outdoors on flat ground?				
Wash and dry your entire body?				
Bend down & pick up clothing from floor?				
Turn regular faucets on and off?				
Get in and out of a car?				

FIGURE 17-3

Modified Health Assessment Questionnaire. *(From T Pincus et al: Arthritis Rheum 26:1346, 1983; with permission.)*

disorders may be associated with systemic features such as fever (SLE, infection), rash (SLE, psoriatic arthritis), nail abnormalities (psoriatic or reactive arthritis), myalgias (fibromyalgia, myopathy), or weakness (polymyositis, neuropathy). In addition, some conditions are associated with involvement of other organ systems including the eyes (Behçet's disease, sarcoidosis, spondyloarthritis), gastrointestinal tract (scleroderma, inflammatory bowel disease), genitourinary tract (reactive arthritis, gonococcemia), or the nervous system (Lyme disease, vasculitis).

Lastly, the examiner should assess the level of pain and physical limitation that accompanies the complaint. The intensity of the patient's pain, stiffness, or weakness can be quantified (0–10) verbally or with the use of a 10-cm visual analogue scale (0 = no pain and 10 = the worst possible pain). Functional limitation and disability should be identified and recorded for future comparisons. There are several validated functional measures that are easily incorporated into the musculoskeletal evaluation, such as the modified Health Assessment Questionnaire (**Fig. 17-3**).

RHEUMATOLOGIC EVALUATION OF THE ELDERLY

The incidence of rheumatic diseases rises with age, such that 58% of those >65 years will have joint complaints. Musculoskeletal disorders in elderly patients are often not diagnosed because the signs and symptoms may be insidious, overlooked, or overshadowed by comorbidities. These difficulties are compounded by the diminished reliability of laboratory testing in the elderly, who often manifest nonpathologic abnormal results. For example, the ESR may be misleadingly elevated, and low-titer positive tests for rheumatoid factor and antinuclear antibodies (ANAs) may be seen in up to 15% of elderly

patients. Although nearly all rheumatic disorders afflict the elderly, certain diseases and drug-induced disorders (Table 17-2) are more common in this age group. The elderly should be approached in the same manner as other patients with musculoskeletal complaints, but with an emphasis on identifying the potential rheumatic consequences of medical comorbidities and therapies. OA, osteoporosis, gout, pseudogout, polymyalgia rheumatica, vasculitis, drug-induced SLE, and chronic salicylate toxicity are all more common in the elderly than in other individuals. The physical examination should identify the nature of the musculoskeletal complaint as well as coexisting diseases that may influence diagnosis and choice of treatment.

PHYSICAL EXAMINATION

The goal of the physical examination is to ascertain the structures involved, the nature of the underlying pathology, the functional consequences of the process, and the presence of systemic or extraarticular manifestations. Knowledge of topographic anatomy is necessary to identify the primary site(s) of involvement and differentiate articular from nonarticular disorders. The musculoskeletal examination depends largely on careful inspection, palpation, and a variety of specific physical maneuvers to elicit diagnostic signs (**Table 17-3**). Although most articulations of the appendicular skeleton can be examined in this manner, adequate inspection and palpation are not possible for many axial (e.g., zygapophyseal) and inaccessible (e.g., sacroiliac or hip) joints. For such joints, there is a greater reliance upon specific maneuvers and imaging for assessment.

Examination of involved and uninvolved joints will determine whether *pain*, *warmth*, *erythema*, or *swelling* is present. The locale and level of pain elicited by palpation or movement should be quantified. One example would be to count the number of tender joints on palpation of 28 easily examined joints [proximal interphalangeals (PIPs), metacarpophalangeals (MCPs), wrists, elbows, shoulders, and knees] (with a range of 0–28). Similarly, the number of swollen joints (0–28) can be counted and recorded. Careful examination should distinguish between true articular swelling (caused by synovial effusion or synovial proliferation) and nonarticular (or periarticular) involvement, which usually extends beyond the normal joint margins. Synovial effusion can be distinguished from synovial hypertrophy or bony hypertrophy by palpation or specific maneuvers. For example, small to moderate knee effusions may be identified by the "bulge sign" or "ballottement of the patellae." Bursal effusions (e.g., effusions of the olecranon or prepatellar bursa) are often focal, periarticular, overlie bony prominences, and are fluctuant with sharply defined borders. Joint *stability* can be assessed by

TABLE 17-3

GLOSSARY OF MUSCULOSKELETAL TERMS

Crepitus
A palpable (less commonly audible) vibratory or crackling sensation elicited with joint motion; fine joint crepitus is common and often insignificant in large joints; coarse joint crepitus indicates advanced cartilaginous and degenerative changes (as in osteoarthritis)

Subluxation
Alteration of joint alignment such that articulating surfaces incompletely approximate each other

Dislocation
Abnormal displacement of articulating surfaces such that the surfaces are not in contact

Range of motion
For diarthrodial joints, the arc of measurable movement through which the joint moves in a single plane

Contracture
Loss of full movement resulting from a fixed resistance caused either by tonic spasm of muscle (reversible) or to fibrosis of periarticular structures (permanent)

Deformity
Abnormal shape or size of a structure; may result from bony hypertrophy, malalignment of articulating structures, or damage to periarticular supportive structures

Enthesitis
Inflammation of the entheses (tendinous or ligamentous insertions on bone)

Epicondylitis
Infection or inflammation involving an epicondyle

palpation and by the application of manual stress. *Subluxation* or *dislocation*, which may be secondary to traumatic, mechanical, or inflammatory causes, can be assessed by inspection and palpation. Joint *swelling or volume* can be assessed by palpation. Distention of the articular capsule usually causes pain and evident swelling. The patient will attempt to minimize the pain by maintaining the joint in the position of least intraarticular pressure and greatest volume, usually partial flexion. For this reason, inflammatory effusions may give rise to flexion contractures. Clinically, this may be detected as fluctuant or "squishy" swelling, voluntary or fixed flexion deformities, or diminished range of motion—especially on extension, when joint volumes are decreased. Active and passive *range of motion* should be assessed in all planes, with contralateral comparison. Serial evaluations of the joints should record the number of tender and swollen joints and the range of motion, using a goniometer to quantify the arc of movement. Each joint should be passively manipulated through its full range of motion (including, as appropriate, flexion, extension, rotation, abduction, adduction, lateral bending, inversion, eversion, supination, pronation, medial/lateral deviation, plantar- or dorsiflexion). Limitation of motion is frequently caused by effusion, pain, deformity, or contracture. If passive motion exceeds active motion, a periarticular process (e.g., tendon rupture or myopathy) should be considered. *Contractures* may reflect antecedent synovial inflammation or trauma. Joint *crepitus* may be felt during palpation or maneuvers and may be especially coarse in OA. Joint *deformity* usually indicates a long-standing or aggressive pathologic process. Deformities may result from ligamentous destruction, soft-tissue contracture, bony enlargement, ankylosis, erosive disease, or subluxation. Examination of the musculature will document strength, atrophy, pain, or spasm. Appendicular muscle weakness should be characterized as proximal or distal. Muscle strength should be assessed by observing the patient's performance (e.g., walking, rising from a chair, grasping, writing). Strength may also be graded on a 5-point scale: 0 for no movement; 1 for trace movement or twitch; 2 for movement with gravity eliminated; 3 for movement against gravity only; 4 for movement against gravity and resistance; and 5 for normal strength. The examiner should assess for often-overlooked nonarticular or periarticular involvement, especially when articular complaints are not supported by objective findings referable to the joint capsule. The identification of soft-tissue/nonarticular pain will prevent unwarranted and often expensive additional evaluations. Specific maneuvers may reveal common nonarticular abnormalities, such as a carpal tunnel syndrome (which can be identified by Tinel's or Phalen's sign). Other examples of soft-tissue abnormalities include olecranon bursitis, epicondylitis (e.g., tennis elbow), enthesitis (e.g., Achilles tendinitis), and trigger points associated with fibromyalgia.

APPROACH TO REGIONAL RHEUMATIC COMPLAINTS

Although all patients should be evaluated in a logical and thorough manner, many cases with focal musculoskeletal complaints are caused by commonly encountered disorders that exhibit a predictable pattern of onset, evolution, and localization; they can often be diagnosed immediately on the basis of limited historic information and selected maneuvers or tests. Although nearly every joint could be approached in this manner, the evaluation of four common involved anatomic regions—the hand, shoulder, hip, and knee—are reviewed here.

HAND PAIN

Focal or unilateral hand pain may result from trauma, overuse, infection, or a reactive or crystal-induced arthritis. By contrast, bilateral hand complaints commonly

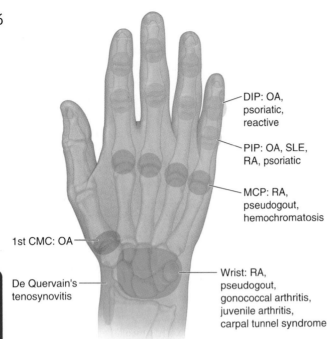

DIP: OA,
psoriatic,
reactive

PIP: OA, SLE,
RA, psoriatic

MCP: RA,
pseudogout,
hemochromatosis

1st CMC: OA

De Quervain's
tenosynovitis

Wrist: RA,
pseudogout,
gonococcal arthritis,
juvenile arthritis,
carpal tunnel syndrome

FIGURE 17-4

Sites of hand or wrist involvement and their potential disease associations. (DIP, distal interphalangeal; OA, osteoarthritis; PIP, proximal interphalangeal; SLE, systemic lupus erythematosus; RA, rheumatoid arthritis; MCP, metacarpophalangeal; CMC, carpometacarpal.) *(From Cush et al, with permission.)*

suggest a degenerative (e.g., OA), systemic, or inflammatory/immune (e.g., RA) etiology. The distribution or pattern of joint involvement is highly suggestive of certain disorders (**Fig. 17-4**). Thus, OA (or degenerative arthritis) may manifest as distal interphalangeal (DIP) and PIP joint pain with bony hypertrophy sufficient to produce Heberden's and Bouchard's nodes, respectively. Pain, with or without bony swelling, involving the base of the thumb (first carpometacarpal joint) is also highly suggestive of OA. By contrast, RA tends to involve the PIP, MCP, intercarpal, and carpometacarpal joints (wrist) with pain, prolonged stiffness, and palpable synovial tissue hypertrophy. Psoriatic arthritis may mimic the pattern of joint involvement seen in OA (DIP and PIP joints), but can be distinguished by the presence of inflammatory signs (erythema, warmth, synovial swelling), with or without carpal involvement, nail pitting or onycholysis. Hemochromatosis should be considered when degenerative changes (bony hypertrophy) are seen at the second and third MCP joints with associated chondrocalcinosis or episodic, inflammatory wrist arthritis.

Soft-tissue swelling over the dorsum of the hand and wrist may suggest an inflammatory extensor tendon tenosynovitis possibly caused by gonococcal infection, gout, or inflammatory arthritis (e.g., RA). The diagnosis

is suggested by local warmth, swelling, or pitting edema and may be confirmed when pain is induced by maintaining the wrist in a fixed, neutral position and flexing the digits distal to the MCP joints to stretch the extensor tendon sheaths.

Focal wrist pain localized to the radial aspect may be caused by De Quervain's tenosynovitis resulting from inflammation of the tendon sheath(s) involving the abductor pollicis longus or extensor pollicis brevis (Fig. 17-4). This commonly results from overuse or follows pregnancy and may be diagnosed with Finkelstein's test. A positive result is present when radial wrist pain is induced after the thumb is flexed and placed inside a clenched fist and the patient actively deviates the hand downward with ulnar deviation at the wrist. Carpal tunnel syndrome is another common disorder of the upper extremity and results from compression of the median nerve within the carpal tunnel. Manifestations include paresthesia in the thumb, second and third fingers, and radial half of the fourth finger and, at times, atrophy of thenar musculature. Carpal tunnel syndrome is commonly associated with pregnancy, edema, trauma, OA, inflammatory arthritis, and infiltrative disorders (e.g., amyloidosis). The diagnosis is suggested by a positive Tinel's or Phalen's sign. With each test, paresthesia in a median nerve distribution is induced or increased by either "thumping" the volar aspect of the wrist (Tinel's sign) or pressing the extensor surfaces of both flexed wrists against each other (Phalen's sign).

SHOULDER PAIN

During the evaluation of shoulder disorders, the examiner should carefully note any history of trauma, fibromyalgia, infection, inflammatory disease, occupational hazards, or previous cervical disease. In addition, the patient should be questioned as to the activities or movement(s) that elicit shoulder pain. Shoulder pain is referred frequently from the cervical spine but may also be referred from intrathoracic lesions (e.g., a Pancoast tumor) or from gall bladder, hepatic, or diaphragmatic disease. Fibromyalgia should be suspected when glenohumeral pain is accompanied by diffuse periarticular (i.e., subacromial, bicipital) pain and tender points (i.e., trapezius or supraspinatus). The shoulder should be put through its full range of motion both actively and passively (with examiner assistance): forward flexion, extension, abduction, adduction, and rotation. Manual inspection of the periarticular structures will often provide important diagnostic information. The examiner should apply direct manual pressure over the subacromial bursa that lies lateral to and immediately beneath the acromion. Subacromial bursitis is a frequent cause of shoulder pain. Anterior to the subacromial bursa, the bicipital tendon traverses the bicipital groove. This tendon is best identified by palpating it in its groove as the patient rotates the humerus internally and externally.

Direct pressure over the tendon may reveal pain indicative of bicipital tendinitis. Palpation of the acromioclavicular joint may disclose local pain, bony hypertrophy, or, uncommonly, synovial swelling. Whereas OA and RA commonly affect the acromioclavicular joint, OA seldom involves the glenohumeral joint, unless there is a traumatic or occupational cause. The glenohumeral joint is best palpated anteriorly by placing the thumb over the humeral head (just medial and inferior to the coracoid process) and having the patient rotate the humerus internally and externally. Pain localized to this region is indicative of glenohumeral pathology. Synovial effusion or tissue is seldom palpable but, if present, may suggest infection, RA, or an acute tear of the rotator cuff.

Rotator cuff tendinitis or tear is a very common cause of shoulder pain. The rotator cuff is formed by the tendons of the supraspinatus, infraspinatus, teres minor, and subscapularis muscles. Rotator cuff tendinitis is suggested by pain on active abduction (but not passive abduction), pain over the lateral deltoid muscle, night pain, and evidence of the impingement sign. This maneuver is performed by the examiner raising the patient's arm into forced flexion while stabilizing and preventing rotation of the scapula. A positive sign is present if pain develops before 180° of forward flexion. A complete tear of the rotator cuff is more common in the elderly and often results from trauma; it may manifest in the same manner as tendinitis but is less common. The diagnosis is also suggested by the drop arm test in which the patient is unable to maintain the arm outstretched once it is passively abducted. If the patient is unable to hold the arm up once 90° of abduction is reached, the test is positive. Tendinitis or tear of the rotator cuff can be confirmed by MRI or ultrasound.

KNEE PAIN

A careful history should delineate the chronology of the knee complaint and whether there are predisposing conditions, trauma, or medications that might underlie the complaint. For example, patellofemoral disease (e.g., OA) may cause anterior knee pain that worsens with climbing stairs. Observation of the patient's gait is also important. The knee should be carefully inspected in the upright (weight-bearing) and prone positions for swelling, erythema, contusion, laceration, or malalignment. The most common form of malalignment in the knee is *genu varum* (bowlegs) or *genu valgum* (knock knees). Bony swelling of the knee joint commonly results from hypertrophic osseous changes seen with disorders such as OA and neuropathic arthropathy. Swelling caused by hypertrophy of the synovium or synovial effusion may manifest as a fluctuant, ballotable, or soft-tissue enlargement in the suprapatellar pouch (suprapatellar reflection of the synovial cavity) or regions lateral and medial to the patella.

Synovial effusions may also be detected by balloting the patella downward toward the femoral groove or by eliciting a "bulge sign." With the knee extended the examiner should manually compress, or "milk," synovial fluid down from the suprapatellar pouch and lateral to the patellae. The application of manual pressure lateral to the patella may cause an observable shift in synovial fluid (bulge) to the medial aspect. The examiner should note that this maneuver is only effective in detecting small to moderate effusions (<100 mL). Inflammatory disorders such as RA, gout, pseudogout, and reactive arthritis may involve the knee joint and produce significant pain, stiffness, swelling, or warmth. A popliteal or *Baker's cyst* is best palpated with the knee partially flexed and is best viewed posteriorly with the patient standing and knees fully extended to visualize popliteal swelling or fullness.

Anserine bursitis is an often missed periarticular cause of knee pain in adults. The pes anserine bursa underlies the semimembranosus tendon and may become inflamed and painful following trauma, overuse, or inflammation. It is often tender in patients with fibromyalgia. Anserine bursitis manifests primarily as point tenderness inferior and medial to the patella and overlies the medial tibial plateau. Swelling and erythema may not be present. Other forms of bursitis may also present as knee pain. The prepatellar bursa is superficial and is located over the inferior portion of the patella. The infrapatellar bursa is deeper and lies beneath the patellar ligament before its insertion on the tibial tubercle.

Internal derangement of the knee may result from trauma or degenerative processes. Damage to the meniscal cartilage (medial or lateral) frequently presents as chronic or intermittent knee pain. Such an injury should be suspected when there is a history of trauma or athletic activity and when the patient relates symptoms of "locking," clicking, or "giving way" of the joint. Pain may be elicited during palpation over the ipsilateral joint line or when the knee is stressed laterally or medially. A positive McMurray test may indicate a meniscal tear. To perform this test, the knee is first flexed at 90°, and the leg is then extended while the lower extremity is simultaneously torqued medially or laterally. A painful click during inward rotation may indicate a lateral meniscus tear, and pain during outward rotation may indicate a tear in the medial meniscus. Lastly, damage to the cruciate ligaments should be suspected with acute onset of pain, possibly with swelling, a history of trauma, or a synovial fluid aspirate that is grossly bloody. Examination of the cruciate ligaments is best accomplished by eliciting a drawer sign. With the patient recumbent, the knee should be partially flexed and the foot stabilized on the examining surface. The examiner should manually attempt to displace the tibia anteriorly or posteriorly with respect to the femur. If anterior movement is detected, then anterior cruciate ligament damage is

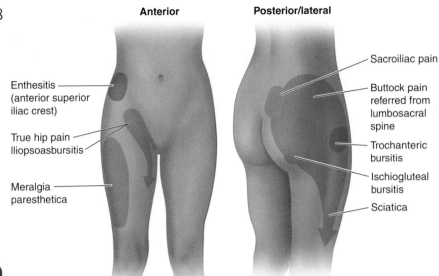

Anterior   **Posterior/lateral**

Enthesitis (anterior superior iliac crest)

True hip pain Iliopsoasbursitis

Meralgia paresthetica

Sacroiliac pain

Buttock pain referred from lumbosacral spine

Trochanteric bursitis

Ischiogluteal bursitis

Sciatica

FIGURE 17-5
Origins of hip pain and dysesthesias.
(From Cush et al, with permission.)

likely. Conversely, significant posterior movement may indicate posterior cruciate damage. Contralateral comparison will assist the examiner in detecting significant anterior or posterior movement.

HIP PAIN

The hip is best evaluated by observing the patient's gait and assessing range of motion. The vast majority of patients reporting "hip pain" localize their pain unilaterally to the posterior or gluteal musculature (Fig. 17-5). Such pain may or may not be associated with low back pain and tends to radiate down the posterolateral aspect of the thigh. This presentation frequently results from degenerative arthritis of the lumbosacral spine and commonly follows a dermatomal distribution with involvement of nerve roots between L5 and S1. Some individuals instead localize their "hip pain" laterally to the area overlying the trochanteric bursa. Because of the depth of this bursa, swelling and warmth are usually absent. Diagnosis of trochanteric bursitis can be confirmed by inducing point tenderness over the trochanteric bursa. Gluteal and trochanteric pain may also indicate underlying fibromyalgia. Range of movement may be limited by pain. Pain in the hip joint is less common and tends to be located anteriorly, over the inguinal ligament; it may radiate medially to the groin or along the anteromedial thigh. Uncommonly, iliopsoas bursitis may mimic true hip joint pain. Diagnosis of iliopsoas bursitis may be suggested by a history of trauma or inflammatory arthritis. Pain associated with iliopsoas bursitis is localized to the groin or anterior thigh and tends to worsen with hyperextension of the hip; many patients prefer to flex and externally rotate the hip to reduce the pain from a distended bursa.

LABORATORY INVESTIGATIONS

The vast majority of musculoskeletal disorders can be easily diagnosed by a complete history and physical examination. An additional objective of the initial encounter is to determine whether additional investigations or immediate therapy are required. A number of features indicate the need for additional evaluation. Monarticular conditions require additional evaluation, as do traumatic or inflammatory conditions and conditions accompanied by neurologic changes or systemic manifestations of serious disease. Finally, individuals with chronic symptoms (>6 weeks), especially when there has been a lack of response to symptomatic measures, are candidates for additional evaluation. The extent and nature of the additional investigation should be dictated by the clinical features and suspected pathologic process. Laboratory tests should be used to confirm a specific clinical diagnosis and not be used to screen or evaluate patients with vague rheumatic complaints. Indiscriminate use of broad batteries of diagnostic tests and radiographic procedures is rarely a useful or cost-effective means to establish a diagnosis.

Besides a complete blood count, including a white blood cell (WBC) and differential count, the routine evaluation should include a determination of an acute-phase reactant such as the ESR or CRP, which can be useful in discriminating inflammatory from noninflammatory disorders. Both are inexpensive and easily obtained and may be elevated with infection, inflammation, autoimmune disorders, neoplasia, pregnancy, renal insufficiency, and advanced age.

Serum uric acid determinations are useful only when gout has been diagnosed and therapy contemplated. Uric acid, the end product of purine metabolism, is primarily excreted in the urine. Serum values range from

238–516 μmol/L (4.0–8.6 mg/dL) in men; the lower values [178–351 μmol/L (3.0–5.9 mg/dL)] seen in women are caused by the uricosuric effects of estrogen. Urinary uric acid levels are normally <750 mg per 24 h. Although hyperuricemia [especially levels >535 μmol/L (9 mg/dL)] is associated with an increased incidence of gout and nephrolithiasis, levels do not correlate with the severity of disease. Uric acid levels (and the risk of gout) may be increased by inborn errors of metabolism (Lesch-Nyhan syndrome), disease states (renal insufficiency, myeloproliferative disease, psoriasis), or drugs (alcohol, cytotoxic therapy, thiazides). Although nearly all patients with gout will demonstrate hyperuricemia at some time during their illness, up to 40% of patients with an acute gouty attack will have normal serum uric acid levels. Monitoring serum uric acid may be useful in assessing the response to hypouricemic therapy or chemotherapy.

Serologic tests for rheumatoid factor, cyclic citrullinated peptide (CCP) antibodies, ANAs, complement levels, Lyme and antineutrophil cytoplasmic antibodies (ANCA), or antistreptolysin O (ASO) titer should be carried out only when there is clinical evidence to suggest an associated diagnosis, as these have poor predictive value when used for screening, especially when the pretest probability is low. Although 4–5% of a healthy population will have positive tests for rheumatoid factor and ANAs, only 1% and <0.4% of the population will have RA or SLE, respectively. IgM rheumatoid factor (autoantibodies against the Fc portion of IgG) is found in 80% of patients with RA and may also be seen in low titers in patients with chronic infections (*tuberculosis*, leprosy); other autoimmune diseases (SLE, Sjögren's syndrome); and chronic pulmonary, hepatic, or renal diseases. When considering RA, anti-CCP antibodies are comparably sensitive but more specific than rheumatoid factor. In RA, the presence of anti-CCP and rheumatoid factor antibodies may indicate a greater risk for more severe, erosive polyarthritis. ANAs are found in nearly all patients with SLE and may also be seen in patients with other autoimmune diseases (polymyositis, scleroderma, antiphospholipid syndrome), drug-induced lupus (resulting from hydralazine, procainamide, quinidine, tetracyclines, tumor necrosis factor inhibitors), chronic liver or renal disorders, and advanced age. Positive ANAs are found in 5% of adults and in up to 14% of elderly or chronically ill individuals. The ANA test is very sensitive but poorly specific for lupus, as <5% of all positive results will be caused by lupus alone. The interpretation of a positive ANA test may depend on the magnitude of the titer and the pattern observed by immunofluorescence microscopy (**Table 17-4**). Diffuse and speckled patterns are least specific, whereas a peripheral, or rim, pattern [related to autoantibodies against double-stranded (native) DNA] is highly specific and suggestive of lupus. Centromeric patterns are seen in patients with limited scleroderma (CREST syndrome) or primary biliary

TABLE 17-4

ANTINUCLEAR ANTIBODY (ANA) PATTERNS AND CLINICAL ASSOCIATIONS

ANA PATTERN	ANTIGEN IDENTIFIED	CLINICAL CORRELATE
Diffuse	Deoxyribonucleo-protein	Nonspecific
	Histones	Drug-induced lupus, lupus
Peripheral (rim)	ds-DNA	50% of SLE (specific)
Speckled	U1-RNP	>90% of MCTD
	Sm	30% of SLE (specific)
	Ro (SS-A)	Sjögren's 60%, SCLE, neonatal lupus, ANA(–) lupus
	La (SS-B)	50% of Sjögren's, 15% lupus
	Scl-70	40% of diffuse scleroderma
	PM-1	Polymyositis (PM), dermatomyositis
	Jo-1	PM w/ pneumonitis + arthritis
Nucleolar	RNA polymerase I, others	40% of PSS
Centromere	Kinetochore	75% CREST (limited scleroderma)

Note: SLE, systemic lupus erythematosus; MCTD, mixed connective tissue disease; SCLE, subacute cutaneous lupus erythematosus; PSS, progressive systemic sclerosis; CREST, calcinosis, *R*aynaud phenomenon, esophageal involvement; *s*clerodactyly; and *t*elangiectasia.

sclerosis, and nucleolar patterns may be seen in patients with diffuse systemic sclerosis or inflammatory myositis.

Aspiration and analysis of synovial fluid are always indicated in acute monarthritis or when an infectious or crystal-induced arthropathy is suspected. Synovial fluid may distinguish between noninflammatory and inflammatory processes by analysis of the appearance, viscosity, and cell count. Tests for synovial fluid glucose, protein, lactate dehydrogenase, lactic acid, or autoantibodies are not recommended as they have no diagnostic value. Normal synovial fluid is clear or a pale straw color and is viscous, primarily because of the high levels of hyaluronate. Noninflammatory synovial fluid is clear, viscous, and amber colored, with a white blood cell count of <2000/μL and a predominance of mononuclear cells. The viscosity of synovial fluid is assessed by expressing fluid from the syringe one drop at a time. Normally, there is a stringing effect, with a long tail behind each synovial drop. Effusions caused by OA or trauma will have normal viscosity. Inflammatory fluid is turbid and yellow, with an increased white cell count (2000–50,000/μL) and a polymorphonuclear leukocyte predominance. Inflammatory fluid has reduced viscosity, diminished hyaluronate, and little or no tail following each drop of synovial fluid. Such effusions are found in RA, gout, and other inflammatory arthritides. Septic fluid is opaque and purulent, with a WBC count usually >50,000/μL, a predominance of polymorphonuclear leukocytes (>75%), and low viscosity. Such effusions are typical of septic arthritis but may occur with RA or gout. In addition, hemorrhagic synovial fluid may be seen with trauma, hemarthrosis, or neuropathic arthritis. An algorithm for synovial fluid aspiration and analysis is shown in **Fig. 17-6.** Synovial fluid should be analyzed immediately for appearance, viscosity, and cell count. Monosodium urate crystals (observed in gout) are seen

by polarized microscopy and are long, needle-shaped, negatively birefringent, and usually intracellular. In chondrocalcinosis and pseudogout, calcium pyrophosphate dihydrate crystals are usually short, rhomboid-shaped, and positively birefringent. Whenever infection is suspected, synovial fluid should be Gram stained and cultured appropriately. If gonococcal arthritis is suspected, immediate plating of the fluid on appropriate culture medium is indicated. Synovial fluid from patients with chronic monarthritis should also be cultured for *M. tuberculosis* and fungi. Last, it should be noted that crystal-induced and septic arthritis occasionally occur together in the same joint.

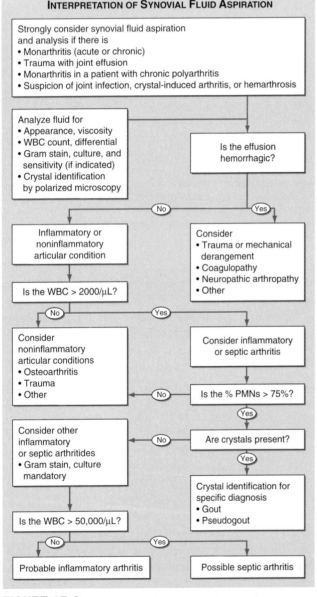

FIGURE 17-6

Algorithmic approach to the use and interpretation of synovial fluid aspiration and analysis. [WBC, white blood cell (count); PMNs, polymorphonuclear (leukocytes).]

DIAGNOSTIC IMAGING IN JOINT DISEASES

Conventional radiography has been a valuable tool in the diagnosis and staging of articular disorders. Plain x-rays are most appropriate when there is a history of trauma, suspected chronic infection, progressive disability, or monarticular involvement; when therapeutic alterations are considered; or when a baseline assessment is desired for what appears to be a chronic process. However, in acute inflammatory arthritis, early radiography is rarely helpful in establishing a diagnosis and may only reveal soft-tissue swelling or juxtaarticular demineralization. As the disease progresses, calcification (of soft tissues, cartilage, or bone), joint space narrowing, erosions, bony ankylosis, new bone formation (sclerosis, osteophytes, or periostitis), or subchondral cysts may develop and suggest specific clinical entities. Consultation with a radiologist will help define the optimal imaging modality, technique, or positioning and prevent the need for further studies.

Additional imaging techniques may possess greater diagnostic sensitivity and facilitate early diagnosis in a limited number of articular disorders, and in selected circumstances and are indicated when conventional radiography is inadequate or nondiagnostic (**Table 17-5**). *Ultrasonography* is useful in the detection of soft-tissue abnormalities that cannot be fully appreciated by clinical examination. Although inexpensive, it is seldom the preferred method of evaluation. The foremost application of ultrasound is in the diagnosis of synovial (Baker's) cysts, although rotator cuff tears and various tendon injuries may be evaluated with ultrasound by an experienced operator. *Radionuclide scintigraphy* provides useful information regarding the metabolic status of bone and, along with radiography, is well suited for total-body assessment of the extent and distribution of skeletal involvement. Radionuclide imaging is a very sensitive, but poorly specific, means of detecting inflammatory or metabolic alterations in bone or periarticular soft-tissue structures. The limited tissue contrast resolution of scintigraphy may obscure the distinction between a bony or periarticular process and may

TABLE 17-5

DIAGNOSTIC IMAGING TECHNIQUES FOR MUSCULOSKELETAL DISORDERS			
METHOD	**IMAGING TIME, h**	**COST**[a]	**CURRENT INDICATIONS**
Ultrasound[b]	<1	+	Synovial cysts Rotator cuff tears Tendon injury
Radionuclide scintigraphy ^{99m}Tc	1–4	++	Metastatic bone survey Evaluation of Paget's disease Acute and chronic osteomyelitis
^{111}In-WBC	24	+++	Acute infection Prosthetic infection Acute osteomyelitis
^{67}Ga	24–48	++++	Acute and chronic infection Acute osteomyelitis
Computed tomography	<1	+++	Herniated intervertebral disk Sacroiliitis Spinal stenosis Spinal trauma Osteoid osteoma Stress fracture
Magnetic resonance imaging	1/2–2	+++++	Avascular necrosis Osteomyelitis Intraarticular derangement and soft-tissue injury Derangements of axial skeleton and spinal cord Herniated intervertebral disk Pigmented villonodular synovitis Inflammatory and metabolic muscle pathology

[a]Relative cost for imaging study.
[b]Results depend on operator.

necessitate the additional use of MRI. Scintigraphy, using ^{99m}Tc, ^{67}Ga, or ^{111}In-labeled WBCs, has been applied to a variety of articular disorders with variable success (Table 17-5). Although [^{99m}Tc] pertechnate or diphosphate scintigraphy (Fig. 17-7) may be useful in identifying osseous infection, neoplasia, inflammation, increased blood flow, bone remodeling, heterotopic bone formation, or avascular necrosis, MRI is preferred in most instances. The poor specificity of ^{99m}Tc scanning has largely limited its use to surveys for bone metastases and Paget's disease of bone. Gallium scanning utilizes ^{67}Ga, which binds serum and cellular transferrin and lactoferrin, and is preferentially taken up by neutrophils, macrophages, bacteria, and tumor tissue (e.g., lymphoma). As such, it is primarily used in the identification of occult infection or malignancy. Scanning with ^{111}In-labeled WBCs has been used to detect osteomyelitis and infectious and inflammatory arthritis. Nevertheless, the use of ^{111}In-labeled WBC or ^{67}Ga scanning has largely been replaced by MRI, except when there is a suspicion of prosthetic joint infections.

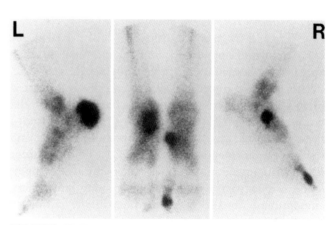

FIGURE 17-7

[^{99m}Tc]diphosphonate scintigraphy of the feet of a 33-year-old black male with reactive arthritis, manifested by sacroiliitis, urethritis, uveitis, asymmetric oligoarthritis, and enthesitis. This bone scan demonstrates increased uptake indicative of enthesitis involving the insertions of the left Achilles tendon, plantar aponeurosis, and right tibialis posterior tendon as well as arthritis of the right first interphalangeal joint.

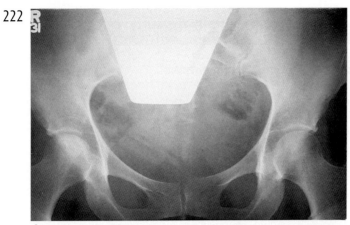

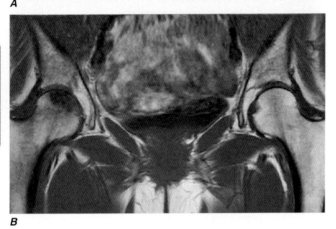

FIGURE 17-8

**Superior sensitivity of MRI in the diagnosis of ost-
eonecrosis of the femoral head.** A 45-year-old woman
receiving high-dose glucocorticoids developed right hip pain.
Conventional x-rays (**A**) demonstrated only mild sclerosis of
the right femoral head. T1-weighted MRI (**B**) demonstrated
low-density signal in the right femoral head, diagnostic of
osteonecrosis.

CT provides detailed visualization of the axial skeleton. Articulations previously considered difficult to visualize by radiography (e.g., zygapophyseal, sacroiliac,
sternoclavicular, hip joints) can be effectively evaluated
using CT. CT has been demonstrated to be useful in the
diagnosis of low back pain syndromes (e.g., spinal stenosis vs. herniated disc), sacroiliitis, osteoid osteoma, and
stress fractures. Helical or spiral CT (with or without
contrast angiography) is a novel technique that is rapid,
cost-effective, and sensitive in diagnosing pulmonary
embolism or obscure fractures, often in the setting of
initially equivocal findings. High-resolution CT can be
advocated in the evaluation of suspected or established
infiltrative lung disease (e.g., scleroderma or rheumatoid
lung). The recent use of hybrid [positron emission
tomography (PET)/CT or single photon emission CT
(SPECT/CT)] scans in metastatic evaluations have

incorporated CT to provide better anatomic localization
of scintigraphic abnormalities.

MRI has significantly advanced the ability to image
musculoskeletal structures. MRI has the advantages of
providing multiplanar images with fine anatomic detail
and contrast resolution (**Fig. 17-8**) that allows for the
superior ability to visualize bone marrow and soft-tissue
periarticular structures. Although more costly with a
longer procedural time than CT, the MRI has become
the preferred technique when evaluating complex musculoskeletal disorders.

MRI can image fascia, vessels, nerve, muscle, cartilage,
ligaments, tendons, pannus, synovial effusions, and bone
marrow. Visualization of particular structures can be
enhanced by altering the pulse sequence to produce
either T1- or T2-weighted spin echo, gradient echo, or
inversion recovery [including short tau inversion recovery (STIR)] images. Because of its sensitivity to changes
in marrow fat, MRI is a sensitive but nonspecific means
of detecting osteonecrosis, osteomyelitis, and marrow
inflammation indicating overlying synovitis or osteitis
(Fig. 17-8). Because of its enhanced soft-tissue resolution, MRI is more sensitive than arthrography or CT in
the diagnosis of soft-tissue injuries (e.g., meniscal and
rotator cuff tears); intraarticular derangements; marrow
abnormalities (osteonecrosis, myeloma); and spinal cord
or nerve root damage or synovitis.

FURTHER READINGS

AVOUAC J et al: Diagnostic and predictive value of anti-cyclic citrullinated protein antibodies in rheumatoid arthritis: A systematic
literature review. Ann Rheum Dis 65(7):845, 2006

CHEN LX et al: Update on identification of pathogenic crystals in
joint fluid. Curr Rheumatol Rep 6:217, 2004

COURTNEY P, DOHERTY M: Joint aspiration and injection and synovial fluid analysis. Best Pract Res Clin Rheumatol 23:161, 2009

CUSH JJ et al: Evaluation of musculoskeletal complaints, in *Rheumatology: Diagnosis and Therapeutics,* 2d ed, JJ Cush, A Kavanaugh,
CM Stein (eds). Philadelphia, Lippincott Williams & Wilkins,
2005, pp 3–20

HOOTMAN JM, HELMICK CG: Projections of US prevalence of arthritis
and associated activity limitations. Arthritis Rheum 54(1):226, 2006

KAVANAUGH A: The utility of immunologic laboratory tests in
patients with rheumatic diseases. Arthritis Rheum 44:2221, 2001

ORY PA: Radiography in the assessment of musculoskeletal conditions. Best Pract Res Clin Rheumatol 17(3):495, 2003

PASCUAL E, DOHERTY M. Aspiration of normal or asymptomatic
pathological joints for diagnosis and research: Indications, technique and success rate. Ann Rheum Dis 68:3, 2009

RUDWALEIT M et al: How to diagnose axial spondyloarthritis early.
Ann Rheum Dis 63(5):535, 2004

SHMERLING RH et al: Synovial fluid tests: What should be ordered?
JAMA 264:1009, 1990

SIVA C et al: Diagnosing acute monoarthritis in adults: A practical
approach for the family physician. Am Fam Physician 68(1):83,
2003

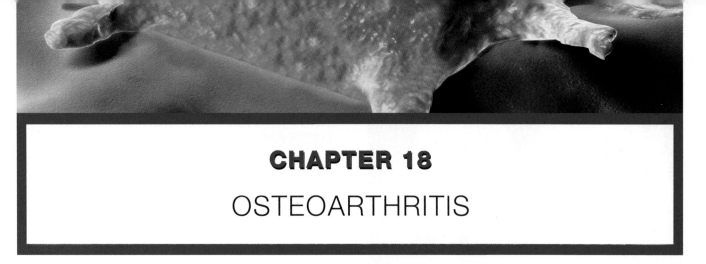

CHAPTER 18

OSTEOARTHRITIS

David T. Felson

Osteoarthritis (OA) is the most common type of arthritis. Its high prevalence, especially in the elderly, and the high rate of disability related to disease make it a leading cause of disability in the elderly. Because of the aging of Western populations and because obesity, a major risk factor, is increasing in prevalence, the occurrence of osteoarthritis is on the rise. In the United States, osteoarthritis prevalence will increase from 66–100% by the year 2020.

OA affects certain joints, yet spares others (**Fig. 18-1**). Commonly affected joints include the cervical and lumbosacral spine, hip, knee, and first metatarsal phalangeal joint (MTP). In the hands, the distal and proximal interphalangeal joints and the base of the thumb are often affected. Usually spared are the wrist, elbow, and ankle. Our joints were designed in an evolutionary sense, when humans were still brachiating apes. We thus develop OA in joints that were ill designed for these tasks, i.e., joints involved in pincer grip in the hands and lower extremity weight-bearing joints. Some joints, like the ankles, may be spared because their articular cartilage may be uniquely resistant to loading stresses.

OA can be diagnosed based on structural abnormalities or on the symptoms these abnormalities evoke. Based on cadaveric studies, structural changes of OA are nearly universal by the elderly years. These include cartilage loss (seen as joint space loss on x-rays) and osteophytes. Many persons with x-ray evidence of OA have no joint symptoms and, while the prevalence of structural abnormalities is of interest in understanding disease

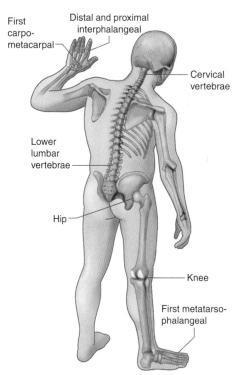

FIGURE 18-1
Joints affected by osteoarthritis.

pathogenesis, what matters more from a clinical and public health perspective is the prevalence of symptomatic OA. Symptoms, usually joint pain, determine disability, visits to clinicians, and disease costs.

223

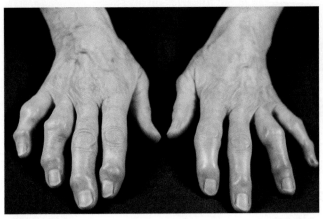

FIGURE 18-2
Severe osteoarthritis of the hands affecting the distal inter-phalangeal joints (Heberden's nodes) and the proximal inter-phalangeal joints (Bouchard's nodes). There is no clear bony enlargement of the other common site in the hands, the thumb base.

Symptomatic OA of the knee (pain on most days of a recent month in a knee plus x-ray evidence of OA in that knee) occurs in ~12% of persons age ≥60 in the United States and 6% of all adults age ≥30. Symptomatic hip OA is roughly one-third as common as disease in the knee. While radiographically evident hand OA and the appearance of bony enlargement in affected hand joints (Fig. 18-2) are extremely common in older persons, most cases are often not symptomatic. Even so, recent studies suggest that symptomatic hand OA occurs in ~10% of elderly individuals and often produces measurable physical functional limitation.

The prevalence of OA correlates strikingly with age. Regardless of how it is defined, OA is uncommon in adults under age 40 and highly prevalent in those over age 60. It is also a disease that, at least in middle-aged and elderly persons, is much more common in women than in men, and sex differences in prevalence increase with age.

X-ray evidence of OA is common in the lower back and neck, but back pain and neck pain have not been tied to findings of OA on x-ray.

DEFINITION

OA is joint failure, a disease in which all structures of the joint have undergone pathologic change, often in concert. The pathologic sine qua non of disease is hyaline articular cartilage loss, present in a focal and, initially, nonuniform manner. This is accompanied by increasing thickness and sclerosis of the subchondral bony plate, by outgrowth of osteophytes at the joint margin, by stretching of the articular capsule, by mild synovitis in many affected joints, and by weakness of muscles bridging the joint. In knees, meniscal degeneration is part of the disease. There are numerous pathways that lead to joint failure, but the initial step is often joint injury in the setting of a failure of protective mechanisms.

JOINT PROTECTIVE MECHANISMS AND THEIR FAILURE

Joint protectors include joint capsule and ligaments, muscle, sensory afferents, and underlying bone. Joint capsule and ligaments serve as joint protectors by providing a limit to excursion, thereby fixing the range of joint motion.

Synovial fluid reduces friction between articulating cartilage surfaces, thereby serving as a major protector against friction-induced cartilage wear. This lubrication function depends on the molecule *lubricin*, a mucinous glycoprotein secreted by synovial fibroblasts whose concentration diminishes after joint injury and in the face of synovial inflammation.

The ligaments, along with overlying skin and tendons, contain mechanoreceptor sensory afferent nerves. These mechanoreceptors fire at different frequencies throughout a joint's range of motion, providing feedback by way of the spinal cord to muscles and tendons. As a consequence, these muscles and tendons can assume the right tension at appropriate points in joint excursion to act as optimal joint protectors, anticipating joint loading.

Muscles and tendons that bridge the joint are key joint protectors. Their co-contractions at the appropriate time in joint movement provide the appropriate power and acceleration for the limb to accomplish its tasks. Focal stress across the joint is minimized by muscle contraction that decelerates the joint before impact and ensures that when joint impact arrives, it is distributed broadly across the joint surface.

The bone underneath the cartilage may also provide a shock-absorbing function, as it may give way subtly to an oncoming impulse load.

Failure of these joint protectors increases the risk of joint injury and OA. For example, in animals, OA develops rapidly when a sensory nerve to the joint is sectioned and joint injury is induced. Similarly, in humans, Charcot arthropathy, which is a severe and rapidly progressive OA, develops when minor joint injury occurs in the presence of posterior column peripheral neuropathy. Another example of joint protector failure is rupture of ligaments, a well-known cause of the early development of OA.

Cartilage and Its Role in Joint Failure

In addition to being a primary target tissue for disease, cartilage also functions as a joint protector. A thin rim of tissue at the ends of two opposing bones, cartilage is lubricated by synovial fluid to provide an almost frictionless surface across which the two bones move. The compressible stiffness of cartilage compared to bone provides the joint with impact-absorbing capacity. Both the smooth frictionless surface and the compressive stiffness

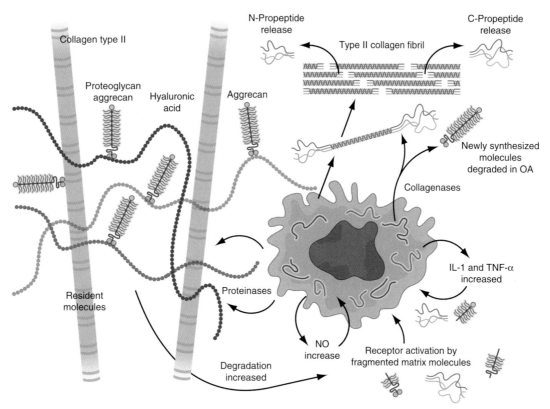

FIGURE 18-3

The chondrocyte and its products, type II collagen, aggrecan and enzymes which degrade these structures along with molecules stimulating chondrocytes. *[From AR Poole et al: Ann Rheum Dis 61 (S): ii78, 2002.]*

of cartilage serve as protective mechanisms preventing joint injury.

Since the earliest changes of OA may occur in cartilage, and abnormalities there can accelerate disease development, understanding the structure and physiology of cartilage is critical to an appreciation of disease pathogenesis. The two major macromolecules in cartilage are type 2 collagen, which provides cartilage its tensile strength, and aggrecan, a proteoglycan macromolecule linked with hyaluronic acid, which consists of highly negatively charged glycosaminoglycans. In normal cartilage, type 2 collagen is woven tightly, constraining the aggrecan molecules in the interstices between collagen strands, forcing these highly negatively charged molecules into close proximity with one another. The aggrecan molecule, through electrostatic repulsion of its negative charges, gives cartilage its compressive stiffness. Chondrocytes, the cells within this avascular tissue, synthesize all elements of the matrix. In addition, they produce enzymes that break down the matrix and cytokines and growth factors, which in turn provide autocrine/paracrine feedback that modulates synthesis of matrix molecules (**Fig. 18-3**). Cartilage matrix synthesis and catabolism are in a dynamic equilibrium influenced by the cytokine and growth factor environment and by mechanical stress. While chondrocytes synthesize numerous enzymes, especially matrix metalloproteinases (MMPs), there are only a few that are critical

in regulating cartilage breakdown. Type 2 cartilage is degraded primarily by MMP-13 (collagenase 3), with other collagenases playing a minor role. Aggrecan degradation is complex but appears to be a consequence, in part, of activation of aggrecanase 1 (ADAMTS-4) and perhaps of MMPs. Both collagenase and aggrecanase act primarily in the territorial matrix surrounding chondrocytes; however, as the osteoarthritic process develops, their activities and effects spread throughout the matrix, especially in the superficial layers of cartilage.

The synovium and chondrocytes synthesize numerous growth factors and cytokines. Chief among them is interleukin (IL) 1, which exerts transcriptional effects on chondrocytes, stimulating production of proteinases and suppressing cartilage matrix synthesis. In animal models of OA, IL-1 blockade prevents cartilage loss. Tumor necrosis factor (TNF) α may play a similar role to that of IL-1. These cytokines also induce chondrocytes to synthesize prostaglandin E_2, nitric oxide, and bone morphogenic protein 2 (BMP-2), which together have complex effects on matrix synthesis and degradation. Nitric oxide inhibits aggrecan synthesis and enhances proteinase activity, whereas BMP-2 is a potent stimulator of anabolic activity. At early stages in the matrix response to injury and in the healthy response to loading, the net effect of cytokine stimulation may be matrix turnover but, ultimately, excess IL-1 triggers a process of matrix degradation. Enzymes in the matrix are held in check by activation inhibitors, including tissue inhibitor of metal-loproteinase (TIMP). Growth factors are also part of this complex network, with insulin–like growth factor type 1 and transforming growth factor β playing prominent roles in stimulating anabolism by chondrocytes.

While healthy cartilage is metabolically sluggish, with slow matrix turnover and a net balance of synthesis and degradation, cartilage in early OA or after an injury is highly metabolically active. In the latter situation, stimulated chondrocytes synthesize enzymes and new matrix molecules, with those enzymes becoming activated in the matrix, causing release of degraded aggrecan and type 2 collagen into cartilage and into the synovial fluid. OA cartilage is characterized by gradual depletion of aggrecan, an unfurling of the tightly woven collagen matrix, and loss of type 2 collagen. With these changes comes increasing vulnerability of cartilage, which no longer has compressive stiffness.

RISK FACTORS

Joint vulnerability and joint loading are the two major factors contributing to the development of OA. On the one hand, a vulnerable joint whose protectors are dysfunctional can develop OA with minimal levels of loading, perhaps even levels encountered during everyday activities. On the other hand, in a young joint with competent protectors, a major acute injury or long-term overloading is necessary to precipitate disease. Risk factors for OA can be understood in terms of their effect either on joint vulnerability or on loading (**Fig. 18–4**).

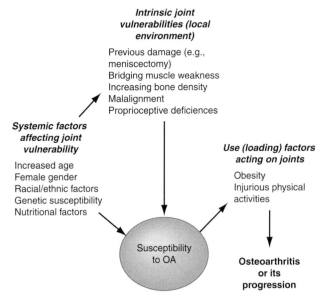

FIGURE 18-4

Risk factors for osteoarthritis either contribute to the susceptibility of the joint (systemic factors or factors in the local joint environment) or they increase risk by the load they put on the joint. Usually a combination of loading and susceptibility factors is required to cause disease or its progression.

Systemic Risk Factors

Age is the most potent risk factor for OA, with prevalence and incidence of disease rising dramatically with age. Radiographic evidence of OA is rare in individuals under age 40; however, in some joints, such as the hands, OA occurs in >50% of persons over age 70. Aging increases joint vulnerability through several mechanisms. Whereas dynamic loading of joints stimulates cartilage matrix by chondrocytes in young cartilage, aged cartilage is less responsive to these stimuli. Indeed, because of the poor responsiveness of older cartilage to such stimulation, cartilage transplant operations are far more challenging in older than in younger persons. Partly because of this failure to synthesize matrix with loading, cartilage thins with age, and thinner cartilage experiences higher shear stress at basal layers and is at greater risk of cartilage damage. Aging also increases the likelihood of failure of major joint protectors. Muscles that bridge the joint become weaker with age and also respond less quickly to oncoming impulses. Sensory nerve input slows with age, retarding the feedback loop of mechanoreceptors to muscles and tendons related to their tension and position. Ligaments stretch with age, making them less able to absorb impulses. A combination of all of these factors works in concert to increase the vulnerability of older joints to OA.

Older women are at high risk of OA in all joints, a risk that emerges as women reach their sixth decade. While hormone loss with menopause may contribute to this risk, there is little understanding of the vulnerability of older women's joints to OA.

Heritability and Genetics

OA is a highly heritable disease, but its heritability varies by joint. Fifty percent of the hand and hip OA in the community is attributable to inheritance, i.e., to disease present in other members of the family. However, the heritable proportion of knee OA is at most 30%, with some studies suggesting no heritability at all. Whereas many people with OA have disease in multiple joints, this "generalized OA" phenotype is rarely inherited and is more often a consequence of aging.

Emerging evidence suggests that persons with genetic mutations in proteins that regulate the transcription of major cartilage molecules are at high risk of OA. One gene implicated is *FRZB*, in which a mutation may put a woman at high risk of hip OA. *FRZB* is a gene for a Frizzle protein that antagonizes an extracellular Wnt ligand, and the Wnt signaling pathway plays a critical role in matrix synthesis and joint development.

Global Considerations

 Hip OA is rare in China and in immigrants from China to the United States. However, OA in the knees is at least as common, if not more so, in

Chinese than in Caucasians from the United States, and knee OA represents a major cause of disability in China. Anatomic differences between Chinese and Caucasian hips may account for much of the difference in prevalence, with Caucasian hips having a higher prevalence of anatomic predispositions to the development of OA. Persons from Africa, but not African Americans, may also have a very low rate of hip OA.

Risk Factors in the Joint Environment

Some risk factors increase vulnerability of the joint through local effects on the joint environment. With changes in joint anatomy, for example, load across the joint is no longer distributed evenly across the joint surface, but rather shows an increase in focal stress. In the hip, three uncommon developmental abnormalities occurring in utero or childhood, congenital dysplasia, Legg-Perthes disease, and slipped femoral capital epiphysis, leave a child with distortions of hip joint anatomy that often lead to OA later in life. Girls are predominantly affected by acetabular dysplasia, a mild form of congenital dislocation, whereas the other abnormalities more often affect boys. Depending on the severity of the anatomic abnormalities, hip OA occurs either in young adulthood (severe abnormalities) or middle age (mild abnormalities).

Major injuries to a joint also can produce anatomic abnormalities that leave the joint susceptible to OA. For example, a fracture through the joint surface often causes OA in joints in which the disease is otherwise rare such as the ankle and the wrist. Avascular necrosis can lead to collapse of dead bone at the articular surface, producing anatomic irregularities and subsequent OA.

Tears of ligaments that protect the joints, such as the anterior cruciate ligament in the knee and the labrum in the hip, can increase joint susceptibility and lead to premature OA. While meniscal tears may increase the risk of OA, meniscectomy operations, including selective ones, increase the risk of later disease, perhaps independent of the tear that led to the operation. Even injuries that do not produce diagnosed joint injuries may increase the risk of OA, perhaps because the structural injury was not detected at the time. For example, in the Framingham study subjects, men with a history of major knee injury, but no surgery, had a 3.5-fold increased risk for subsequent knee OA.

Another source of anatomic abnormality is malalignment across the joint (**Fig. 18-5**). This factor has been best studied in the knee, which is the fulcrum of the longest lever arm in the body. Varus (bowlegged) knees with OA are at exceedingly high risk of cartilage loss in the medial or inner compartment of the knee, whereas valgus (knock kneed) malalignment predisposes to rapid cartilage loss in the lateral compartment. Malalignment causes this effect by decreasing contact area during loading, increasing stress on a focal area or cartilage, which

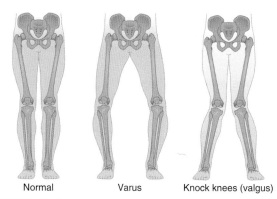

Normal   Varus   Knock knees (valgus)

FIGURE 18-5
The two types of limb malalignment in the frontal plane: varus, in which the stress is placed across the medial compartment of the knee joint, and valgus, which places excess stress across the lateral compartment of the knee.

then breaks down. There is evidence that malalignment in the knee not only causes cartilage loss but leads to underlying bone damage, producing bone marrow lesions seen on MRI.

While it is likely that the weakness in muscles bridging a joint increases the risk of OA in that joint, there is no definitive evidence in this regard.

Patients with knee OA have impaired proprioception across their knees, and this may predispose them to further disease progression. The role of bone in serving as a shock absorber for impact load is not well understood, but persons with increased bone density are at high risk of OA, suggesting that the resistance of bone to impact during joint use may play a role in disease development.

Loading Factors

Obesity

Three to six times body weight is exerted across the knee during single leg stance. Any increase in weight may be multiplied by this factor to reveal the excess force across the knee in overweight persons during walking. Obesity is a well-recognized and potent risk factor for the development of knee OA and, less so, for hip OA. Obesity precedes the development of disease and is not just a consequence of the inactivity present in those with disease. Obesity is a stronger risk factor for disease in women than in men, and in women, the relationship of weight to the risk of disease is linear, so that with each increase in weight, there is a commensurate increase in risk. Weight loss in women lowers the risk of developing symptomatic disease. Not only is obesity a risk factor for OA in weight-bearing joints, but obese persons have more severe symptoms from the disease.

Obesity's effect on the development and progression of disease is mediated mostly through the increased loading in weight-bearing joints that occurs in overweight persons. However, a modest association of obesity with an increased risk of hand OA suggests that there may be a systemic metabolic factor circulating in obese persons that affects disease risk also.

Repeated Use of Joint

There are two categories of repetitive joint use: occupational use and leisure time physical activities. Workers performing repetitive tasks as part of their occupations for many years are at high risk of developing OA in the joints they use repeatedly. For example, farmers are at high risk for hip OA, miners have high rates of OA in knees and spine, and shipyard and dockyard workers have a higher prevalence of disease in knees and fingers than do office workers. Even within a textile mill, women whose jobs required fine pincer grip [increasing the stress across the interphalangeal (IP) joints] had much more distal IP (DIP) joint OA than women of the same age whose jobs required repeated power grip, a motion that does not stress the DIP joints. Workers whose jobs require regular knee bending or lifting or carrying heavy loads have a high rate of knee OA. One reason why workers may get disease is that during long days at work, their muscles may gradually become exhausted, no longer serving as effective joint protectors.

While exercise is a major element of the treatment of OA, certain types of exercise may paradoxically increase the risk of disease. While recreational runners are not at increased risk of knee OA, studies suggest that they do have a modest increased risk of disease in the hip. However, persons who have already sustained major knee injuries are at increased risk of progressive knee OA as a consequence of running. Compared to nonrunners, elite runners (professional runners and those on Olympic teams) have high risks of both knee and hip OA. Given the widespread recommendation to adopt a healthier, more exercise-filled lifestyle; longitudinal epidemiologic studies of exercise contain cautionary notes. For example, women with increased levels of physical activity, either as teenagers or at age 50, had a higher risk of developing symptomatic hip disease later in life than women who were sedentary. Other athletic activities that pose high risks of joint injury, such as football, may thereby predispose to OA.

PATHOLOGY

The pathology of OA provides evidence of the panarticular involvement of disease. Cartilage initially shows surface fibrillation and irregularity. As disease progresses, focal erosions develop there, and these eventually extend down to the subjacent bone. With further progression, cartilage erosion down to bone expands to involve a larger proportion of the joint surface, even though OA remains a focal disease with nonuniform loss of cartilage (Fig. 18-6).

After an injury to cartilage, chondrocytes undergo mitosis and clustering. While the metabolic activity of

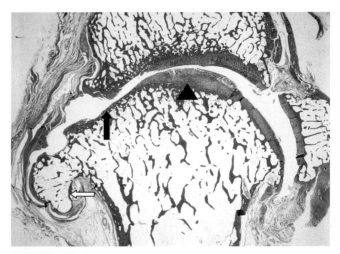

FIGURE 18-6
Pathologic changes of osteoarthritis in a toe joint. Note the nonuniform loss of cartilage (*arrowhead* vs *solid arrow*), the increased thickness of the subchondral bone envelope (*solid arrow*), and the osteophyte (*open arrow*). *(From the American College of Rheumatology slide collection.)*

these chondrocyte clusters is high, the net effect of this activity is to promote proteoglycan depletion in the matrix surrounding the chondrocytes. This is because the catabolic activity is greater than the synthetic. As disease develops, collagen matrix becomes damaged, the negative charges of proteoglycans get exposed, and cartilage swells from ionic attraction to water molecules. Because in damaged cartilage proteoglycans are no longer forced into close proximity, cartilage does not bounce back after loading as it did when healthy, and cartilage becomes vulnerable to further injury. Chondrocytes at the basal level of cartilage undergo apoptosis.

With loss of cartilage come alterations in subchondral bone. Stimulated by growth factors and cytokines, osteoclasts and osteoblasts in the subchondral bony plate, just underneath cartilage, become activated. Bone formation produces a thickening and stiffness of the subchondral plate that occurs even before cartilage ulcerates. Trauma to bone during joint loading may be the primary factor driving this bone response, with healing from injury (including microcracks) producing stiffness. Small areas of osteonecrosis usually exist in joints with advanced disease. Bone death may also be caused by bone trauma with shearing of microvasculature, leading to a cutoff of vascular supply to some bone areas.

At the margin of the joint, near areas of cartilage loss, osteophytes form. These start as outgrowths of new cartilage and, with neurovascular invasion from the bone, this cartilage ossifies. Osteophytes are an important radiographic hallmark of OA. In malaligned joints, osteophytes grow larger on the side of the joint subject to the most loading stress (e.g., in varus knees, osteophytes grow larger on the medial side).

The synovium produces lubricating fluids that minimize shear stress during motion. In healthy joints, the synovium consists of a single discontinuous layer filled with fat and containing two types of cells—macrophages and fibroblasts—but, in OA, it can sometimes become edematous and inflamed. There is a migration of macrophages from the periphery into the tissue, and cells lining the synovium proliferate. Enzymes secreted by the synovium digest cartilage matrix that has been sheared from the surface of the cartilage.

Additional pathologic changes occur in the capsule, which stretches, becomes edematous, and can become fibrotic.

The pathology of OA is not identical across joints. In hand joints with severe OA, for example, there are often cartilage erosions in the center of the joint probably produced by bony pressure from the opposite side of the joint. Bone remodeling is a prominent feature of hand OA, in part because of the thin cartilage in each hand joint. In hand OA, pathology has also been noted in ligament site insertions, which may help propagate disease.

Basic calcium phosphate and calcium pyrophosphate dihydrate crystals are present microscopically in most joints with end-stage OA. Their role in osteoarthritic cartilage is unclear, but their release from cartilage into the joint space and joint fluid likely triggers synovial inflammation, which can, in turn, produce release of enzymes and trigger nociceptive stimulation.

SOURCES OF PAIN

Because cartilage is aneural, cartilage loss in a joint is not accompanied by pain. Thus, pain in OA likely arises from structures outside the cartilage. Innervated structures in the joint include the synovium, ligaments, joint capsule, muscles, and subchondral bone. Most of these are not visualized by x-ray, and the severity of x-ray changes in OA correlates poorly with pain severity.

Based on MRI studies in osteoarthritic knees comparing those with and without pain, and on studies mapping tenderness in unanesthetized joints, likely sources of pain include synovial inflammation, joint effusions, and bone marrow edema. Modest synovitis develops in many but not all osteoarthritic joints. Some diseased joints have no synovitis, whereas others have synovial inflammation that approaches the severity of joints with rheumatoid arthritis (Chap. 5). The presence of synovitis on MRI is correlated with the presence and severity of knee pain. Capsular stretching from fluid in the joint stimulates nociceptive fibers there, inducing pain. Increased focal loading as part of the disease not only damages cartilage but probably also injures the underlying bone. As a consequence, bone marrow edema appears on the MRI; histologically, this edema may signal the presence of microcracks and scar, which are the consequences of trauma. These lesions may stimulate bone nociceptive fibers. Also, hemostatic

pressure within bone rises in OA, and the increased pressure itself may stimulate nociceptive fibers, causing pain. Lastly, osteophytes themselves may be a source of pain. When osteophytes grow, neurovascular innervation penetrates through the base of the bone into the cartilage and into the developing osteophyte.

Pain may arise from outside the joint also, including bursae near the joints. Common sources of pain near the knee are anserine bursitis and iliotibial band syndrome.

CLINICAL FEATURES

Joint pain from OA is activity related. Pain comes on either during or just after joint use and then gradually resolves. Examples include knee or hip pain with going up or down stairs, pain in weight-bearing joints when walking, and, for hand OA, pain after cooking. Early in disease, pain is episodic, triggered often by a day or two of overactive use of a diseased joint, such as a person with knee OA taking a long run and noticing a few days of pain thereafter. As disease progresses, the pain becomes continuous and even begins to be bothersome at night. Stiffness of the affected joint may be prominent, but morning stiffness is usually brief (<30 min).

In knees, buckling may occur, in part due to weakness of muscles crossing the joint. Mechanical symptoms, such as buckling, catching, or locking, could also signify internal derangement, such as meniscal tears, and need to be evaluated. In the knee, pain with activities requiring knee flexion, such as stair climbing and arising from a chair, often emanates from the patellofemoral compartment of the knee, which does not actively articulate until the knee is bent ~35°.

OA is the most common cause of chronic knee pain in persons over age 45, but the differential diagnosis is long. Inflammatory arthritis is likely if there is prominent morning stiffness and many other joints are affected. Bursitis occurs commonly around knees and hips. A physical examination should focus on whether tenderness is over the joint line (at the junction of the two bones around which the joint is articulating) or is outside of it. Anserine bursitis, medial and distal to the knee, is an extremely common cause of chronic knee pain that may respond to a glucocorticoid injection. Prominent nocturnal pain in the absence of end-stage OA merits a distinct workup. For hip pain, OA can be detected by loss of internal rotation on passive movement, and pain isolated to an area lateral to the hip joint usually reflects the presence of trochanteric bursitis.

No blood tests are routinely indicated for workup of patients with OA unless symptoms and signs suggest inflammatory arthritis. Examination of the synovial fluid is often more helpful diagnostically than an x-ray. If the synovial fluid white count is >1000/μL, inflammatory arthritis or gout or pseudogout are likely, the latter two being also identified by the presence of crystals.

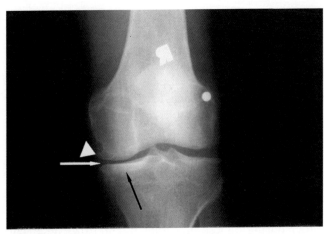

FIGURE 18-7

X-ray of knee with medial osteoarthritis. Note the narrowed joint space on medial side of the joint only (*white arrow*), the sclerosis of the bone in the medial compartment providing evidence of cortical thickening (*black arrow*), and the osteophytes in the medial femur (*white wedge*).

X-rays are indicated to evaluate chronic hand pain and hip pain thought to be due to OA, as the diagnosis is often unclear without confirming radiographs. For knee pain, x-rays should be obtained if symptoms or signs are not typical of OA or if knee pain persists after effective treatment. In OA, radiographic findings (**Fig. 18-7**) correlate poorly with the presence and severity of pain. Further, radiographs may be normal in early disease as they are insensitive to cartilage loss and other early findings.

While MRI may reveal the extent of pathology in an osteoarthritic joint, it is not indicated as part of the diagnostic workup. Findings such as meniscal tears in cartilage and bone lesions occur in most patients with OA in the knee, but almost never warrant a change in therapy.

℞ **Treatment:**
OSTEOARTHRITIS

The goals of the treatment of OA are to alleviate pain and minimize loss of physical function. To the extent that pain and loss of function are consequences of inflammation, of weakness across the joint, and of laxity and instability, the treatment of OA involves addressing each of these impairments. Comprehensive therapy consists of a multimodality approach including nonpharmacologic and pharmacologic elements.

Patients with mild and intermittent symptoms may need only reassurance or nonpharmacologic treatments. Patients with ongoing, disabling pain are likely to need both nonpharmaco- and pharmacotherapy.

Treatments for knee OA have been more completely evaluated than those for hip and hand OA or for disease in other joints. Thus, while the principles of treatment are identical for OA in all joints, we shall focus below on the treatment of knee OA, noting specific recommendations for disease in other joints, especially when they differ from those for disease in the knee.

NONPHARMACOTHERAPY Since OA is a mechanically driven disease, the mainstay of treatment involves altering loading across the painful joint and improving the function of joint protectors so they can better distribute load across the joint. Ways of lessening focal load across the joint include:

1. Avoiding activities that overload the joint, as evidenced by their causing pain;
2. Improving the strength and conditioning of muscles that bridge the joint, so as to optimize their function; and
3. Unloading the joint, either by redistributing load within the joint with a brace or a splint or by unloading the joint during weight bearing with a cane or a crutch.

The simplest effective treatment for many patients is to avoid activities that precipitate pain. For example, for the middle-aged patient whose long-distance running brings on symptoms of knee OA, a less demanding form of weight-bearing activity may alleviate all symptoms. For an older person whose daily constitutionals up and down hills bring on knee pain, routing the constitutional away from hills might eliminate symptoms.

Each pound of weight increases the loading across the knee three- to sixfold. Weight loss may have a commensurate multiplier effect, unloading both knees and hips. Thus, weight loss, especially if substantial, may lessen symptoms of knee and hip OA.

In hand joints affected by OA, splinting, by limiting motion, often minimizes pain for patients with involvement either in the base of the thumb or in the DIP or proximal IP joints. With an appropriate splint, function can often be preserved. Weight-bearing joints such as knees and hips can be unloaded by using a cane in the hand opposite to the affected joint for partial weight bearing. A physical therapist can help teach the patient how to use the cane optimally, including ensuring that its height is optimal for unloading. Crutches or walkers can serve a similar beneficial function.

Exercise Osteoarthritic pain in knees or hips during weight bearing results in lack of activity and poor mobility and, because OA is so common, the inactivity that results represents a public health concern, increasing the risk of cardiovascular disease and of obesity. Aerobic capacity is poor in most elders with symptomatic knee OA, worse than others of the same age.

The development of weakness in muscles that bridge osteoarthritic joints is multifactorial in etiology. First, there is a decline in strength with age. Second, with limited mobility comes disuse muscle atrophy. Third, patients with painful knee or hip OA alter their gait so as to lessen loading across the affected joint, and this further diminishes muscle use. Fourth, "arthrogenous inhibition" may occur, whereby contraction of muscles bridging the joint is inhibited by a nerve afferent feedback loop emanating in a swollen and stretched joint capsule; this prevents maximal attainment of voluntary maximal strength. Since adequate muscle strength and conditioning are critical to joint protection, weakness in a muscle that bridges a diseased joint makes the joint more susceptible to further damage and pain. The degree of weakness correlates strongly with the severity of joint pain and the degree of physical limitation. One of the cardinal elements of the treatment of OA is to improve the functioning of muscles surrounding the joint.

At least for knee OA, trials have shown that exercise lessens pain and improves physical function. Most effective exercise regimens consist of aerobic and/or resistance training, the latter of which focuses on strengthening muscles across the joint. Exercises are likely to be effective, especially if they train muscles for the activities a person performs daily. Some exercises may actually increase pain in the joint; these should be avoided, and the regimen needs to be individualized to optimize effectiveness and minimize discomfort. Range-of-motion exercises, which do not strengthen muscles, and isometric exercises that strengthen muscles, but not through range of motion, are unlikely to be effective by themselves. Isokinetic and isotonic strengthening (strengthening that occurs when a person flexes or extends the knees against resistance) have been shown consistently to be efficacious. Low-impact exercises, including water aerobics and water resistance training, are often better tolerated by patients than exercises involving impact loading, such as running or treadmill exercises. A patient should be referred to an exercise class or to a therapist who can create an individualized regimen, and then an individualized home-based regimen can be crafted.

There is no strong evidence that patients with hip or hand OA benefit from therapeutic exercise, although for any patient with OA, individualized exercise programs should be tried. Adherence to exercise over the long term is the major challenge to an exercise prescription. In trials involving patients with knee OA who are interested in exercise treatment, a third to over a half of patients stopped exercising by 6 months. Less than 50% continued regular exercise at 1 year. The strongest predictor of continued exercise in a patient is a previous personal history of successful exercise. Physicians should reinforce the exercise prescription at each clinic visit, help the patient recognize barriers to ongoing exercise, and identify convenient times for exercise to be done routinely. The combination of exercise with calorie restriction is especially effective in lessening pain.

One clinical trial has suggested that, among those with very early OA, participating in a strengthening and multimodality exercise program led to improvement in cartilage biochemistry, as evidenced by MRI imaging. There is little other evidence, however, that strengthening or other exercise has an effect on joint structure.

Correction of Malalignment Malalignment in the frontal plane (varus-valgus) markedly increases the stress across the joint, which can lead to progression of disease and to pain and disability (Fig. 18-5). Correcting malalignment, either surgically or with bracing, can relieve pain in persons whose knees are maligned. Malalignment develops over years as a consequence of gradual anatomic alterations of the joint and bone, and correcting it is often very challenging. One way is with a fitted brace, which takes an often varus osteoarthritic knee and straightens it by putting valgus stress across the knee. Unfortunately, many patients are unwilling to wear a realigning knee brace; plus, in patients with obese legs, braces may slip with usage and lose their realigning effect. They are indicated for willing patients who can learn to put them on correctly and on whom they do not slip.

Other ways of correcting malalignment across the knee include the use of orthotics in footwear. Unfortunately, while they may have modest effects on knee alignment, trials have heretofore not demonstrated efficacy of a lateral wedge orthotic vs placebo wedges.

Pain from the patellofemoral compartment of the knee can be caused by tilting of the patella or patellar malalignment with the patella riding laterally (or less often, medially) in the femoral trochlear groove. Using a brace to realign the patella, or tape to pull the patella back into the trochlear sulcus or reduce its tilt, has been shown, when compared to placebo taping in clinical trials, to lessen patellofemoral pain. However, patients may find it difficult to apply tape, and skin irritation from the tape is common. Commercial patellar braces may be a solution, but they have not been tested.

While their effect on malalignment is questionable, neoprene sleeves pulled to cover the knee lessen pain and are easy to use and popular among patients. The explanation for their therapeutic effect on pain is unclear.

In patients with knee OA, acupuncture produces modest pain relief compared to placebo needles and may be an adjunctive treatment.

PHARMACOTHERAPY While nonpharmacologic approaches to therapy constitute its mainstay, pharmacotherapy serves an important adjunctive role in OA

TABLE 18-1

PHARMACOLOGIC TREATMENT FOR OSTEOARTHRITIS

TREATMENT	DOSAGE	COMMENTS
Acetaminophen	Up to 1 g qid	Prolongs half-life of warfarin
NSAIDs[a]		Take with food. High rates of gastrointestinal side effects, including ulcers and bleeding, occur. Patients at high risk for gastrointestinal side effects should also take either a proton-pump inhibitor or misoprostol.[b] There is an increased concern about side effects (gastrointestinal or bleeding) when taken with acetylsalicylic acid. Can also cause edema and renal insufficiency.
Naproxen	375–500 mg bid	
Salsalate	1500 mg bid	
Ibuprofen	600–800 mg 3–4 times a day	
Cyclooxygenase-2 inhibitors	100–200 mg/d	High doses are associated with an increased risk of myocardial infarction and stroke. Can cause edema and renal insufficiency.
Celecoxib		
Opiates	Various	Common side effects include dizziness, sedation, nausea or vomiting, dry mouth, constipation, urinary retention, and pruritus. Respiratory and central nervous system depression can occur.
Capsaicin	0.025–0.075% cream 3–4 times a day	Can irritate mucous membranes.
Intraarticular injections		
Hyaluronans	Varies from 3 to 5 weekly injections depending on preparation	Mild to moderate pain at injection site.
Steroids		Controversy exists re: efficacy.

[a]NSAIDs denotes nonsteroidal anti-inflammatory drugs.
[b]Patients at high risk include those with previous gastrointestinal events, persons ≥60 years, and persons taking glucocorticoids. Trials have shown the efficacy of proton-pump inhibitors and misoprostol in the prevention of ulcers and bleeding. Misoprostol is associated with a high rate of diarrhea and cramping; therefore, proton-pump inhibitors are more widely used to reduce NSAID-related gastrointestinal symptoms.
Source: Adapted from Felson, 2006.

treatment. Available drugs are administered using oral, topical, and intraarticular routes.

Acetaminophen, Nonsteroidal Anti-inflammatory Drugs (NSAIDs), and COX-2 Inhibitors

Acetaminophen (paracetamol) is the initial analgesic of choice for patients with OA in the knee, hip, or hands. For some patients, it is adequate to control symptoms, in which case more toxic drugs such as NSAIDs can be avoided. Doses up to 1 g four times daily can be used (Table 18-1).

NSAIDs are the most popular drugs to treat osteoarthritic pain. In clinical trials, NSAIDs produce ~30% greater improvement in pain than high-dose acetaminophen. Occasional patients treated with NSAIDs experience dramatic pain relief, whereas others experience little improvement. Initially, NSAIDs should be taken on an "as needed" basis because side effects are less frequent with low intermittent doses, which may be highly efficacious. If occasional medication use is insufficiently effective, then daily treatment with NSAIDs is indicated, with an anti-inflammatory dose selected (Table 18-1). Patients should be reminded to take low-dose aspirin and NSAIDs at different times to eliminate drug interactions.

NSAIDs have substantial and frequent side effects, the most common of which is upper gastrointestinal (GI) toxicity, including dyspepsia, nausea, bloating, GI bleeding, and ulcer disease. Some 30–40% of patients experience upper GI side effects so severe as to require discontinuation of medication. Strategies to avoid or minimize the risk of NSAID-related GI side effects include:

- Take medications after food.
- Avoid use of two NSAIDs.
- Use a relatively safe NSAID. In terms of GI toxicity, meta-analyses have suggested that nonacetylated salicylates, ibuprofen and nabumetone, are among the safer NSAIDs; more dangerous ones include piroxicam, ketorolac, and ketoprofen.
- For persons at high risk of GI bleeding and/or complications, prescribe a gastroprotective agent (Table 18-1).

Major NSAID-related GI side effects can occur in patients who do not complain of upper GI symptoms. In one study of patients hospitalized for GI bleeding, 81% had no premonitory symptoms.

There are other common side effects of NSAIDs, including the tendency to develop edema, because of prostaglandin inhibition of afferent blood supply to glomeruli in the kidneys and, for similar reasons, a predilection toward reversible renal insufficiency. Blood pressure may increase modestly in some NSAID-treated patients.

Alternative anti-inflammatory medications are cyclooxygenase-2 (COX-2) inhibitors. While their rate of GI side effects may be less than for conventional NSAIDs, their risk of causing edema and renal insufficiency is similar. In addition, COX-2 inhibitors, especially at high doses, increase the risk of myocardial infarction and of stroke. This is because selective COX-2 inhibitors reduce prostaglandin I_2 production by vascular endothelium, but do not inhibit platelet thromboxane A_2 production, leading to an increased risk of intravascular thrombosis.

Intraarticular Injections: Glucocorticoids and Hyaluronic Acid Since synovial inflammation is likely to be a major cause of pain in patients with OA, local anti-inflammatory treatments administered intraarticularly may be effective in ameliorating pain, at least temporarily. Glucocorticoid injections provide such efficacy, but work better than placebo injections for only 1 or 2 weeks. This may be because the disease remains mechanically driven and, when a person begins to use the joint, the loading factors that induce pain return. Glucocorticoid injections are useful to get patients over acute flares of pain and may be especially indicated if the patient has coexistent OA and crystal deposition disease, especially from calcium pyrophosphate dihydrate crystals (Chap. 19). There is no evidence that repeated glucocorticoid injections into the joint are dangerous.

Hyaluronic acid injections can be given for treatment of symptoms in knee and hip OA, but there is controversy as to whether they have efficacy vs. placebo (Table 18-1).

Optimal therapy for OA is often achieved by trial and error, with each patient having idiosyncratic responses to specific treatments. When medical therapies have failed and the patient has an unacceptable reduction in their quality of life and ongoing pain and disability, then at least for knee and hip OA, total joint arthroplasty is indicated.

SURGERY For knee OA, several operations are available. Among the most popular surgeries, at least in the United States, is arthroscopic debridement and lavage. A well-done randomized trial evaluating this operation showed that its efficacy was no greater than that of sham surgery for relief of pain or disability. There is controversy as to whether mechanical symptoms such as buckling, which are extremely common in patients with knee OA, respond to arthroscopic debridement. While buckling is usually due to muscle weakness, a history of a recent injury, along with knee catching or locking, may suggest that a meniscal tear is contributing to this symptom. In such cases arthroscopic debridement with partial meniscal resection might be warranted.

For patients with knee OA isolated to the medial compartment, operations to realign the knee to lessen medial loading can relieve pain. These include a high tibial osteotomy, in which the tibia is broken just below the tibial plateau and realigned so as to load the lateral, nondiseased compartment, or a unicompartmental replacement with realignment. Each surgery may provide the patient with years of pain relief before they require a total knee replacement.

Ultimately, when the patient with knee or hip OA has failed medical treatment modalities and remains in pain, with limitations of physical function that compromise the quality of life, the patient should be referred for total knee or hip arthroplasty. These are highly efficacious operations that relieve pain and improve function in the vast majority of patients. Currently, failure rates are ~1% per year, although these rates are higher in obese patients. The chance of surgical success is greater in centers where at least 50 such operations are performed yearly or with surgeons who perform a similar number annually. The timing of knee or hip replacement is critical. If the patient suffers for many years until their functional status has declined substantially, with considerable muscle weakness, postoperative functional status may not improve to a level achieved by others who underwent operation earlier in their disease course.

Cartilage Regeneration Chondrocyte transplantation has not been found to be efficacious in OA, perhaps because OA includes pathology of joint mechanics, which is not corrected by chondrocyte transplants. Similarly, abrasion arthroplasty (chondroplasty) has not been well studied for efficacy in OA, but it produces fibrocartilage in place of damaged hyaline cartilage. Both of these surgical attempts to regenerate and reconstitute articular cartilage may be more likely to be efficacious early in disease when joint malalignment and many of the other noncartilage abnormalities that characterize OA have not yet developed.

FURTHER READINGS

BENNELL K, HINMAN R: Exercise as a treatment for osteoarthritis. Curr Opin Rheumatol 17:634, 2005

BRADLEY JD et al: Comparison of an anti-inflammatory dose of ibuprofen, an analgesic dose of ibuprofen, and acetaminophen in the treatment of patients with osteoarthritis of the knee. N Engl J Med 325:87, 1991

BRANDT K et al (eds): *Osteoarthritis*, 2d ed. Oxford, Oxford University Press, 2003

CLEGG DO et al: Glucosamine, chondroitin sulfate, and the two in combination for painful knee osteoarthritis. N Engl J Med 354:795, 2006

ENGLUND M et al: Meniscal tear in knees without surgery and the development of radiographic osteoarthritis among middle-aged and elderly persons: The Multicenter Osteoarthritis Study. Arthritis Rheum 60:831, 2009

FELSON DT: Osteoarthritis of the knee. N Engl J Med 354:841, 2006

———: Developments in the clinical understanding of osteoarthritis. Arthritis Res Ther 11:203, 2009

——— et al: Knee buckling: Prevalence, risk factors, and associated limitations in function. Ann Intern Med 147:534, 2007

——— et al: The effects of impaired joint position sense on the development and progression of pain and structural damage in knee osteoarthritis. Arthritis Rheum 61:1070, 2009

KIRKLEY A et al: A randomized trial of arthroscopic surgery for osteoarthritis of the knee. N Engl J Med 359:1097, 2008

KROHN K: Footwear alterations and bracing as treatments for knee osteoarthritis. Curr Opin Rheumatol 17:653, 2005

LO G et al: Intraarticular hyaluronic acid in treatment of knee osteoarthritis. A meta-analysis. JAMA 290:3115, 2003

MOSELEY JB et al: A controlled trial of arthroscopic surgery for osteoarthritis of the knee. N Engl J Med 347:81, 2002

NIU J et al: Is obesity a risk factor for progressive radiographic knee osteoarthritis? Arthritis Rheum 61:329, 2009

PSATY BM, FURBER CD: Cox-2 inhibitors—Lessons in drug safety. N Engl J Med 352:1133, 2005

REICHENBACH S et al: Meta-analysis: Chondroitin for osteoarthritis of the knee or hip. Ann Intern Med 146:580, 2007

ROZENDAAL RM et al: Effect of glucosamine sulfate on hip osteoarthritis: A randomized trial. Ann Intern Med 148:268, 2008

SAWITZKE AD et al: The effect of glucosamine and/or chondroitin sulfate on the progression of knee osteoarthritis: A report from the glucosamine/chondroitin arthritis intervention trial. Arthritis Rheum 58:3183, 2008

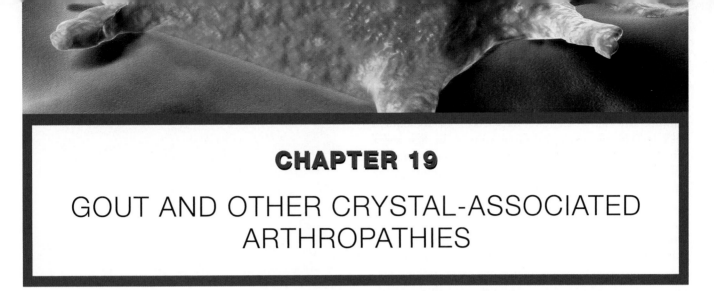

CHAPTER 19

GOUT AND OTHER CRYSTAL-ASSOCIATED ARTHROPATHIES

H. Ralph Schumacher ■ Lan X. Chen

The use of polarizing light microscopy during synovial fluid analysis in 1961 by McCarty and Hollander and the subsequent application of other crystallographic techniques, such as electron microscopy, energy-dispersive elemental analysis, and x-ray diffraction, have allowed investigators to identify the roles of different microcrystals, including monosodium urate (MSU), calcium pyrophosphate dihydrate (CPPD), calcium apatite (apatite), and calcium oxalate (CaOx), in inducing acute or chronic arthritis or periarthritis. The clinical events that result from deposition of MSU, CPPD, apatite, and CaOx have many similarities but also important differences. Prior to the use of crystallographic techniques in rheumatology, much of what was considered to be gouty arthritis in fact was not. Because of often similar clinical presentations, the need to perform synovial fluid analysis to distinguish the type of crystal involved must be emphasized. Polarized light microscopy alone can identify most typical crystals; apatite, however, is an exception. Aspiration and analysis of effusions are also important to assess the possibility of infection. Apart from the identification of specific microcrystalline materials or organisms, synovial fluid characteristics in crystal-associated diseases are nonspecific, and synovial fluid can be inflammatory or noninflammatory. A list of possible

TABLE 19-1

MUSCULOSKELETAL MANIFESTATIONS OF CRYSTAL-INDUCED ARTHRITIS	
Acute mono- or polyarthritis	Destructive arthropathies
Bursitis	Pseudo-rheumatoid
Tendinitis	arthritis
Enthesitis	Pseudo-ankylosing
Tophaceous deposits	spondylitis
Peculiar type of osteoarthritis	Spinal stenosis
Synovial osteochondromatosis	Crown dens syndrome
	Carpal tunnel syndrome
	Tendon rupture

musculoskeletal manifestations of crystal-associated arthritis is shown in **Table 19-1**.

GOUT

Gout is a metabolic disease most often affecting middle-aged to elderly men and postmenopausal women. It is the result of an increased body pool of urate with hyperuricemia. It is typically characterized by episodic acute and chronic arthritis, due to deposition of MSU crystals in joints and connective tissue tophi, and the risk for deposition in kidney interstitium or uric acid nephrolithiasis.

Acute arthritis is the most frequent early clinical manifestation of gout. Usually, only one joint is affected initially, but polyarticular acute gout can occur in subsequent episodes. The metatarsophalangeal joint of the first toe is often involved, but tarsal joints, ankles, and knees are also commonly affected. Especially in elderly patients or in advanced disease, finger joints may be involved. Inflamed Heberden's or Bouchard's nodes may be a first manifestation of gouty arthritis. The first episode of acute gouty arthritis frequently begins at night with dramatic joint pain and swelling. Joints rapidly become warm, red, and tender, with a clinical appearance that often mimics cellulitis. Early attacks tend to subside spontaneously within 3–10 days, and most patients have intervals of varying length with no residual symptoms until the next episode. Several events may precipitate acute gouty arthritis: dietary excess, trauma, surgery, excessive ethanol ingestion, hypouricemic therapy, and serious medical illnesses such as myocardial infarction and stroke.

After many acute mono- or oligoarticular attacks, a proportion of gouty patients may present with a chronic nonsymmetric synovitis, causing potential confusion with rheumatoid arthritis (Chap. 5). Less commonly, chronic gouty arthritis will be the only manifestation and, more rarely, the disease will manifest only as periarticular tophaceous deposits in the absence of synovitis. Women represent only 5–20% of all patients with gout. Premenopausal gout is rare; it is seen mostly in individuals with a strong family history of gout. Kindreds of precocious gout in young females caused by decreased renal urate clearance and renal insufficiency have been described. Most women with gouty arthritis are postmenopausal and elderly, have osteoarthritis and arterial hypertension causing mild renal insufficiency, and are usually receiving diuretics.

Laboratory Diagnosis

Even if the clinical appearance strongly suggests gout, the diagnosis should be confirmed by needle aspiration of acutely or chronically involved joints or tophaceous deposits. Acute septic arthritis, several of the other crystalline-associated arthropathies, palindromic rheumatism, and psoriatic arthritis may present with similar clinical features. During acute gouty attacks, strongly birefringent needle-shaped MSU crystals with negative elongation are typically seen both intracellularly and extracellularly (**Fig. 19-1**). Synovial fluid cell counts are elevated from 2000 to 60,000/μL. Effusions appear cloudy due to the increased numbers of leukocytes. Large amounts of crystals occasionally produce a thick pasty or chalky joint fluid. Bacterial infection can coexist with urate crystals in synovial fluid; if there is any suspicion of septic arthritis, joint fluid must also be cultured.

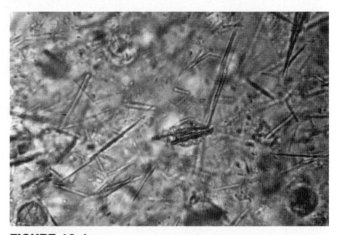

FIGURE 19-1

Extracellular and intracellular monosodium urate crystals, as seen in a fresh preparation of synovial fluid, illustrate needle- and rod-shaped strongly negative birefringent crystals (compensated polarized light microscopy; 400×).

MSU crystals can also often be demonstrated in the first metatarsophalangeal joint and in knees not acutely involved with gout. Arthrocentesis of these joints is a useful technique to establish the diagnosis of gout between attacks.

Serum uric acid levels can be normal or low at the time of the acute attack, as inflammatory cytokines can be uricosuric and effective initiation of hypouricemic therapy can precipitate attacks. This limits the value of serum uric acid determinations for the diagnosis of gout. Nevertheless, serum urate levels are almost always elevated at some time and are important to use to follow the course of hypouricemic therapy. A 24-h urine collection for uric acid can, in some cases, be useful in assessing the risk of stones, in elucidating overproduction or underexcretion of uric acid, and in deciding if it might be appropriate to use a uricosuric therapy. Excretion of >800 mg of uric acid per 24 h on a regular diet suggests that causes of overproduction of purine should be considered. Urinalysis, serum creatinine, hemoglobin, white blood cell (WBC) count, liver function tests, and serum lipids should be obtained because of possible pathologic sequelae of gout and other associated diseases requiring treatment, and as baselines because of possible adverse effects of gout treatment.

Radiographic Features

Early in the disease radiographic studies may only confirm clinically evident swelling. Cystic changes, well-defined erosions with sclerotic margins (often with overhanging bony edges), and soft-tissue masses are characteristic radiographic features of advanced chronic tophaceous gout.

℞ Treatment: GOUT

ACUTE GOUTY ARTHRITIS The mainstay of treatment during an acute attack is the administration of anti-inflammatory drugs such as nonsteroidal anti-inflammatory drugs (NSAIDs), colchicine, or glucocorticoids. NSAIDs are most often used in individuals without complicating comorbid conditions. Both colchicine and NSAIDs may be poorly tolerated and dangerous in the elderly and in the presence of renal insufficiency and gastrointestinal disorders. In attacks involving one or two joints, intraarticular glucocorticoid injections may be preferable and effective. Ice pack applications and rest of the involved joints can be helpful. Colchicine given orally is a traditional and effective treatment, if used early in the attack. One to two 0.6-mg tablets can be given every 6–8 h over several days with subsequent tapering. This is generally better tolerated than the formerly advised hourly regimen. The drug must be stopped promptly at the first sign of loose stools, and symptomatic treatment must be given for the diarrhea. Intravenous colchicine is occasionally used, e.g., as pre- or postoperative prophylaxis in 1- to 2-mg doses when patients cannot take medications orally. Life-threatening colchicine toxicity and sudden death have been described with the administration of >4 mg/d IV. The IV colchicine should be given slowly through an established venous line over 10 min in a soluset. The total dose should never exceed 4 mg.

NSAIDs given in full anti-inflammatory doses are effective in ~90% of patients, and the resolution of signs and symptoms usually occurs in 5–8 days. The most effective drugs are any of those with a short half-life and include indomethacin, 25–50 mg tid; ibuprofen, 800 mg tid; or diclofenac, 50 mg tid. Oral glucocorticoids such as prednisone, 30–50 mg/d as the initial dose and gradually tapered with the resolution of the attack, can be effective in polyarticular gout. For single or few involved joints intraarticular triamcinolone acetonide, 20–40 mg, or methylprednisolone, 25–50 mg, have been effective and well tolerated. Adrenocorticotropic hormone (ACTH) as an intramuscular injection of 40–80 IU in a single dose or every 12 h for 1–2 days can be effective in patients with acute polyarticular refractory gout or in those with a contraindication for using colchicine or NSAIDs.

HYPOURICEMIC THERAPY Ultimate control of gout requires correction of the basic underlying defect, the hyperuricemia. Attempts to normalize serum uric acid to <300–360 μmol/L (5.0–6.0 mg/dL) to prevent recurrent gouty attacks and eliminate tophaceous deposits entail a commitment to long-term hypouricemic regimens and medications that generally are required for life. Hypouricemic therapy should be considered when, as in most patients, the hyperuricemia cannot be corrected by simple means (control of body weight, low-purine diet, increase in liquid intake, limitation of ethanol use, and avoidance of diuretics). The decision to initiate hypouricemic therapy is usually made taking into consideration the number of acute attacks (urate lowering may be cost-effective after two attacks), serum uric acid levels [progression is more rapid in patients with serum uric acid >535 μmol/L (>9.0 mg/dL)], patient's willingness to commit to lifelong therapy, or presence of uric acid stones. Urate-lowering therapy should be initiated in any patient who already has tophi or chronic gouty arthritis. Uricosuric agents, such as probenecid, can be used in patients with good renal function who underexcrete uric acid, with <600 mg in a 24-h urine sample. Urine volume must be maintained by ingestion of 1500 mL of water every day. Probenecid can be started at a dosage of 250 mg twice daily and increased gradually as needed up to 3 g in order to maintain a serum uric acid level <300 μmol/L (5 mg/dL). Probenecid is generally not effective in patients with serum creatinine levels of >177 μmol/L (2.0 mg/dL). These patients may require allopurinol or benzbromarone (not available in the United States). The latter is another uricosuric drug that is more effective in patients with renal failure. Recent reports have identified that losartan, fenofibrate, and amlodipine have some mild uricosuric effects.

The xanthine oxidase inhibitor allopurinol is by far the most commonly used hypouricemic agent and is the best drug to lower serum urate in overproducers, urate stone formers, and patients with renal disease. It can be given in a single morning dose, 100–300 mg initially and increasing up to 800 mg if needed. In patients with chronic renal disease, the initial allopurinol dosage should be lower and adjusted depending on the serum creatinine concentration; for example, with a creatinine clearance of 10 mL/min, one would generally use 100 mg every other day. Doses can gradually be increased to reach the target urate level; however, more studies are needed to provide exact guidance. Patients with frequent acute attacks may also require lower initial doses to prevent exacerbations. Toxicity of allopurinol has been recognized increasingly in patients with renal failure who use thiazide diuretics and in those patients allergic to penicillin and ampicillin. The most serious side effects include skin rash with progression to life-threatening toxic epidermal necrolysis, systemic vasculitis, bone marrow suppression, granulomatous hepatitis, and renal failure. Patients with mild cutaneous reactions to allopurinol can reconsider the use of a uricosuric agent or undergo an attempt at desensitization to allopurinol. A treatment option for allopurinol-sensitive patients is febuxostat, a new specific xanthine oxidase inhibitor, which is approved for the chronic management of hyperuricemia in patients with gout. In contrast to allopurinol, febuxostat does not require dosage adjustment based on level of renal function. The recommended starting dose of febuxostat is 40 mg once a day, and for patients who do not achieve a serum uric acid level of less than 6 mg/dL after 2 weeks, the dose can be increased to 80 mg daily. Similar to allopurinol, febuxostat has important interactions with azathioprine, mercaptopurine, and theophylline in which concomitant administration could increase plasma concentrations of these drugs resulting in severe toxicity. Urate-lowering drugs are generally not initiated during acute attacks, but after the patient is stable and low-dose colchicine has been initiated to decrease the risk of flares that often occur with urate lowering. Colchicine prophylaxis in doses of 0.6 mg one to two times daily is usually continued, along with the hypouricemic therapy, until the patient is normouricemic and without gouty attacks for 6 months or as long as tophi are present. A new urate-lowering drug undergoing investigation is a PEGylated uricase.

CPPD DEPOSITION DISEASE

PATHOGENESIS

The deposition of CPPD crystals in articular tissues is most common in the elderly, occurring in 10–15% of persons aged 65–75 years and 30–50% of those >85 years. In most cases this process is asymptomatic, and the cause of CPPD deposition is uncertain. Because >80% of patients are >60 years and 70% have preexisting joint damage from other conditions, it is likely that biochemical changes in aging or diseased cartilage favor crystal nucleation. In patients with CPPD arthritis there is an increased production of inorganic pyrophosphate and decreased levels of pyrophosphatases in cartilage extracts. Mutations in the ANKH gene described in both familial and sporadic cases can increase elaboration and extracellular transport of pyrophosphate. The increase in pyrophosphate production appears to be related to enhanced activity of adenosine triphosphate (ATP) pyrophosphohydrolase and 5'-nucleotidase, which catalyze the reaction of ATP to adenosine and pyrophosphate. This pyrophosphate could combine with calcium to form CPPD crystals in matrix vesicles or on collagen fibers. There are decreased levels of cartilage glycosaminoglycans that normally inhibit and regulate crystal nucleation. In vitro studies have demonstrated that transforming growth factor β_1 and epidermal growth factor both stimulate the production of pyrophosphate by articular cartilage and thus may contribute to the deposition of CPPD crystals.

Release of CPPD crystals into the joint space is followed by the phagocytosis of these crystals by

TABLE 19-2

CONDITIONS ASSOCIATED WITH CALCIUM PYROPHOSPHATE DIHYDRATE DISEASE

Aging
  Disease-associated
  Primary hyperparathyroidism
  Hemochromatosis
  Hypophosphatasia
  Hypomagnesemia
  Chronic gout
  Postmeniscectomy
Epiphyseal dysplasias
Hereditary: Slovakian-Hungarian, Spanish, Spanish-American (Argentinian,[a] Colombian, and Chilean), French,[a] Swedish, Dutch, Canadian, Mexican-American, Italian-American,[a] German-American, Japanese, Tunisian, Jewish, English[a]

[a]Mutations in the ANKH gene.

monocyte-macrophages and neutrophils, which respond by releasing chemotactic and inflammatory substances.

A minority of patients with CPPD arthropathy have metabolic abnormalities or hereditary CPPD disease (Table 19-2). These associations suggest that a variety of different metabolic products may enhance CPPD deposition either by directly altering cartilage or inhibiting inorganic pyrophosphatases. Included among these conditions are hyperparathyroidism, hemochromatosis, hypophosphatasia, and hypomagnesemia. The presence of CPPD arthritis in individuals <50 years old should lead to consideration of these metabolic disorders and inherited forms of disease, including those identified in a variety of ethnic groups (Table 19-2). Genomic DNA studies performed on different kindreds have shown a possible location of genetic defects on chromosome 8q or on chromosome 5p in a region that expresses the gene of the membrane pyrophosphate channel (ANKH gene). Mutations as noted above described in the ANKH gene in kindreds with CPPD arthritis can increase extracellular pyrophosphate and induce CPPD crystal formation. Investigation of younger patients with CPPD deposition should include inquiry for evidence of familial aggregation and evaluation of serum calcium, phosphorus, alkaline phosphatase, magnesium, serum iron, and transferrin.

CLINICAL MANIFESTATIONS

CPPD arthropathy may be asymptomatic, acute, subacute, or chronic or cause acute synovitis superimposed on chronically involved joints. Acute CPPD arthritis was originally termed *pseudogout* by McCarty and coworkers because of its striking similarity to gout. Other clinical manifestations of CPPD deposition include (1) induction or enhancement of peculiar forms of osteoarthritis; (2) induction of severe destructive disease that may radiographically mimic neuropathic arthritis; (3) production of symmetric proliferative synovitis, clinically similar to rheumatoid arthritis and frequently seen in familial forms with early onset; (4) intervertebral disk and ligament calcification with restriction of spine mobility, mimicking ankylosing spondylitis (also seen in hereditary forms); and (5) rarely spinal stenosis (most commonly seen in the elderly) (Table 19-1).

The knee is the joint most frequently affected in CPPD arthropathy. Other sites include the wrist, shoulder, ankle, elbow, and hands. Rarely, the temporomandibular joint and ligamentum flavum of the spinal canal are involved. Clinical and radiographic evidence indicates that CPPD deposition is polyarticular in at least two-thirds of patients. When the clinical picture resembles that of slowly progressive osteoarthritis, diagnosis may be difficult. Joint distribution may provide important clues suggesting CPPD disease. For example, primary osteoarthritis rarely involves a metacarpophalangeal, wrist, elbow, shoulder, or ankle joint. If radiographs reveal punctate and/or linear radiodense deposits in fibrocartilaginous joint menisci or articular hyaline cartilage (*chondrocalcinosis*), the diagnostic likelihood of CPPD disease is further enhanced. *Definitive diagnosis* requires demonstration of typical crystals in synovial fluid or articular tissue (**Fig. 19-2**). In the absence of joint effusion or indications to obtain a synovial biopsy, chondrocalcinosis is presumptive of CPPD deposition. One exception is chondrocalcinosis due to CaOx in some patients with chronic renal failure.

Acute attacks of CPPD arthritis may be precipitated by trauma. Rapid diminution of serum calcium concentration, as may occur in severe medical illness or after surgery (especially parathyroidectomy), can also lead to pseudogout attacks.

In as many as 50% of cases, episodes of CPPD-induced inflammation are associated with low-grade fever and, on occasion, temperatures as high as 40°C. Whether or not radiographic proof of chondrocalcinosis is evident in the involved joint(s), synovial fluid analysis with microbial cultures is essential to rule out the possibility of infection. In fact, infection in a joint with any microcrystalline deposition process can lead to crystal shedding and subsequent synovitis from both crystals and microorganisms. Synovial fluid in acute CPPD disease has inflammatory characteristics. The leukocyte count can range from several thousand cells to 100,000 cells/μL, the mean being about 24,000 cells/μL and the predominant cell being the neutrophil. Polarized light microscopy usually reveals rhomboid, square, or rod-like crystals with weak positive birefringence inside tissue fragments and fibrin clots and in neutrophils (Fig. 19-2). CPPD crystals may coexist with MSU and apatite in some cases.

℞ Treatment:
CPPD DEPOSITION DISEASE

Untreated acute attacks may last a few days to as long as a month. Treatment by joint aspiration and NSAIDs or by intraarticular glucocorticoid injection may result in return to prior status in ≤10 days. For patients with frequent recurrent attacks of pseudogout, daily prophylactic treatment with low doses of colchicine may be helpful in decreasing the frequency of the attacks. Severe polyarticular attacks usually require short courses of glucocorticoids. Unfortunately, there is no effective way to remove CPPD deposits from cartilage and synovium. Uncontrolled studies suggest that the administration of antimalarial agents or even methotrexate may be helpful in controlling persistent synovitis. Patients with progressive destructive large-joint arthropathy may require joint replacement.

CALCIUM APATITE DEPOSITION DISEASE

PATHOGENESIS

Apatite is the primary mineral of normal bone and teeth. Abnormal accumulation can occur in areas of tissue damage (dystrophic calcification), in hypercalcemic or hyperparathyroid states (metastatic calcification), and in certain conditions of unknown cause (Table 19-3). In chronic renal failure, hyperphosphatemia can contribute to extensive apatite deposition both in and around joints. Familial aggregation is rarely seen; no association with *ANKH* mutations has been described thus far. Apatite crystals are deposited primarily on matrix vessels.

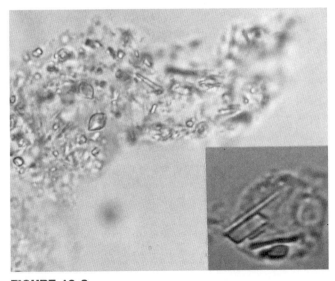

FIGURE 19-2

Intracellular and extracellular calcium pyrophosphate dihydrate crystals, as seen in a fresh preparation of synovial fluid, illustrate rectangular, rod-shaped, and rhomboid weakly positive birefringent crystals (compensated polarized light microscopy; 400×).

TABLE 19-3

CONDITIONS ASSOCIATED WITH APATITE DEPOSITION DISEASE
Aging
Osteoarthritis
Hemorrhagic shoulder effusions in the elderly (Milwaukee shoulder)
Destructive arthropathy
Tendinitis, bursitis
Tumoral calcinosis (sporadic cases)
Disease-associated
Hyperparathyroidism
Milk-alkali syndrome
Renal failure/long-term dialysis
Connective tissue diseases (e.g., systemic sclerosis, idiopathic myositis, SLE)
Heterotopic calcification following neurologic catastrophes (e.g., stroke, spinal cord injury)
Heredity
Bursitis, arthritis
Tumoral calcinosis
Fibrodysplasia ossificans progressiva

Note: SLE, systemic lupus erythematosus.

Incompletely understood alterations in matrix proteoglycans, phosphatases, hormones, and cytokines can probably influence crystal formation.

Apatite aggregates are commonly present in synovial fluid in an extremely destructive chronic arthropathy of the elderly that occurs most often in shoulders (Milwaukee shoulder) and in a similar process in hips, knees, and erosive osteoarthritis of fingers. Joint destruction is associated with damage to cartilage and supporting structures, leading to instability and deformity. Progression tends to be indolent, and synovial fluid leukocyte counts are usually <2000/μL. Symptoms range from minimal to severe pain and disability that may lead to joint replacement surgery. Whether severely affected patients merely represent an extreme synovial tissue response to the apatite crystals that are so common in osteoarthritis is uncertain. Synovial lining cell cultures exposed to apatite (or CPPD) crystals markedly increase the release of collagenases and neutral proteases, underscoring the destructive potential of abnormally stimulated synovial lining cells.

CLINICAL MANIFESTATIONS

Periarticular or articular deposits may occur and may be associated with acute reversible inflammation and/or chronic damage to the joint capsule, tendons, bursa, or articular surfaces. The most common sites of apatite deposition include bursae and tendons in and/or around the knees, shoulders, hips, and fingers. Clinical manifestations include asymptomatic radiographic abnormalities, acute synovitis, bursitis, tendinitis, and chronic destructive arthropathy. Although the true incidence of apatite arthritis is not known, 30–50% of patients with osteoarthritis have apatite microcrystals in their synovial fluid. Such crystals can frequently be identified in clinically stable osteoarthritic joints, but they are more likely to come to attention in persons experiencing acute or subacute worsening of joint pain and swelling. The synovial fluid leukocyte count in apatite arthritis is usually low (<2000/μL), despite dramatic symptoms, with predominance of mononuclear cells.

DIAGNOSIS

Intra- and/or periarticular calcifications with or without erosive, destructive, or hypertrophic changes may be seen on radiographs (**Fig. 19-3**). These should be distinguished from the linear calcifications typical of CPPD deposition disease.

Definitive diagnosis of apatite arthropathy depends on identification of crystals from synovial fluid or tissue (Fig. 19-3). Individual crystals, which generally contain mostly carbonate substituted apatite, are very small and can be seen only by electron microscopy. Clumps of crystals may appear as 1- to 20-μm shiny intra- or extracellular non-birefringent globules or aggregates that stain purplish with Wright's stain and bright red with alizarin red S. Absolute identification depends on electron microscopy with energy-dispersive elemental analysis, x-ray diffraction, or infrared spectroscopy, but these are usually not required in clinical diagnosis.

> ℞ **Treatment:**
> ## CALCIUM APATITE DEPOSITION DISEASE
>
> Treatment of apatite arthritis or periarthritis is nonspecific. Acute attacks of bursitis or synovitis may be self-limiting, resolving in days to several weeks. Aspiration of effusions and the use of either NSAIDs or oral colchicine for 2 weeks or intra- or periarticular injection of a depot glucocorticoid appear to shorten the duration and intensity of symptoms. Periarticular apatite deposits may be resorbed with resolution of attacks. Agents to lower serum phosphate levels may lead to resorption of deposits in renal failure patients receiving hemodialysis. In patients with underlying severe destructive articular changes, response to medical therapy is usually less rewarding.

CaOx DEPOSITION DISEASE

PATHOGENESIS

Primary oxalosis is a rare hereditary metabolic disorder. Enhanced production of oxalic acid may result from at least two different enzyme defects, leading to hyperoxalemia and deposition of calcium oxalate crystals in

Nongonococcal Bacterial Arthritis

Epidemiology

Although hematogenous infections with virulent organisms such as *S. aureus*, *H. influenzae*, and pyogenic streptococci occur in healthy persons, there is an underlying host predisposition in many cases of septic arthritis. Patients with rheumatoid arthritis have the highest incidence of infective arthritis (most often secondary to *S. aureus*) because of chronically inflamed joints; glucocorticoid therapy; and frequent breakdown of rheumatoid nodules, vasculitic ulcers, and skin overlying deformed joints. Diabetes mellitus, glucocorticoid therapy, hemodialysis, and malignancy all carry an increased risk of infection with *S. aureus* and gram-negative bacilli. Tumor necrosis factor (TNF) inhibitors (etanercept and infliximab), increasingly used for the treatment of rheumatoid arthritis, predispose to mycobacterial infections and possibly to other pyogenic bacterial infections and could be associated with septic arthritis in this population. Pneumococcal infections complicate alcoholism, deficiencies of humoral immunity, and hemoglobinopathies. Pneumococci, *Salmonella*, and *H. influenzae* cause septic arthritis in persons infected with HIV. Persons with primary immunoglobulin deficiency are at risk for mycoplasmal arthritis, which results in permanent joint damage if treatment with tetracycline and IV immunoglobulin (IVIg) replacement is not administered promptly. IV drug users acquire staphylococcal and streptococcal infections from their own flora and acquire pseudomonal and other gram-negative infections from drugs and injection paraphernalia.

Clinical Manifestations

Some 90% of patients present with involvement of a single joint—most commonly the knee; less frequently the hip; and still less often the shoulder, wrist, or elbow. Small joints of the hands and feet are more likely to be affected after direct inoculation or a bite. Among IV drug users, infections of the spine, sacroiliac joints, or sternoclavicular joints (Fig. 20-1) are more common than infections of the appendicular skeleton. Polyarticular infection is most common among patients with rheumatoid arthritis and may resemble a flare of the underlying disease.

The usual presentation consists of moderate to severe pain that is uniform around the joint, effusion, muscle spasm, and decreased range of motion. Fever in the range of 38.3°–38.9°C (101°–102°F) and sometimes higher is common but may be lacking, especially in persons with rheumatoid arthritis, renal or hepatic insufficiency, or conditions requiring immunosuppressive therapy. The inflamed, swollen joint is usually evident on examination except in the case of a deeply situated joint, such as the hip, shoulder, or sacroiliac joint. Cellulitis, bursitis, and acute osteomyelitis, which may produce a similar clinical picture, should be distinguished from septic

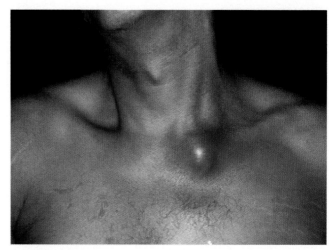

FIGURE 20-1

Acute septic arthritis of the sternoclavicular joint. A man in his 40s with a history of cirrhosis presented with a new onset of fever and lower neck pain. He had no history of IV drug use or previous catheter placement. Jaundice and a painful swollen area over his left sternoclavicular joint were evident on physical exam. Cultures of blood drawn at admission grew group B *Streptococcus*. The patient recovered after treatment with IV penicillin. *(Courtesy of Francisco M. Marty, MD, Brigham & Women's Hospital, Boston; with permission.)*

arthritis by their greater range of motion and less-than-circumferential swelling. A focus of extraarticular infection, such as a boil or pneumonia, should be sought. Peripheral-blood leukocytosis with a left shift and elevation of the erythrocyte sedimentation rate (ESR) or C-reactive protein level are common.

Plain radiographs show evidence of soft-tissue swelling, joint-space widening, and displacement of tissue planes by the distended capsule. Narrowing of the joint space and bony erosions indicate advanced infection and a poor prognosis. Ultrasound is useful for detecting effusions in the hip, and CT or MRI can demonstrate infections of the sacroiliac joint, the sternoclavicular joint, and the spine very well.

Laboratory Findings

Specimens of peripheral blood and synovial fluid should be obtained before antibiotics are administered. Blood cultures are positive in up to 50–70% of *S. aureus* infections but are less frequently positive in infections due to other organisms. The synovial fluid is turbid, serosanguineous, or frankly purulent. Gram-stained smears confirm the presence of large numbers of neutrophils. Levels of total protein and lactate dehydrogenase in synovial fluid are elevated, and the glucose level is depressed; however, these findings are not specific for infection, and measurement of these levels is not necessary to make the diagnosis. The synovial fluid should be examined for crystals, because gout and pseudogout can resemble septic arthritis clinically, and infection and crystal-induced disease occasionally occur together. Organisms are seen on synovial fluid smears in nearly three-quarters of infections with *S. aureus* and streptococci and in 30–50% of infections due to gram-negative and other bacteria. Cultures of synovial fluid are positive in >90% of cases. Inoculation of synovial fluid into bottles containing liquid media for blood cultures increases the yield of culture, especially if the pathogen is a fastidious organism or the patient is taking an antibiotic. Although not yet widely available, PCR-based assays for bacterial DNA will also be useful for the diagnosis of partially treated or culture-negative bacterial arthritis.

SECTION III

Disorders of the Joints and Adjacent Tissues

℞ Treatment:
NONGONOCOCCAL BACTERIAL ARTHRITIS

Prompt administration of systemic antibiotics and drainage of the involved joint can prevent destruction of cartilage, postinfectious degenerative arthritis, joint instability, or deformity. Once samples of blood and synovial fluid have been obtained for culture, empirical antibiotics should be given that are directed against bacteria visualized on smears or against the pathogens that are likely, given the patient's age and risk factors. Initial therapy should consist of the IV administration of bactericidal agents; direct instillation of antibiotics into the joint is not necessary to achieve adequate levels in synovial fluid and tissue. An IV third-generation cephalosporin such as cefotaxime (1 g every 8 h) or ceftriaxone (1–2 g every 24 h) provides adequate empirical coverage for most community-acquired infections in adults when smears show no organisms. Either oxacillin or nafcillin (2 g every 4 h) is used if there are gram-positive cocci on the smear. If methicillin-resistant *S. aureus* is a possible pathogen (e.g., when it is widespread in the community or in hospitalized patients), IV vancomycin (1 g every 12 h) should be given. In addition, an aminoglycoside or third-generation cephalosporin should be given to IV drug users or other patients in whom *Pseudomonas aeruginosa* may be the responsible agent.

Definitive therapy is based on the identity and antibiotic susceptibility of the bacteria isolated in culture. Infections due to staphylococci are treated with oxacillin, nafcillin, or vancomycin for 4 weeks. Pneumococcal and streptococcal infections due to penicillin-susceptible organisms respond to 2 weeks of therapy with penicillin G (2 million units IV every 4 h); infections caused by *H. influenzae* and by strains of *Streptococcus pneumoniae* that are resistant to penicillin are treated with cefotaxime or ceftriaxone for 2 weeks. Most enteric gram-negative infections can be cured in 3–4 weeks by a second- or third-generation cephalosporin given IV or by

a fluoroquinolone, such as levofloxacin (500 mg IV or PO every 24 h). *P. aeruginosa* infection should be treated for at least 2 weeks with a combination regimen of an aminoglycoside plus either an extended-spectrum penicillin, such as mezlocillin (3 g IV every 4 h), or an antipseudomonal cephalosporin, such as ceftazidime (1 g IV every 8 h). If tolerated, this regimen is continued for an additional 2 weeks; alternatively, a fluoroquinolone, such as ciprofloxacin (750 mg PO twice daily), is given by itself or with the penicillin or cephalosporin in place of the aminoglycoside.

Timely drainage of pus and necrotic debris from the infected joint is required for a favorable outcome. Needle aspiration of readily accessible joints such as the knee may be adequate if loculations or particulate matter in the joint does not prevent its thorough decompression. Arthroscopic drainage and lavage may be employed initially or within several days if repeated needle aspiration fails to relieve symptoms, decrease the volume of the effusion and the synovial white cell count, and clear bacteria from smears and cultures. In some cases, arthrotomy is necessary to remove loculations and débride infected synovium, cartilage, or bone. Septic arthritis of the hip is best managed with arthrotomy, particularly in young children, in whom infection threatens the viability of the femoral head. Septic joints do not require immobilization except for pain control before symptoms are alleviated by treatment. Weight bearing should be avoided until signs of inflammation have subsided, but frequent passive motion of the joint is indicated to maintain full mobility. While addition of glucocorticoids to antibiotic treatment improves the outcome of *S. aureus* arthritis in experimental animals, no clinical trials have yet evaluated this approach in humans.

Gonococcal Arthritis

▉ Epidemiology

Although its incidence has declined in recent years, gonococcal arthritis has accounted for up to 70% of episodes of infectious arthritis in persons <40 years of age in the United States. Arthritis due to *N. gonorrhoeae* is a consequence of bacteremia arising from gonococcal infection or, more frequently, from asymptomatic gonococcal mucosal colonization of the urethra, cervix, or pharynx. Women are at greatest risk during menses and during pregnancy and overall are two to three times more likely than men to develop disseminated gonococcal infection (DGI) and arthritis. Persons with complement deficiencies, especially of the terminal components, are prone to recurrent episodes of gonococcemia. Strains of gonococci that are most likely to cause DGI include those that produce transparent colonies in culture, have the type IA outer-membrane protein, or are of the AUH–auxotroph type.

Clinical Manifestations and Laboratory Findings

The most common manifestation of DGI is a syndrome of fever, chills, rash, and articular symptoms. Small numbers of papules that progress to hemorrhagic pustules develop on the trunk and the extensor surfaces of the distal extremities. Migratory arthritis and tenosynovitis of the knees, hands, wrists, feet, and ankles are prominent. The cutaneous lesions and articular findings are believed to be the consequence of an immune reaction to circulating gonococci and immune-complex deposition in tissues. Thus, cultures of synovial fluid are consistently negative, and blood cultures are positive in <45% of patients. Synovial fluid may be difficult to obtain from inflamed joints and usually contains only 10,000–20,000 leukocytes/μL.

True gonococcal septic arthritis is less common than the DGI syndrome and always follows DGI, which is unrecognized in one-third of patients. A single joint, such as the hip, knee, ankle, or wrist, is usually involved. Synovial fluid, which contains >50,000 leukocytes/μL, can be obtained with ease; the gonococcus is only occasionally evident in gram-stained smears, and cultures of synovial fluid are positive in <40% of cases. Blood cultures are almost always negative.

Because it is difficult to isolate gonococci from synovial fluid and blood, specimens for culture should be obtained from potentially infected mucosal sites. Cultures and gram-stained smears of skin lesions are occasionally positive. All specimens for culture should be plated onto Thayer-Martin agar directly or in special transport media at the bedside and transferred promptly to the microbiology laboratory in an atmosphere of 5% CO_2, as generated in a candle jar. PCR-based assays are extremely sensitive in detecting gonococcal DNA in synovial fluid. A dramatic alleviation of symptoms within 12–24 h after the initiation of appropriate antibiotic therapy supports a clinical diagnosis of the DGI syndrome if cultures are negative.

Rx Treatment: GONOCOCCAL ARTHRITIS

Initial treatment consists of ceftriaxone (1 g IV or IM every 24 h) to cover possible penicillin-resistant organisms. Once local and systemic signs are clearly resolving and if the sensitivity of the isolate permits, the 7-day course of therapy can be completed with an oral agent such as ciprofloxacin (500 mg twice daily) if sensitivity allows. If penicillin-susceptible organisms are isolated, amoxicillin (500 mg three times daily) may be used. Suppurative arthritis usually responds to needle aspiration of involved joints and 7–14 days of antibiotic treatment. Arthroscopic lavage or arthrotomy is rarely required. Patients with DGI should be treated for *Chlamydia*

trachomatis infection unless this infection is ruled out by appropriate testing.

It is noteworthy that arthritis symptoms similar to those seen in DGI occur in meningococcemia. A dermatitis-arthritis syndrome, purulent monarthritis, and reactive polyarthritis have been described. All respond to treatment with IV penicillin.

SPIROCHETAL ARTHRITIS

Lyme Disease

Lyme disease due to infection with the spirochete *Borrelia burgdorferi* causes arthritis in up to 70% of persons who are not treated. Intermittent arthralgias and myalgias—but not arthritis—occur within days or weeks of inoculation of the spirochete by the *Ixodes* tick. Later, there are three patterns of joint disease: (1) Fifty percent of untreated persons experience intermittent episodes of monarthritis or oligoarthritis involving the knee and/or other large joints. The symptoms wax and wane without treatment over months, and each year 10–20% of patients report loss of joint symptoms. (2) Twenty percent of untreated persons develop a pattern of waxing and waning arthralgias. (3) Ten percent of untreated patients develop chronic inflammatory synovitis resulting in erosive lesions and destruction of the joint. Serologic tests for IgG antibodies to *B. burgdorferi* are positive in >90% of persons with Lyme arthritis, and a PCR-based assay detects *Borrelia* DNA in 85%.

Rx Treatment: LYME ARTHRITIS

Lyme arthritis generally responds well to therapy. A regimen of oral doxycycline (100 mg twice daily for 30 days), oral amoxicillin (500 mg four times daily for 30 days), or parenteral ceftriaxone (2 g/d for 2–4 weeks) is recommended. Patients who do not respond to a total of 2 months of oral therapy or 1 month of parenteral therapy are unlikely to benefit from additional antibiotic therapy and are treated with anti-inflammatory agents or synovectomy. Failure of therapy is associated with host features such as the HLA-DR4 genotype, persistent reactivity to OspA (outer-surface protein A), and the presence of hLFA-1 (human leukocyte function–associated antigen 1), which cross-reacts with OspA.

Syphilitic Arthritis

Articular manifestations occur in different stages of syphilis. In early congenital syphilis, periarticular swelling and immobilization of the involved limbs (Parrot's pseudoparalysis) complicate osteochondritis of long bones. Clutton's joint, a late manifestation of congenital syphilis that typically develops between the ages of 8 and 15 years, is caused by chronic painless synovitis with effusions of large joints, particularly the knees and elbows. Secondary syphilis may be associated with arthralgias; with symmetric arthritis of the knees and ankles and occasionally of the shoulders and wrists; and with sacroiliitis. The arthritis follows a subacute to chronic course with a mixed mononuclear and neutrophilic synovial-fluid pleocytosis (typical cell counts, 5000–15,000/μL). Immunologic mechanisms may contribute to the arthritis, and symptoms usually improve rapidly with penicillin therapy. In tertiary syphilis, Charcot's joint is a result of sensory loss due to tabes dorsalis. Penicillin is not helpful in this setting.

MYCOBACTERIAL ARTHRITIS

Tuberculous arthritis accounts for ~1% of all cases of tuberculosis and for 10% of extrapulmonary cases. The most common presentation is chronic granulomatous monarthritis. An unusual syndrome, Poncet's disease, is a reactive symmetric form of polyarthritis that affects persons with visceral or disseminated tuberculosis. No mycobacteria are found in the joints, and symptoms resolve with antituberculous therapy.

Unlike tuberculous osteomyelitis, which typically involves the thoracic and lumbar spine (50% of cases), tuberculous arthritis primarily involves the large weight-bearing joints, in particular the hips, knees, and ankles, and only occasionally involves smaller non–weight-bearing joints. Progressive monarticular swelling and pain develop over months or years, and systemic symptoms are seen in only half of all cases. Tuberculous arthritis occurs as part of a disseminated primary infection or through late reactivation, often in persons with HIV infection or other immunocompromised hosts. Coexistent active pulmonary tuberculosis is unusual.

Aspiration of the involved joint yields fluid with an average cell count of 20,000/μL, with ~50% neutrophils. Acid-fast staining of the fluid yields positive results in fewer than one-third of cases, and cultures are positive in 80%. Culture of synovial tissue taken at biopsy is positive in ~90% of cases and shows granulomatous inflammation in most. DNA amplification methods such as PCR can shorten the time to diagnosis to 1 or 2 days. Radiographs reveal peripheral erosions at the points of synovial attachment, periarticular osteopenia, and eventually joint-space narrowing. Therapy for tuberculous arthritis is the same as that for tuberculous pulmonary disease, requiring the administration of multiple agents for 6–9 months. Therapy is more prolonged in immunosuppressed individuals, such as those infected with HIV.

Various atypical mycobacteria found in water and soil may cause chronic indolent arthritis. Such disease results from trauma and direct inoculation associated with farming, gardening, or aquatic activities. Smaller joints, such as the digits, wrists, and knees, are usually involved. Involvement of tendon sheaths and bursae is typical. The mycobacterial species involved include *Mycobacterium marinum*, *M. avium-intracellulare*, *M. terrae*, *M. kansasii*, *M. fortuitum*, and *M. chelonae*. In persons who have HIV infection or are receiving immunosuppressive therapy, hematogenous spread to the joints has been reported for *M. kansasii*, *M. avium-intracellulare*, and *M. haemophilum*. Diagnosis usually requires biopsy and culture, and therapy is based on antimicrobial susceptibility patterns.

FUNGAL ARTHRITIS

Fungi are an unusual cause of chronic monarticular arthritis. Granulomatous articular infection with the endemic dimorphic fungi *Coccidioides immitis*, *Blastomyces dermatitidis*, and (less commonly) *Histoplasma capsulatum* (**Fig. 20-2**) results from hematogenous seeding or direct extension from bony lesions in persons with disseminated disease. Joint involvement is an unusual complication of sporotrichosis (infection with *Sporothrix schenckii*) among gardeners and other persons who work with soil or sphagnum moss. Articular sporotrichosis is six times more common among men than among women, and alcoholics and other debilitated hosts are at risk for polyarticular infection.

Candida infection involving a single joint—usually the knee, hip, or shoulder—results from surgical procedures, intraarticular injections, or (among critically ill patients with debilitating illnesses, such as diabetes mellitus or hepatic or renal insufficiency, and patients receiving immunosuppressive therapy) hematogenous spread. *Candida* infections in IV drug users typically involve the spine, sacroiliac joints, or other fibrocartilaginous joints. Unusual cases of arthritis due to *Aspergillus* species, *Cryptococcus neoformans*, *Pseudallescheria boydii*, and the dematiaceous fungi have also resulted from direct inoculation or disseminated hematogenous infection in immunocompromised persons.

The synovial fluid in fungal arthritis usually contains 10,000–40,000 cells/μL, with ~70% neutrophils. Stained specimens and cultures of synovial tissue often confirm the diagnosis of fungal arthritis when studies of synovial fluid give negative results. Treatment consists of drainage and lavage of the joint and systemic administration of an antifungal agent directed at a specific pathogen. The doses and duration of therapy are the same as for disseminated disease. Intraarticular instillation of amphotericin B has been used in addition to IV therapy.

VIRAL ARTHRITIS

Viruses produce arthritis by infecting synovial tissue during systemic infection or by provoking an immunologic reaction that involves joints. As many as 50% of

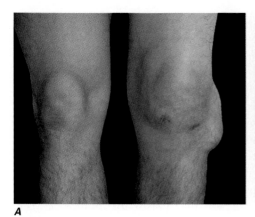
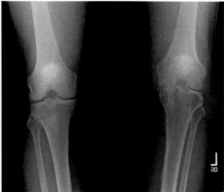
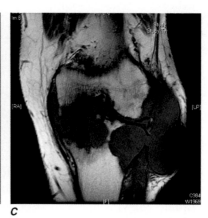

A

B

C

FIGURE 20-2

Chronic arthritis caused by *Histoplasma capsulatum* in the left knee. **A.** A man in his 60s from El Salvador presented with a history of progressive knee pain and difficulty walking for several years. He had undergone arthroscopy for a meniscal tear 7 years before presentation (without relief) and had received several intraarticular glucocorticoid injections. The patient developed significant deformity of the knee over time, including a large effusion in the lateral aspect. **B.** An x-ray of the knee showed multiple abnormalities, including severe medial femorotibial joint-space narrowing, several large subchondral cysts within the tibia and the patellofemoral compartment, a large suprapatellar joint effusion, and a large soft-tissue mass projecting laterally over the knee. **C.** MRI further defined these abnormalities and demonstrated the cystic nature of the lateral knee abnormality. Synovial biopsies demonstrated chronic inflammation with giant cells, and cultures grew *H. capsulatum* after 3 weeks of incubation. All clinical cystic lesions and the effusion resolved after 1 year of treatment with itraconazole. The patient underwent a left total knee replacement for definitive treatment. *(Courtesy of Francisco M. Marty, MD, Brigham & Women's Hospital, Boston; with permission.)*

women report persistent arthralgias and 10% report frank arthritis within 3 days of the rash that follows natural infection with rubella virus and within 2–6 weeks after receipt of live-virus vaccine. Episodes of symmetric inflammation of fingers, wrists, and knees uncommonly recur for >1 year, but a syndrome of chronic fatigue, low-grade fever, headaches, and myalgias can persist for months or years. IVIg has been helpful in selected cases. Self-limited monarticular or migratory polyarthritis may develop within 2 weeks of the parotitis of mumps; this sequela is more common among men than women. Approximately 10% of children and 60% of women develop arthritis after infection with parvovirus B19. In adults, arthropathy sometimes occurs without fever or rash. Pain and stiffness, with less prominent swelling (primarily of the hands but also of the knees, wrists, and ankles), usually resolve within weeks, although a small proportion of patients develop chronic arthropathy.

About 2 weeks before the onset of jaundice, up to 10% of persons with acute hepatitis B develop an immune complex–mediated, serum sickness–like reaction with maculopapular rash, urticaria, fever, and arthralgias. Less common developments include symmetric arthritis involving the hands, wrists, elbows, or ankles, and morning stiffness that resembles a flare of rheumatoid arthritis. Symptoms resolve at the time jaundice develops. Many persons with chronic hepatitis C infection report persistent arthralgia or arthritis, both in the presence and in the absence of cryoglobulinemia. Painful arthritis involving larger joints often accompanies the fever and rash of several arthropod-borne viral infections, including those caused by chikungunya, O'nyong-nyong, Ross River, Mayaro, and Barmah Forest viruses. Symmetric arthritis involving the hands and wrists may occur during the convalescent phase of infection with lymphocytic choriomeningitis virus. Patients infected with an enterovirus frequently report arthralgias, and echovirus has been isolated from patients with acute polyarthritis.

Several arthritis syndromes are associated with HIV infection. Reactive arthritis with painful lower-extremity oligoarthritis often follows an episode of urethritis in HIV-infected persons. HIV-associated reactive arthritis appears to be extremely common among persons with the HLA-B27 haplotype, but sacroiliac joint disease is unusual and is seen mostly in the absence of HLA-B27. Up to one-third of HIV-infected persons with psoriasis develop psoriatic arthritis. Painless monarthropathy and persistent symmetric polyarthropathy occasionally complicate HIV infection. Chronic persistent oligoarthritis of the shoulders, wrists, hands, and knees occurs in women infected with human T cell lymphotropic virus type I. Synovial thickening, destruction of articular cartilage, and leukemic-appearing atypical lymphocytes in synovial fluid are characteristic, but progression to T-cell leukemia is unusual.

PARASITIC ARTHRITIS

Arthritis due to parasitic infection is rare. The guinea worm *Dracunculus medinensis* may cause destructive joint lesions in the lower extremities as migrating gravid female worms invade joints or cause ulcers in adjacent soft tissues that become secondarily infected. Hydatid cysts infect bones in 1–2% of cases of infection with *Echinococcus granulosus*. The expanding destructive cystic lesions may spread to and destroy adjacent joints, particularly the hip and pelvis. In rare cases, chronic synovitis has been associated with the presence of schistosomal eggs in synovial biopsies. Monarticular arthritis in children with lymphatic filariasis appears to respond to therapy with diethylcarbamazine, even in the absence of microfilariae in synovial fluid. Reactive arthritis has been attributed to hookworm, *Strongyloides*, *Cryptosporidium*, and *Giardia* infection in case reports, but confirmation is required.

POSTINFECTIOUS OR REACTIVE ARTHRITIS

Reactive arthritis (Chap. 9), a reactive polyarthritis, develops several weeks after ~1% of cases of nongonococcal urethritis and 2% of enteric infections, particularly those due to *Yersinia enterocolitica*, *Shigella flexneri*, *Campylobacter jejuni*, and *Salmonella* species. Only a minority of these patients have the other findings of classic reactive arthritis, including urethritis, conjunctivitis, uveitis, oral ulcers, and rash. This triad of arthritis, urethritis, and conjunctivitis was formerly known as Reiter's syndrome, which is an eponym now of historical interest only. Studies have identified microbial DNA or antigen in synovial fluid or blood, but the pathogenesis of this condition is poorly understood.

Reactive arthritis is most common among young men (except after *Yersinia* infection) and has been linked to the HLA-B27 locus as a potential genetic predisposing factor. Patients report painful, asymmetric oligoarthritis affecting mainly the knees, ankles, and feet. Low-back pain is common, and radiographic evidence of sacroiliitis is found in patients with long-standing disease. Most patients recover within 6 months, but prolonged recurrent disease is more common in cases following chlamydial urethritis. Antiinflammatory agents help to relieve symptoms, but the role of prolonged antibiotic therapy in eliminating microbial antigen from the synovium is controversial.

Migratory polyarthritis and fever constitute the usual presentation of acute rheumatic fever in adults (Chap. 6). This presentation is distinct from that of poststreptococcal reactive arthritis, which also follows infections with group A *Streptococcus* but is not migratory, lasts beyond the typical 3-week maximum of acute rheumatic fever, and responds poorly to aspirin.

INFECTIONS IN PROSTHETIC JOINTS

Infection complicates 1–4% of total joint replacements. The majority of infections are acquired intraoperatively or immediately postoperatively as a result of wound breakdown or infection; less commonly, these joint infections develop later after joint replacement and are the result of hematogenous spread or direct inoculation. The presentation may be acute, with fever, pain, and local signs of inflammation, especially in infections due to *S. aureus*, pyogenic streptococci, and enteric bacilli. Alternatively, infection may persist for months or years without causing constitutional symptoms when less virulent organisms, such as coagulase-negative staphylococci or diphtheroids, are involved. Such indolent infections are usually acquired during joint implantation and are discovered during evaluation of chronic unexplained pain or after a radiograph shows loosening of the prosthesis; the ESR and C-reactive protein level are usually elevated in such cases.

The diagnosis is best made by needle aspiration of the joint; accidental introduction of organisms during aspiration must be meticulously avoided. Synovial fluid pleocytosis with a predominance of polymorphonuclear leukocytes is highly suggestive of infection, since other inflammatory processes uncommonly affect prosthetic joints. Culture and Gram's stain usually yield the responsible pathogen. Use of special media for unusual pathogens such as fungi, atypical mycobacteria, and *Mycoplasma* may be necessary if routine and anaerobic cultures are negative.

℞ Treatment:
PROSTHETIC JOINT INFECTIONS

Treatment includes surgery and high doses of parenteral antibiotics, which are given for 4–6 weeks because bone is usually involved. In most cases, the prosthesis must be replaced to cure the infection. Implantation of a new prosthesis is best delayed for several weeks or months because relapses of infection occur most commonly within this time frame. In some cases, reimplantation is not possible, and the patient must manage without a joint, with a fused joint, or even with amputation. Cure of infection without removal of the prosthesis is occasionally possible in cases that are due to streptococci or pneumococci and that lack radiologic evidence of loosening of the prosthesis. In these cases, antibiotic therapy must be initiated within several days of the onset of infection, and the joint should be drained vigorously either by open arthrotomy or arthroscopically. In selected patients who prefer to avoid the high morbidity associated with joint removal and reimplantation, suppression of the infection with antibiotics may be a reasonable goal. A high cure rate with retention of the prosthesis has been reported when the combination of oral rifampin and ciprofloxacin is given for 3–6 months to persons with staphylococcal prosthetic joint infection of short duration. This approach, which is based on the ability of rifampin to kill organisms adherent to foreign material and in the stationary growth phase, requires confirmation in prospective trials.

Prevention

To avoid the disastrous consequences of infection, candidates for joint replacement should be selected with care. Rates of infection are particularly high among patients with rheumatoid arthritis, persons who have undergone previous surgery on the joint, and persons with medical conditions requiring immunosuppressive therapy. Perioperative antibiotic prophylaxis, usually with cefazolin, and measures to decrease intraoperative contamination, such as laminar flow, have lowered the rates of perioperative infection to <1% in many centers. After implantation, measures should be taken to prevent or rapidly treat extraarticular infections that might give rise to hematogenous spread to the prosthesis. The effectiveness of prophylactic antibiotics for the prevention of hematogenous infection following dental procedures has not been demonstrated; in fact, viridans streptococci and other components of the oral flora are extremely unusual causes of prosthetic joint infection. Accordingly, the American Dental Association and the American Academy of Orthopaedic Surgeons do not recommend antibiotic prophylaxis for most dental patients with total joint replacements. They do, however, recommend prophylaxis for patients who may be at high risk of hematogenous infection, including those with inflammatory arthropathies, immunosuppression, Type 1 diabetes mellitus, joint replacement within 2 years, previous prosthetic joint infection, malnourishment, or hemophilia. The recommended regimen is amoxicillin (2 g PO) 1 h before dental procedures associated with a high incidence of bacteremia. Clindamycin (600 mg PO) is suggested for patients allergic to penicillin.

ACKNOWLEDGMENT

The contributions of James H. Maguire and the late Scott J. Thaler to this chapter in earlier editions of Harrison's Principles of Internal Medicine are gratefully acknowledged.

FURTHER READINGS

AMERICAN DENTAL ASSOCIATION; AMERICAN ACADEMY OF ORTHOPAEDIC SURGEONS: Antibiotic prophylaxis for dental patients with total joint replacements. J Am Dent Assoc 134:895, 2003

ARLIEVSKY N et al: Septic arthritis with osteomyelitis due to *Streptococcus pneumoniae* in human immunodeficiency virus–infected children. Clin Infect Dis 27:898, 1998

ATKINS BL et al: Prospective evaluation of criteria for microbiological diagnosis of prosthetic-joint infection at revision arthroplasty. The OSIRIS Collaborative Study Group. J Clin Microbiol 36:2932, 1998

AVILES RJ et al: Poststreptococcal reactive arthritis in adults: A case series. Mayo Clin Proc 75:144, 2000

BARDIN T: Gonococcal arthritis. Best Pract Res Clin Rheumatol 17:201, 2003

BAS S, VISCHER TL: *Chlamydia trachomatis* antibody detection and diagnosis of reactive arthritis. Br J Rheumatol 37:1054, 1998

BERBARI EF et al: Prosthetic joint infection due to *Mycobacterium tuberculosis*: A case series and review of the literature. Am J Orthop 27:219, 1998

———— et al: Risk factors for prosthetic joint infection: Case-control study. Clin Infect Dis 27:1247, 1998

BERMAN A et al: Human immunodeficiency virus infection associated arthritis: Clinical characteristics. J Rheumatol 26:1158, 1999

BLEVINS FT et al: Septic arthritis following arthroscopic meniscus repair: A cluster of three cases. Arthroscopy 15:35, 1999

BRANDT CM et al: *Staphylococcus aureus* prosthetic joint infection treated with debridement and prosthesis retention. Clin Infect Dis 24:914, 1997

———— et al: *Staphylococcus aureus* prosthetic joint infection treated with prosthesis removal and delayed reimplantation arthroplasty. Mayo Clin Proc 74:553, 1999

BROWER AC: Septic arthritis. Radiol Clin North Am 34:293, 1996

CIMMINO MA: Recognition and management of bacterial arthritis. Drugs 54:50, 1997

CROCKARELL JR et al: Treatment of infection with debridement and retention of the components following hip arthroplasty. J Bone Joint Surg Am 80:1306, 1998

CUCKLER JM et al: Diagnosis and management of the infected total joint arthroplasty. Orthop Clin North Am 22:523, 1991

CUCURULL E, ESPINOZA LR: Gonococcal arthritis. Rheum Dis Clin North Am 24:305, 1998

CUELLAR ML: HIV infection–associated inflammatory musculoskeletal disorders. Rheum Dis Clin North Am 24:403, 1998

CUNNINGHAM R et al: Clinical and molecular aspects of the pathogenesis of *Staphylococcus aureus* bone and joint infections. J Med Microbiol 44:157, 1996

DONATTO KC: Orthopedic management of septic arthritis. Rheum Dis Clin North Am 24:275, 1998

DRANGSHOLT MT: Current concepts review. Prophylactic use of antibiotics for procedures after total joint replacement. J Bone Joint Surg Am 80:1394, 1998

EUSTACE SJ et al: Lyme arthropathy. Radiol Clin North Am 34:454, 1996

FEDER HM JR et al: A critical appraisal of "chronic Lyme disease." N Engl J Med 357:1422, 2007

FISMAN DN et al: Clinical effectiveness and cost-effectiveness of 2 management strategies for infected total hip arthroplasty in the elderly. Clin Infect Dis 32:419, 2001

FRANSSILA R, HEDMAN K: Infection and musculoskeletal conditions: Viral causes of arthritis. Best Pract Res Clin Rheumatol 20:1139, 2006

FRANZ A et al: Mycoplasmal arthritis in patients with primary immunoglobulin deficiency: Clinical features and outcome in 18 patients. Br J Rheumatol 36:661, 1997

GARCÍA-DE LA TORRE I, NAVA-ZAVALA A. Gonococcal and nongonococcal arthritis. Rheum Dis Clin North Am 35:63, 2009

GARDNER GC, WEISMAN MH: Pyarthrosis in patients with rheumatoid arthritis: A report of 13 cases and a review of the literature from the past 40 years. Am J Med 88:503, 1990

GILLESPIE WJ: Prevention and management of infection after total joint replacement. Clin Infect Dis 25:1310, 1997

GOLDENBERG DL: Septic arthritis. Lancet 351:197, 1998

GROSS DM et al: Identification of LFA-1 as a candidate autoantigen in treatment-resistant Lyme arthritis. Science 281:703, 1998

HANSSEN AD, OSMON DR: The use of prophylactic antimicrobial agents during and after hip arthroplasty. Clin Orthop 369:124, 1999

HARRINGTON JT: Mycobacterial and fungal arthritis. Curr Opin Rheumatol 10:335, 1998

HOEFFEL DP et al: Molecular diagnostics for the detection of musculoskeletal infection. Clin Orthop 360:37, 1999

HUGHES RA, KEAT AC: Reiter's syndrome and reactive arthritis: A current view. Semin Arthritis Rheum 24:190, 1994

IKE RW: Bacterial arthritis. Curr Opin Rheumatol 10:330, 1998

KEAT A: Reactive arthritis. Adv Exp Med Biol 455:201, 1999

KEATING MR, STECKELBERG JM: Editorial response: Orthopedic prosthesis salvage. Clin Infect Dis 29:296, 1999

KOCAR IH et al: *Clostridium difficile* infection in patients with reactive arthritis of undetermined etiology. Scand J Rheumatol 27:357, 1998

LANE SMP: Intra-articular corticosteroids in septic arthritis: Beneficial or barmy? Ann Rheum Dis 59:240, 2000

LAPORTE DM et al: Infections associated with dental procedures in total hip arthroplasty. J Bone Joint Surg Br 81:56, 1999

LEE YH et al: Cryoglobulinaemia and rheumatic manifestations in patients with hepatitis C virus infection. Ann Rheum Dis 57:728, 1998

LENTINO JR: Prosthetic joint infections: Bane of orthopedists, challenge for infectious disease specialists. Clin Infect Dis 36:1157, 2003

LIEBLING MR et al: Identification of *Neisseria gonorrhoeae* in synovial fluid using the polymerase chain reaction. Arthritis Rheum 37:702, 1994

LOSSOS IS et al: Septic arthritis of the glenohumeral joint. A report of 11 cases and review of the literature. Medicine (Baltimore) 77:177, 1998

LOUIE JS, LIEBLING MR: The polymerase chain reaction in infectious and post-infectious arthritis. A review. Rheum Dis Clin North Am 24:227, 1998

MAGANTI RM et al: Therapy insight: The changing spectrum of rheumatic disease in HIV infection. Nat Clin Pract Rheumatol 4:428, 2008

MARIANI BD, TUAN RS: Advances in the diagnosis of infection in prosthetic joint implants. Mol Med Today 4:207, 1998

MATHEWS CJ, COAKLEY G. Septic arthritis: Current diagnostic and therapeutic algorithm. Curr Opin Rheumatol 20:457, 2008

McCALLUM RM et al: Arthritis syndromes associated with human T cell lymphotropic virus type I infection. Med Clin North Am 81:261, 1997

MEDINA RODRIGUEZ F: Rheumatic manifestations of human immunodeficiency virus infection. Rheum Dis Clin North Am 29:145, 2003

MEEHAN AM et al: Outcome of penicillin-susceptible streptococcal prosthetic joint infection treated with debridement and retention of the prosthesis. Clin Infect Dis 36:845, 2003

MITCHELL LA et al: Chronic rubella vaccine–associated arthropathy. Arch Intern Med 153:2268, 1993

NILSSON IM et al: Alpha-toxin and gamma-toxin jointly promote *Staphylococcus aureus* virulence in murine septic arthritis. Infect Immun 67:1045, 1999

NOLLA JM et al: Group B *Streptococcus* (*Streptococcus agalactiae*) pyogenic arthritis in nonpregnant adults. Medicine 82:119, 2003

PANDEY R et al: An assessment of the histological criteria used to diagnose infection in hip revision arthroplasty tissues. J Clin Pathol 52:118, 1999

PINALS RS: Polyarthritis and fever. N Engl J Med 330:769, 1994

PURVIS RS et al: Sporotrichosis presenting as arthritis and subcutaneous nodules. J Am Acad Dermatol 28:879, 1993

REGINATO AJ: Syphilitic arthritis and osteitis. Rheum Dis Clin North Am 19:379, 1993

RODRIGUEZ JA et al: Incisional cellulitis after total hip replacement. J Bone Joint Surg Br 80:876, 1998

ROSS JJ et al: Pneumococcal septic arthritis: Review of 190 cases. Clin Infect Dis 36:319, 2003

SACK K: Monarthritis: Differential diagnosis. Am J Med 102:30S, 1997

SCHATTNER A, VOSTI KL: Bacterial arthritis due to beta-hemolytic streptococci of serogroups A, B, C, F, and G. Analysis of 23 cases and a review of the literature. Medicine 77:122, 1998

SEGRETI J et al: Prolonged suppressive antibiotic therapy for infected orthopedic prostheses. Clin Infect Dis 27:711, 1998

SHIRTLIFF ME, MADER JT: Acute septic arthritis. Clin Microbiol Rev 15:527, 2002

SHMERLING RH et al: Synovial fluid tests: What should be ordered? JAMA 264:1009, 1990

SIEPER J et al: No benefit of long-term ciprofloxacin treatment in patients with reactive arthritis and undifferentiated oligoarthritis: A three-month, multicenter, double-blind, randomized, placebo-controlled study. Arthritis Rheum 42:1386, 1999

SILVEIRA LH et al: *Candida* arthritis. Rheum Dis Clin North Am 19:427, 1993

SPANGEHL MJ et al: Prospective analysis of preoperative and intraoperative investigations for the diagnosis of infection at the sites of two hundred and two revision total hip arthroplasties. J Bone Joint Surg Am 81:672, 1999

STEERE A: Lyme disease. N Engl J Med 345:115, 2001

STENGEL D et al: Systematic review and meta-analysis of antibiotic therapy for bone and joint infections. Lancet Infect Dis 1:175, 2001

TARKOWSKI A: Infection and musculoskeletal conditions: Infectious arthritis. Best Pract Res Clin Rheumatol 20:1029, 2006

TATTEVIN P et al: Prosthetic joint infection: When can prosthesis salvage be considered? Clin Infect Dis 29:292, 1999

THOMAS MG et al: Adhesion of *Staphylococcus aureus* to collagen is not a major virulence determinant for septic arthritis, osteomyelitis, or endocarditis. J Infect Dis 179:291, 1999

TOBIN EH: Prosthetic joint infections: Controversies and clues. Lancet 353:770, 1999

TSUKAYAMA DT et al: Infection after total hip arthroplasty. A study of the treatment of one hundred and six infections. J Bone Joint Surg Am 78:512, 1996

TUNNEY MM et al: Improved detection of infection in hip replacements. A currently underestimated problem. J Bone Joint Surg Br 80:568, 1998

van der HEIJDEN IM et al: Detection of bacterial DNA in serial synovial samples obtained during antibiotic treatment from patients with septic arthritis. Arthritis Rheum 42:2198, 1999

van ELSACKER-NIELE AM, KROES AC: Human parvovirus B19: Relevance in internal medicine. Neth J Med 54:221, 1999

VASSILOPOULOS D, CALABRESE LH. Virally associated arthritis 2008: clinical, epidemiologic, and pathophysiologic considerations. Arthritis Res Ther 10:215, 2008

VON ESSEN R: Culture of joint specimens in bacterial arthritis. Impact of blood culture bottle utilization. Scand J Rheumatol 26:293, 1997

WAHL MJ: Myths of dental-induced prosthetic joint infections. Clin Infect Dis 20:1420, 1995

SECTION III

Disorders of the Joints and Adjacent Tissues

WALDMAN BJ et al: Total knee arthroplasty infections associated with dental procedures. Clin Orthop 343:164, 1997

WISE CM et al: Gonococcal arthritis in an era of increasing penicillin resistance. Presentations and outcomes in 41 recent cases (1985–1991). Arch Intern Med 154:2690, 1994

WUORELA M, GRANFORS K: Infectious agents as triggers of reactive arthritis. Am J Med Sci 316:264, 1998

WYSENBEEK AJ et al: Treatment of staphylococcal septic arthritis in rabbits by systemic antibiotics and intra-articular corticosteroids. Ann Rheum Dis 57:687, 1998

YTTERBERG SR: Viral arthritis. Curr Opin Rheumatol 11:275, 1999

ZABRISKIE JB et al: The arthritogenic properties of microbial antigens. Their implications in disease states. Rheum Dis Clin North Am 24:211, 1998

ZAVASKY DM, SANDE MA: Reconsideration of rifampin: A unique drug for a unique infection. JAMA 279:1575, 1998

ZIMMERLI W et al: Role of rifampin for treatment of orthopedic implant–related staphylococcal infections: A randomized controlled trial. Foreign-Body Infection (FBI) Study Group. JAMA 279:1537, 1998

——— et al: Prosthetic-joint infections. N Engl J Med 351:145, 2004

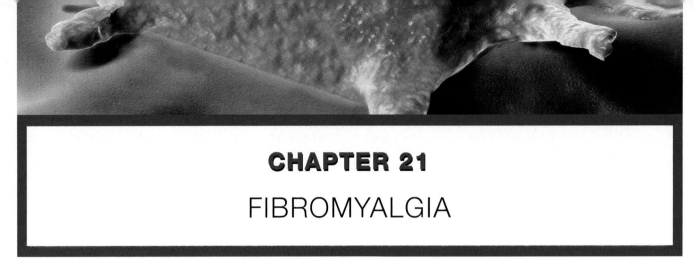

CHAPTER 21

FIBROMYALGIA

Carol A. Langford ■ Bruce C. Gilliland[†]

Fibromyalgia is a commonly encountered disorder characterized by chronic widespread musculoskeletal pain, stiffness, paresthesia, disturbed sleep, and easy fatigability along with multiple painful tender points, which are widely and symmetrically distributed. Fibromyalgia affects predominantly women in a ratio of 9:1 compared to men. This disorder is found in most countries, in most ethnic groups, and in all types of climates. The prevalence of fibromyalgia in the general population of a community in the United States using the 1990 American College of Rheumatology (ACR) classification criteria (see below) was reported to be 3.4% in women and 0.5% in men. Contrary to some previous reports, fibromyalgia was not found to be present mainly in young women but, rather, to be most prevalent in women ≥50 years. The prevalence increased with age, being 7.4% in women between the ages of 70 and 79. Although not common, fibromyalgia also occurs in children. The reported prevalence of fibromyalgia in some rheumatology clinics has been as high as 20%. Most patients present with fibromyalgia between the ages of 30–50 years.

PATHOGENESIS

Several causative mechanisms for fibromyalgia have been postulated to explain abnormal pain perception. Several abnormalities of the central nervous system have been

suggested. Disturbed sleep has been implicated as a factor in the pathogenesis. Nonrestorative sleep or awakening unrefreshed has been observed in most patients with fibromyalgia. Sleep electroencephalographic studies in patients with fibromyalgia have shown disruption of normal stage 4 sleep [non–rapid eye movement (NREM) sleep] by many repeated α-wave intrusions. The idea that stage 4 sleep deprivation has a role in causing this disorder was supported by the observation that symptoms of fibromyalgia developed in normal subjects whose stage 4 sleep was disrupted artificially by induced α-wave intrusions. This sleep disturbance, however, has been demonstrated in healthy individuals; in emotionally distressed individuals; and in patients with sleep apnea, fever, osteoarthritis, or rheumatoid arthritis. Low levels of serotonin metabolites have been reported in the cerebrospinal fluid (CSF) of patients with fibromyalgia, suggesting that a deficiency of serotonin, a neurotransmitter that regulates pain and NREM sleep, might also be involved in the pathogenesis of fibromyalgia. Fibromyalgia patients as a group have been reported by some investigators to have reduced levels of growth hormone, which is important for muscle repair and strength. Growth hormone is secreted normally during stage 4 sleep, which is disturbed in patients with fibromyalgia. The reduction of growth hormone may explain the extended periods of muscle pain following exertion in these patients. The level of the neurotransmitter substance P has been reported to be increased in the CSF of fibromyalgia patients and may play a role in spreading muscle pain. Patients with fibromyalgia have a decreased

---

[†]Deceased. A contributor to *Harrison's Principles of Internal Medicine* since the 11th edition, Dr. Gilliland passed away on February 17, 2007.

cortisol response to stress. Low urinary free cortisol and a diminished cortisol response to corticotropin-releasing hormone suggest an abnormal hypothalamic-pituitary-adrenal axis. Autonomic dysfunction has also been suggested to play a role in the pathogenesis of fibromyalgia. Some patients experience orthostatic hypotension on tilt-table testing and may have increased resting supine heart rates. Disturbances of the autonomic and peripheral nervous system may also account for the dry eyes and mouth and the cold sensitivity and Raynaud's-like symptoms seen in patients with fibromyalgia. Single photon emission computed tomography (SPECT) imaging has demonstrated reduced blood flow to the thalamus, caudate nucleus, and pontine tectum, which are areas in the brain involved in the signaling, integration, and modulation of pain. Patients with fibromyalgia have been shown to perceive stimuli such as heat or pressure as painful with less degree of stimulation than normal individuals. The actual threshold for detecting stimuli appears to be similar in both patients and normal subjects. Studies have also suggested that patients with fibromyalgia may have psychophysiologic abnormalities in their ability to inhibit irrelevant somatosensory stimulation.

Many patients with fibromyalgia have psychological abnormalities; there has been disagreement as to whether some of these abnormalities represent reactions to the chronic pain or whether the symptoms of fibromyalgia are a reflection of psychiatric disturbance. Approximately 30% of patients fit a psychiatric diagnosis, the most common being depression, anxiety, somatization, and hypochondriasis. Studies have also shown a high prevalence of sexual and physical abuse and eating disorders. However, fibromyalgia also occurs in patients without significant psychiatric problems.

Since patients experience pain from muscle and musculotendinous sites, many studies have been done to examine muscle, both structurally and physiologically. Inflammation or diagnostic muscle abnormalities have not been found. Evidence indicates deconditioning of muscles, and patients experience a greater degree of postexertional pain than do unaffected persons. A better understanding of fibromyalgia awaits further studies.

CLINICAL MANIFESTATIONS

Symptoms are generalized musculoskeletal aching and stiffness and fatigue. Patients may complain of low back pain, which may radiate into the buttocks and legs. Others complain of pain and tightness in the neck and across the upper posterior shoulders. Patients complain of muscle pain after even mild exertion, and some degree of pain is always present. The pain has been described as a burning or gnawing pain or as soreness, stiffness, or aching. Pain may begin in one region, such as the shoulders, neck, or lower back (Chap. 22) before it eventually becomes widespread. Patients may complain of joint pain and perceive

that their joints are swollen; however, joint examination yields normal findings. Stiffness is generally present on arising in the morning; usually it improves during the day, but in some patients it lasts all day. Patients may complain of numbness of their hands and feet. They may also feel colder overall than others in the home, and some may experience Raynaud's-like phenomena or actual Raynaud's phenomenon. Patients complain of feeling fatigued and exhausted and wake up tired. They also awaken frequently at night and have trouble falling back to sleep. Patients may experience cognitive impairment with difficulty thinking and loss of short-term memory. Headaches, including migraine type, are also common symptoms. Others experience episodes of light-headedness, dizziness, anxiety, or depression. Symptoms are made worse by stress or anxiety; cold, damp weather; and overexertion. Patients often feel better during warmer weather and vacations.

The characteristic feature on physical examination is the demonstration of specific sites or points, which are more tender or painful than the same sites in normal individuals. The ACR Criteria for Fibromyalgia defines 18 tender points (Fig. 21-1). These points of tenderness are remarkably constant in location. A moderate and consistent degree of pressure should be used in digital

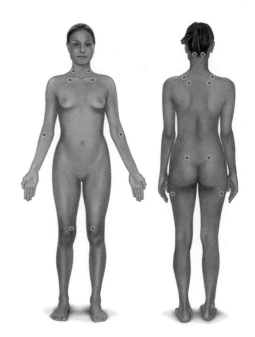

FIGURE 21-1

Tender points in fibromyalgia. Suboccipital muscle insertion at base of skull; anterior aspect of intertransverse process spaces at C5–7; midpoint of upper border of trapezius muscle; above scapular spine near medial border of scapula; second costochondral junction; lateral epicondyle; upper outer quadrant of buttocks; posterior aspect of trochanteric prominence; medial fat pad of knee (all bilateral). *(From the brochure "Fibromyalgia," Arthritis Information, Advice and Guidance, Disease Series. Used by permission of the Arthritis Foundation.)*

palpation of these tender points. As a guideline to reduce variability in the interpretation of point tenderness, the amount of force applied should be 4 kg (~9 lb), which is the degree of force required to just blanch the examiner's thumbnail. This amount of pressure does not produce significant tenderness or pain in normal subjects. Some workers recommend that the tender site be palpated using a rolling motion, which may be more effective in eliciting the tenderness. The tender sites can also be examined using a dolorimeter, which is a spring-loaded pressure gauge; however, digital palpation appears to be as effective and accurate. Some investigators have quantitated the degree of tenderness or pain, but the number of tender point sites is more diagnostic. Some patients are tender all over, although still more tender or painful at the specific tender point sites.

Skinfold tenderness may be present, particularly over the upper scapular region. Subcutaneous nodules may be felt at sites of tenderness. Nodules in similar locations are present in normal persons but are not tender.

Fibromyalgia may be triggered by emotional stress, infections and other medical illness, surgery, hypothyroidism, and trauma. It has appeared in some patients with hepatitis C infection, HIV infection, parvovirus B19 infection, or Lyme disease. In the latter situation, fibromyalgia may persist despite adequate antibiotic treatment for Lyme disease, and especially anxious patients may believe that they still have Lyme disease. Disorders commonly associated with fibromyalgia include irritable bowel syndrome, irritable bladder, headaches (including migraine headaches), dysmenorrhea, premenstrual syndrome, restless legs syndrome, temporomandibular joint pain, noncardiac chest pain, Raynaud's phenomenon, and sicca syndrome.

The course of fibromyalgia is variable. Symptoms wax and wane in some patients, while in others pain and fatigue are persistent regardless of therapy. Studies from tertiary medical centers indicate a poor prognosis for most patients. The prognosis may be better in community-treated patients. In a community-based study reported after 2 years of treatment, 24% of patients were in remission, and 47% no longer fulfilled the ACR criteria for fibromyalgia.

DIAGNOSIS

Fibromyalgia is diagnosed by a history of widespread musculoskeletal pain present for at least 3 months and the demonstration of significant tenderness or pain in at least 11 of the 18 tender point sites on digital palpation (Fig. 21-1). The ACR criteria are useful for standardizing the diagnosis; however, not all patients with fibromyalgia meet these criteria (Table 21-1). Some patients have fewer tender sites and more regional pain and may be considered to have fibromyalgia.

The musculoskeletal and neurologic examinations are normal in fibromyalgia patients, and there are no laboratory

TABLE 21-1

THE AMERICAN COLLEGE OF RHEUMATOLOGY 1990 CRITERIA FOR THE CLASSIFICATION OF FIBROMYALGIA[a]

1. History of widespread pain. Pain is considered widespread when all of the following are present:
   a. Pain in the left side of the body
   b. Pain in the right side of the body
   c. Pain above the waist
   d. Pain below the waist
   e. Axial skeletal pain (cervical spine or anterior chest or thoracic spine or low back)
2. Pain on digital palpation in at least 11 of the following 18 tender point sites (see Fig. 20-1):
   a. Occiput: bilateral, at the suboccipital muscle insertion
   b. Low cervical: bilateral, at the anterior aspect of the intertransverse spaces at C5–7
   c. Trapezius: bilateral, at the midpoint of the upper border
   d. Supraspinatus: bilateral, at the origin, above the scapular spine near the medial border
   e. Second rib: bilateral, at the second costochondral junction, just lateral to the junction on the upper surface
   f. Lateral epicondyle: bilateral, 2 cm distal to the epicondyle
   g. Gluteal: bilateral, in the upper outer quadrant of the buttock
   h. Greater trochanter: bilateral, posterior to the trochanteric prominence
   i. Knee: bilateral, at the medial fat pad proximal to the joint line

Digital palpation should be performed with a moderate degree of pressure. For a tender point to be considered positive, the subject must state that the palpation was painful. "Tender" is not to be considered painful.

[a]For purposes of classification, patients will be said to have fibromyalgia if both criteria are satisfied. Widespread pain must have been present for at least 3 months. The presence of a second clinical disorder does not exclude the diagnosis of fibromyalgia.
Source: Modified from F Wolfe et al: Arthritis Rheum 33:171, 1990.

abnormalities. Fibromyalgia may occur in patients with rheumatoid arthritis, systemic lupus erythematosus (SLE), other connective tissue diseases, or other medical illness. A distinction is no longer made between primary and secondary fibromyalgia (concomitant with other disease), as the signs and symptoms are similar. Fibromyalgia and chronic fatigue syndrome have many similarities. Both are associated with fatigue, abnormal sleep, musculoskeletal pain, impaired memory and concentration, and psychiatric conditions such as less severe forms of depression and anxiety. Patients with chronic fatigue syndrome, however, are more likely to have symptoms suggesting a viral illness. These include mild fever, sore throat, and pain in the axillary and anterior and posterior cervical lymph nodes. The onset of chronic fatigue syndrome is usually sudden; patients are usually able to date the onset. While many patients with chronic fatigue syndrome have tender or painful points, the diagnosis does not require their presence. Patients with fibromyalgia may be misdiagnosed with SLE or Sjögren's syndrome as these disorders have in common symptoms of musculoskeletal pain, dry eyes, cold hands, and fatigue. The antinuclear antibody (ANA) test may also be positive. The frequency of a positive ANA test in fibromyalgia patients, however, is the same as sex- and aged-matched normal controls. The predictive value of a positive ANA test in patients without characteristic symptoms and objective features of a connective tissue disease is quite low. Discretion is advised before ordering an ANA test. Patients with fibromyalgia may complain of muscle weakness, but on muscle strength testing, they have "giveaway" weakness secondary to pain. Proximal muscle weakness and elevated muscle enzymes distinguish patients with polymyositis. Polymyalgia rheumatica is distinguished from fibromyalgia in an elderly patient by the presence of more proximal muscle stiffness and pain and an elevated erythrocyte sedimentation rate. Patients should be evaluated for hypothyroidism, which may have symptoms similar to fibromyalgia or may accompany fibromyalgia. Disturbed sleep, musculoskeletal pain, and fatigue occur in patients with sleep apnea and restless legs syndrome. A distinguishing feature of sleep apnea is the presence of significant daytime somnolence. These patients should be referred to a sleep laboratory for evaluation and treatment. Myofascial pain syndrome, which involves an area such as the shoulder or neck, may represent a localized form of fibromyalgia (Chap. 22). Some patients with this syndrome progress to fibromyalgia.

The diagnosis of fibromyalgia has taken on a more complex significance in regard to labor and industry issues. This has become a significant issue since it has been reported that 10–25% of patients are not able to work in any capacity, while others require modification of their work. Disability evaluation in fibromyalgia is controversial. The diagnosis of fibromyalgia is not accepted by all. It is hard to evaluate patients' perceptions of their inability to function. The determination of tender points can also be subjective, on the part of both the physician and the patient, particularly when issues of compensation are pending. Patients also encounter difficulty in having their illness recognized as a disability. Physicians have been placed in the inappropriate role of assessing the patient's disability. Physicians are not in a position to quantitate disability at the workplace; that is better done by a work evaluation specialist. Better instruments are clearly needed for measuring disability, particularly in patients with fibromyalgia.

℞ Treatment: FIBROMYALGIA

Patients should be informed that they have a condition that is not crippling, deforming, or degenerative, and that treatment is available. Pregabalin, a calcium channel alpha$_2$-delta-subunit ligand with analgesic, anxiolytic, and antiepileptic activity, has had demonstrated efficacy for reducing symptoms of pain, disturbed sleep, and fatigue in patients with fibromyalgia. Duloxetine, a serotonin/norepinephrine reuptake inhibitor, has shown benefit for the management of symptoms associated with fibromyalgia in patients with or without major depressive disorder. Milnacipran, a dual norepinephrine and serotonin reuptake inhibitor, was also recently approved by the Food and Drug Administration for the treatment of fibromyalgia.

The use of tricyclics such as amitriptyline (10–50 mg), nortriptyline (10–75 mg), and doxepin (10–25 mg) or a pharmacologically similar drug, cyclobenzaprine (10–40 mg), 1–2 h before bedtime will give the patient restorative sleep (stage 4 sleep), resulting in clinical improvement. Patients should be started on a low dose, which is increased gradually as needed. Side effects of these tricyclics and cyclobenzaprine limit their use; these include constipation, dry mouth, weight gain, drowsiness, and difficulty thinking. Trazodone or zolpidem also improves sleep quality. In patients with restless legs syndrome, clonazepam may be effective. Depression and anxiety should next be treated with appropriate drugs and, when indicated, with psychiatric counseling.

Fluoxetine, sertraline, paroxetine, citalopram, or other newer selective serotonin reuptake inhibitors can be used as antidepressants. Other useful antidepressants are trazodone and venlafaxine. Alprazolam and lorazepam are effective for anxiety. Patients may also benefit by regular aerobic exercises, which are started after patients begin to have improved sleep and less pain and fatigue. Exercise should be of a low-impact type and begun at a low level. Eventually the patient should be exercising 20–30 min, 3–4 days a week. Regular stretching exercises are also very important. Salicylates or other nonsteroidal anti-inflammatory drugs (NSAIDs) only partially improve symptoms. Glucocorticoids have been of little benefit and should not be used in these patients. Opiate analgesics should be avoided. For pain, acetaminophen or tramadol may be useful. Also, gabapentin (300–1200 mg/d in divided doses) may reduce pain. Local measures such as heat, massage, injection of tender sites with steroids or lidocaine, and acupuncture provide only temporary relief of symptoms. Other therapies that may help to varying degrees include biofeedback, behavioral modification, hypnotherapy, and stress management and relaxation response training. Life stresses should be identified and discussed with the patient, and the patient should be provided with help on how to cope with these stresses. Patients may benefit from a multidisciplinary team approach involving a mental health professional, a physical therapist, and a physical medicine and rehabilitation specialist. Group therapy may be beneficial.

258 Patients should be well educated about their disorder and taught the importance of self-help. There are patient support groups in many communities. While treatment of fibromyalgia is effective in some patients, others continue to have chronic disease, which is relieved only partially if at all.

FURTHER READINGS

ABELES M et al: Update on fibromyalgia therapy. Am J Med 121:555, 2008

ARNOLD LM et al: A double-blind, multicenter trial comparing duloxetine with placebo in the treatment of fibromyalgia patients with or without major depressive disorder. Arthritis Rheum 50:2974, 2004

BRADLEY LA, ALARCON GS: Fibromyalgia, in *Arthritis and Allied Conditions*, 15th ed, WJ Koopman (ed). Philadelphia, Lippincott Williams & Wilkins, 2005, pp 1869–1910

BURKHAM J: Fibromyalgia, in *Kelley's Textbook of Rheumatology*, 7th ed, ED Harris et al (eds). Philadelphia, Saunders, 2005, pp 522–536

BUSCH A et al: Exercise for treating fibromyalgia syndrome (Cochrane Review). Cochrane Database Syst Rev 2002; CD003786

CROFFORD LJ : Pain management in fibromyalgia. Curr Opin Rheumatol 20:246, 2008

——— et al: Pregabalin for the treatment of fibromyalgia syndrome: Results of a randomized, double-blind, placebo-controlled trial. Arthritis Rheum 52:1264, 2005

GOLDENBERG DL: Fibromyalgia syndrome a decade later: What have we learned? Arch Intern Med 159:777, 1999

———: Fibromyalgia and related syndromes, in *Rheumatology*, 3d ed, MC Hochberg et al (eds). Philadelphia, Mosby, 2003, pp 701–712

———: Pharmacological treatment of fibromyalgia and other chronic musculoskeletal pain. Best Pract Res Clin Rheumatol 21:499, 2007

GOWANS SE et al: Six-month and one-year follow-up of 23 weeks of aerobic exercise for individuals with fibromyalgia. Arthritis Rheum 51:890, 2004

HÄUSER W et al: Efficacy of multicomponent treatment in fibromyalgia syndrome: A meta-analysis of randomized controlled clinical trials. Arthritis Rheum 61:216, 2009

MEASE PJ et al: A randomized, double-blind, placebo-controlled, phase III trial of pregabalin in the treatment of patients with fibromyalgia. J Rheumatol 35:502, 2008

——— et al: The efficacy and safety of milnacipran for treatment of fibromyalgia. A randomized, double-blind, placebo-controlled trial. J Rheumatol 36:398, 2009

TOFFERI JK et al: Treatment of fibromyalgia with cyclobenzaprine: A meta-analysis. Arthritis Rheum 51:9, 2004

UÇEYLER N et al: A systematic review on the effectiveness of treatment with antidepressants in fibromyalgia syndrome. Arthritis Rheum 59:1279, 2008

WOLFE F et al: The prevalence and characteristics of fibromyalgia in the general population. Arthritis Rheum 38:19, 1995

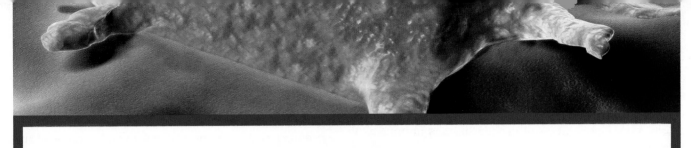

CHAPTER 22

ARTHRITIS ASSOCIATED WITH SYSTEMIC DISEASE AND OTHER ARTHRITIDES

Carol A. Langford ■ Bruce C. Gilliland[†]

ARTHRITIS ASSOCIATED WITH SYSTEMIC DISEASE

ARTHROPATHY OF ACROMEGALY

Acromegaly is the result of excessive production of growth hormone by an adenoma in the anterior pituitary gland. Middle-aged persons are most often affected. The excessive secretion of growth hormone along with insulin-like growth factor I stimulates proliferation of cartilage, periarticular connective tissue, and bone, resulting in several musculoskeletal abnormalities, including osteoarthritis, back pain, muscle weakness, and carpal tunnel syndrome.

An arthropathy resembling osteoarthritis is a common feature, affecting most often the knees, shoulders, hips, and hands. Single or multiple joints may be affected. The overgrowth of cartilage initially produces widening of the joint space. The newly synthesized cartilage is not developed in an organized manner, making it susceptible to fissuring, ulceration, and destruction. Ligamental laxity of the joint resulting from the growth of connective tissue also contributes to the development of osteoarthritis. With breakdown and loss of cartilage,

the joint space narrows, and subchondral sclerosis and osteophytes appear on radiographs. Joint examination reveals marked crepitus and hypermobility. Joint fluid is noninflammatory. Calcium pyrophosphate dihydrate crystals are found in the cartilage in some cases of acromegaly arthropathy and, when shed into the joint, can produce attacks of pseudogout. Chondrocalcinosis may also be observed radiographically. Approximately half of the patients with acromegaly experience back pain, which is predominantly lumbosacral. Hypermobility of the spine may be a contributing factor in back pain. Radiograph of the spine shows normal or increased intervertebral disk spaces, hypertrophic anterior osteophytes, and ligamental calcification. These changes are similar to those observed in patients with diffuse idiopathic skeletal hyperostosis. Dorsal kyphosis in conjunction with elongation of the ribs contributes to the development of the barrel chest seen in acromegalic patients. The hands and feet become enlarged owing to soft-tissue proliferation. The fingers are thickened and have spade-like distal tufts. One-third of patients have a thickened heel pad. Approximately 25% of patients have Raynaud's phenomenon.

Carpal tunnel syndrome occurs in about half of patients. The median nerve is compressed by the excessive growth of connective tissue in the carpal tunnel. The median nerve also becomes enlarged. Patients with

---

[†]Deceased. A contributor to *Harrison's Principles of Internal Medicine* since the 11th edition, Dr. Gilliland passed away on February 17, 2007.

acromegaly also develop proximal muscle weakness, which is thought to be caused by the effect of growth hormone on muscle. Results of muscle enzyme assays and electromyography are normal. Muscle biopsy specimens show muscle fibers of varying size and no inflammatory changes.

ARTHROPATHY OF HEMOCHROMATOSIS

Hemochromatosis is a disorder of iron storage. Excessive amounts of iron are absorbed from the intestine, leading to iron deposition in parenchymal cells, which results in tissue damage and impairment of organ function. Symptoms of hemochromatosis usually begin between the ages of 40 and 60 but can occur earlier. Arthritis, which occurs in 20–40% of patients, usually begins after the age of 50 and may be the first clinical feature of hemochromatosis. The arthropathy is an osteoarthritis-like disorder affecting the small joints of the hands, followed later by larger joints such as knees, ankles, shoulders, and hips. The second and third metacarpophalangeal joints of both hands are often the first joints affected; they can provide an important clue to the possibility of hemochromatosis. Patients experience stiffness and pain. Morning stiffness usually lasts less than half an hour. The affected joints are enlarged and mildly tender. Synovial tissue is not appreciably increased. Radiographs show irregular narrowing of the joint space, subchondral sclerosis, and subchondral cysts. There is juxtaarticular proliferation of bone, with frequent hook-like osteophytes. The synovial fluid is noninflammatory. The synovium shows mild to moderate proliferation of lining cells, fibrosis, and a low number of inflammatory cells, which are mononuclear. In approximately half of patients, there is evidence of calcium pyrophosphate deposition disease (CPPD), and patients may experience episodes of pseudogout. Iron can be demonstrated in the lining cells of the synovium and also in chondrocytes.

Iron may damage the articular cartilage in several ways. Iron catalyzes superoxide-dependent lipid peroxidation, which may play a role in joint damage. In animal models, ferric iron has been shown to interfere with collagen formation. Iron has also been shown to increase the release of lysosomal enzymes from cells in the synovial membrane. Iron may also play a role in the development of chondrocalcinosis. Iron inhibits synovial tissue pyrophosphatase in vitro and, therefore, may inhibit pyrophosphatase in vivo, resulting in chondrocalcinosis. Iron in synovial cells may also inhibit the clearance of calcium pyrophosphate from the joint.

℞ Treatment:
ARTHROPATHY OF HEMOCHROMATOSIS

The treatment of hemochromatosis is repeated phlebotomy. Unfortunately, this treatment has little effect on the arthritis, which, along with chondrocalcinosis, usually continues to progress. Treatment of the arthritis consists of administration of acetaminophen and nonsteroidal anti-inflammatory drugs (NSAIDs). Acute pseudogout attacks are treated with higher doses of an NSAID or a short course of glucocorticoids. Placement of a hip or knee prosthesis has been successful in advanced disease.

HEMOPHILIC ARTHROPATHY

Hemophilia is a sex-linked recessive genetic disorder characterized by the absence or deficiency of factor VIII (hemophilia A, or classic hemophilia) or factor IX (hemophilia B, or Christmas disease). Hemophilia A is by far the more common type, constituting 85% of cases. Spontaneous hemarthrosis is a common problem with both types of hemophilia and can lead to a chronic deforming arthritis. The frequency and severity of hemarthrosis are related to the degree of clotting factor deficiency. Hemarthrosis is not common in other inherited disorders of coagulation, such as von Willebrand disease or factor V deficiency.

Hemarthrosis becomes evident after 1 year of age, when the child begins to walk and run. In order of frequency, the joints most commonly affected are the knees, ankles, elbows, shoulders, and hips. Small joints of the hands and feet are occasionally involved.

In the initial stage of arthropathy, hemarthrosis produces a warm, tensely swollen, and painful joint. The patient holds the affected joint in flexion and guards against any movement. Blood in the joint remains liquid because of the absence of intrinsic clotting factors and the absence of tissue thromboplastin in the synovium. The blood in the joint space is resorbed over a period of a week or longer, depending on the size of the hemarthrosis. Joint function usually returns to normal or baseline in about 2 weeks.

Recurrent hemarthrosis leads to the development of a chronic arthritis. The involved joints remain swollen, and flexion deformities develop. In the later stages of arthropathy, joint motion is restricted and function is severely limited. Joint ankylosis, subluxation, and laxity are features of end-stage disease.

Bleeding into muscle and soft tissue also causes musculoskeletal disorders. When bleeding into the iliopsoas muscle occurs, the hip is held in flexion because of the pain, resulting in a hip flexion contracture. Rotation of the hip is preserved, which distinguishes this problem from intraarticular hemorrhage. Expansion of the hematoma may place pressure on the femoral nerve, resulting in a femoral neuropathy. Another problem is shortening of the heel cord secondary to bleeding into the gastrocnemius. Hemorrhage into a closed compartment space, such as the volar compartment in the forearm, can result in muscle necrosis, neuropathy, and flexion deformities of the wrist and fingers. When bleeding involves periosteum or bone, a pseudotumor forms. These occur distal to the elbows or knees in children and improve with treatment of the hemophilia. Surgical removal is indicated if the pseudotumor continues to enlarge. In adults, they occur in the femur and pelvis and are usually refractory to treatment. When bleeding occurs in muscle, cysts may develop within the muscle. Needle aspiration of a cyst is contraindicated because it can induce bleeding.

Septic arthritis can occur in hemophilia and is difficult at times to distinguish from acute hemarthrosis on physical examination. Whenever there is suspicion of an infected joint, the joint should be aspirated immediately, the fluid cultured, and the patient started on antibiotics that provide broad coverage until the results of the culture are known. The patient should be infused with the deficient clotting factor before the joint is tapped to decrease the risk of further bleeding.

Radiographs of joints reflect the stage of disease. In early stages there is only capsule distention; later, juxtaarticular osteopenia, marginal erosions, and subchondral cysts develop. In late disease, the joint space is narrowed and there is bony overgrowth. The changes are similar to those observed in osteoarthritis. Unique features of hemophilic arthropathy are widening of the femoral intercondylar notch, enlargement of the proximal radius, and squaring of the distal end of the patella.

Recurrent hemarthrosis produces synovial hyperplasia and hypertrophy. A pannus covers the cartilage. Cartilage is damaged by collagenase and other degradative enzymes released by mononuclear cells in the overlying synovium. Hemosiderin is found in synovial lining cells, the subsynovium, and chondrocytes and may also play a role in cartilage destruction.

℞ **Treatment: HEMARTHROSIS**

The treatment of hemarthrosis is initiated with the immediate infusion of factor VIII or IX at the first sign of joint or muscle hemorrhage. The patient is placed at bed rest, with the involved joint in as much extension as the patient can tolerate. Analgesic doses of an NSAID and local icing may help with the pain. NSAIDs can be given safely for short periods even though they have a stabilizing effect on platelets. Studies have shown no significant abnormalities in platelet function or bleeding time in hemophiliacs receiving ibuprofen. The cyclooxygenase-2 inhibitors do not interfere with platelet function and can be safely given for pain where their use is felt to be safe and indicated based upon the risks versus benefits. Synovectomy, open or arthroscopic, may be indicated in patients with chronic synovial proliferation and recurrent

hemarthrosis. Hypertrophied synovium is very vascular and subject to bleeding. Both types of synovectomy reduce the number of hemarthroses and slow the roentgenographic progression of hemophilic arthropathy. Open surgical synovectomy, however, is associated with some loss of range of motion. Radiosynovectomy with either yttrium 90 silicate or phosphorus 31 colloid also has been effective and may be a useful alternative when surgical synovectomy is not practical. Total joint replacement is indicated for severe joint destruction and incapacitating pain. Because of the young age of hemophilic patients, total-joint prostheses may need to be replaced more than once during their lives.

ARTHROPATHIES ASSOCIATED WITH HEMOGLOBINOPATHIES

Sickle Cell Disease

Sickle cell disease is associated with several musculoskeletal abnormalities (Table 22-1). Children under the age of 5 may develop diffuse swelling, tenderness, and warmth of the hands and feet lasting from 1 to 3 weeks. The condition, referred to as *sickle cell dactylitis* or *hand-foot syndrome*, has also been observed in sickle cell disease and sickle cell thalassemia. Dactylitis is believed to result from infarction of the bone marrow and cortical bone leading to periostitis and soft-tissue swelling. Radiographs show periosteal elevation, subperiosteal new bone formation, and areas of radiolucency and increased density involving the metacarpals, metatarsals, and proximal phalanges. These bone changes disappear after several months. The syndrome leaves little or no residual damage. Because hematopoiesis ceases in the small bones of hands and feet with age, the syndrome is rarely seen after age 4 or 5 and does not occur in adults.

Sickle cell crisis is often associated with periarticular pain and joint effusions. The joint and periarticular area are warm and tender. Knees and elbows are most often affected, but other joints can be involved. Joint effusions are noninflammatory, with white cell counts $<1000/\mu L$; mononuclear cells predominate. There have been a few reports of sterile inflammatory effusion with high cell counts consisting of mostly polymorphonuclear white

TABLE 22-1

MUSCULOSKELETAL ABNORMALITIES IN SICKLE CELL DISEASE	
Sickle cell dactylitis	Avascular necrosis
Joint effusions in sickle cell crises	Bone changes secondary to marrow hyperplasia
Osteomyelitis	
Infarction of bone	Septic arthritis
Infarction of bone marrow	Gouty arthritis

cells. Synovial biopsies have shown mild lining cell proliferation and microvascular thrombosis. Scintigraphic studies have shown decreased marrow uptake adjacent to the involved joint. The joint effusion and periarticular pain are considered to be the result of ischemia and infarction of the synovium and adjacent bone and bone marrow. The treatment is that for sickle cell crisis.

Patients with sickle cell disease may also develop osteomyelitis, which commonly involves the long tubular bones. These patients are particularly susceptible to bacterial infections, especially *Salmonella* infections, which are found in more than half of cases. The most common isolate is *S. typhimurium*. Radiographs of the involved site show periosteal elevation initially, followed by disruption of the cortex. Treatment of the infection results in healing of the bone lesion. Sickle cell disease is also associated with bone infarction resulting from thrombosis secondary to the sickling of red cells. Bone infarction also occurs in hemoglobin sickle cell disease and sickle cell thalassemia. The bone pain in sickle cell crisis is due to bone and bone marrow infarction. In children, infarction of the epiphyseal growth plate interferes with normal growth of the affected extremity. Radiographically, infarction of the bone cortex results in periosteal elevation and irregular thickening of the bone cortex. Infarction in the bone marrow leads to lysis, fibrosis, and new bone formation.

Avascular necrosis of the head of the femur is seen in ~5% of patients. It also occurs in the humeral head and less commonly in the distal femur, tibial condyles, distal radius, vertebral bodies, and other juxtaarticular sites. The mechanism for avascular necrosis is most likely the same as for bone infarction. Subchondral hemorrhage may play a role in the deterioration of articular cartilage. Irregularity of the femoral head or of other bone surfaces affected by avascular necrosis eventually results in degenerative joint disease. Radiograph of the affected joint may show patchy radiolucency and density followed by flattening of the bone. MRI is a sensitive technique for detecting early avascular necrosis as well as bone infarction elsewhere. Total hip replacement and placement of prostheses in other joints may improve function and relieve pain in those patients with severe joint destruction.

Septic arthritis is occasionally encountered in sickle cell disease (Chap. 20). Multiple joints may be infected. Joint infection may result from hematogenous spread or from spread of contiguous osteomyelitis. Microorganisms identified include *Staphylococcus aureus*, *Streptococcus*, *Escherichia coli*, and *Salmonella*. The latter is not seen as frequently in septic arthritis as it is in osteomyelitis. Acute gouty arthritis is uncommon in sickle cell disease, even though 40% of patients are hyperuremic. Hyperuricemia is due to overproduction of uric acid secondary to increased red cell turnover. Attacks may be polyarticular.

The bone marrow hyperplasia in sickle cell disease results in widening of the medullary cavities, thinning of the cortices, and coarse trabeculations and central cupping of the vertebral bodies. These changes are also seen to a lesser degree in hemoglobin sickle cell disease and sickle cell thalassemia. In normal individuals, red marrow is located mostly in the axial skeleton, but in sickle cell disease, red marrow is found in the bones of the extremities and even in the tarsal and carpal bones. Vertebral compression may lead to dorsal kyphosis, and softening of the bone in the acetabulum may result in protrusio acetabuli.

Thalassemia

β-Thalassemia is a congenital disorder of hemoglobin synthesis characterized by impaired production of β chains. Bone and joint abnormalities occur in β-thalassemia, being most common in the major and intermedia groups. In one study, ~50% of patients with β-thalassemia had evidence of symmetric ankle arthropathy, characterized by a dull aching pain aggravated by weight bearing. The onset was most often in the second or third decade of life. The degree of ankle pain in these patients varied. Some patients experienced self-limited ankle pain, which occurred only after strenuous physical activity and lasted several days to weeks. Other patients had chronic ankle pain, which became worse with walking. Symptoms eventually abated in a few patients. Compression of the ankle, calcaneus, or forefoot was painful in some patients. Synovial fluid from two patients was noninflammatory. Radiographs of ankle showed osteopenia, widened medullary spaces, thin cortices, and coarse trabeculations. These findings were largely the result of bone marrow expansion. The joint space was preserved. Specimens of bone from three patients revealed osteomalacia, osteopenia, and microfractures. Increased osteoblasts as well as increased foci of bone resorption were present on the bone surface. Iron staining was found in the bone trabeculae, in osteoid, and in the cement line. Synovium showed hyperplasia of lining cells, which contained deposits of hemosiderin. This arthropathy was considered to be related to the underlying bone pathology. The role of iron overload or abnormal bone metabolism in the pathogenesis of this arthropathy is not known. The arthropathy was treated with analgesics and splints. Patients were also transfused to decrease hematopoiesis and bone marrow expansion.

Patients with β-thalassemia major and intermedia also have involvement of other joints, including the knees, hips, and shoulders. Acquired hemochromatosis with arthropathy has been described in a patient with thalassemia. Gouty arthritis and septic arthritis can occur. Avascular necrosis is not a feature of thalassemia because there is no sickling of red cells leading to thrombosis and infarction.

β-Thalassemia minor (trait) is also associated with joint manifestations. Chronic seronegative oligoarthritis affecting predominantly ankles, wrists, and elbows has been described. These patients had mild persistent synovitis without large effusions. Joint erosions were not seen. Recurrent episodes of an acute asymmetric arthritis have also been reported; episodes last less than a week and may affect knees, ankles, shoulders, elbows, wrists, and metacarpal phalangeal joints. The mechanism for this arthropathy is unknown. Treatment with nonsteroidal drugs was not particularly effective.

MUSCULOSKELETAL DISORDERS ASSOCIATED WITH HYPERLIPIDEMIA

Musculoskeletal manifestations may be the first indication of a hereditary disorder of lipoprotein metabolism. Patients with familial hypercholesterolemia (previously referred to as *type II hyperlipoproteinemia*) may have recurrent migratory polyarthritis involving knees and other large peripheral joints and, to a lesser degree, peripheral small joints. In a few patients, the arthritis is monarticular. Fever may accompany the arthritis. Pain ranges from moderate to very severe to incapacitating. The involved joints can be warm, erythematous, swollen, and tender. Arthritis usually has a sudden onset, lasts from a few days to 2 weeks, and does not cause joint damage. Episodes may suggest acute gout attacks. Several attacks occur per year. Synovial fluid from involved joints is not inflammatory and contains few white cells and no crystals. Joint involvement may actually represent inflammatory periarthritis or peritendinitis and not intraarticular disease. The recurrent, transient nature of the arthritis may suggest rheumatic fever, especially since patients with hyperlipoproteinemia have an elevated erythrocyte sedimentation rate and a falsely elevated antistreptolysin O titer. Patients may also experience Achilles tendinitis, which can be very painful. Attacks of tendinitis come on gradually and last only a few days. Fever is not present. Patients may be asymptomatic between attacks. During an attack the Achilles tendon is warm, erythematous, swollen, and tender to palpation. Achilles tendinitis and other joint manifestations often precede the appearance of xanthomas and may be the first clinical indication of hyperlipoproteinemia. Attacks of tendinitis may occur following treatment with a lipid-lowering drug. Patients can also have tendinous xanthomas in the Achilles, patellar, and extensor tendons of the hands and feet. Xanthomas have also been reported in the peroneal tendon, the plantar aponeurosis, and the periosteum overlying the distal tibia. These xanthomas are located within tendon fibers. Tuberous xanthomas are soft subcutaneous masses located over the extensor surfaces of the elbows, knees, and hands, as well as on the buttocks. They appear in childhood in homozygous patients and after the age of 30 in heterozygous patients. Patients with elevated plasma levels of very low-density lipoprotein (VLDL) and triglyceride (previously referred to as *type IV hyperlipoproteinemia*) may also have a mild inflammatory arthritis affecting large and small peripheral joints, usually in an asymmetric pattern with only a few joints involved at a time. The onset of arthritis is usually in middle age. Arthritis may be persistent or recurrent, with episodes lasting a few days to weeks. Joint pain is severe in some patients. Patients may experience morning stiffness. Joint tenderness and periarticular hyperesthesia may also be present, as may synovial thickening. Joint fluid is usually noninflammatory and without crystals but may have increased white blood cell counts with predominantly mononuclear cells. The fluid is occasionally lactescent. Radiographs may show juxtaarticular osteopenia and cystic lesions. Large bone cysts have been noted in a few patients. Xanthoma and bone cysts are also observed in other lipoprotein disorders. The pathogenesis of arthritis in patients with familial hypercholesterolemia or with elevated levels of VLDL and triglyceride is not well understood. Salicylates, other NSAIDs, or analgesics usually provide relief of symptoms. Clinical improvement may also occur in patients treated with lipid-lowering agents; however, patients treated with an HMG-CoA reductase inhibitor may experience myalgias, and a few patients may develop polymyositis or even rhabdomyolysis. Myositis has also been reported with the use of niacin.

OTHER ARTHRITIDES

NEUROPATHIC JOINT DISEASE

Neuropathic joint disease (Charcot's joint) is a progressive destructive arthritis associated with loss of pain sensation, proprioception, or both. In addition, normal muscular reflexes that modulate joint movement are decreased. Without these protective mechanisms, joints are subjected to repeated trauma, resulting in progressive cartilage and bone damage. Neuropathic arthropathy was first described by Jean-Martin Charcot in 1868 in patients with tabes dorsalis. The term *Charcot's joint* is commonly used interchangeably with *neuropathic joint*. Today, diabetes mellitus is the most frequent cause of neuropathic joint disease (**Fig. 22-1**). A variety of other disorders are associated with neuropathic arthritis including leprosy, yaws, syringomyelia, meningomyelocele, congenital indifference to pain, peroneal muscular atrophy (Charcot-Marie-Tooth disease), and amyloidosis. An arthritis resembling neuropathic joint disease is seen in patients who have received frequent intraarticular glucocorticoid injections into a weight-bearing joint and in patients with CPPD. The distribution of joint involvement depends on the underlying neurologic disorder (**Table 22-2**). In tabes dorsalis, knees, hips, and

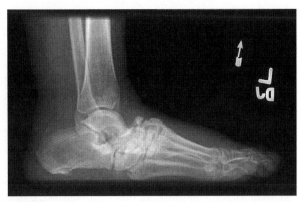

FIGURE 22-1

Charcot arthropathy associated with diabetes mellitus.
Lateral foot radiograph demonstrating complete loss of the
arch due to bony fragmentation and dislocation in the mid-
foot. *(Courtesy of Andrew Neckers, MD, and Jean Schils,
MD; with permission.)*

ankles are most commonly affected; in syringomyelia,
the glenohumeral joint, elbow, and wrist; and in diabetes
mellitus, the tarsal and tarsometatarsal joints.

Pathology and Pathophysiology

The pathologic changes in the neuropathic joint are
similar to those found in the severe osteoarthritic joint.
There is fragmentation and eventual loss of articular cartilage with eburnation of the underlying bone. Osteophytes are found at the joint margins. With more
advanced disease, erosions are present on the joint surface. Fractures, devitalized bone, and intraarticular loose
bodies may be present. Microscopic fragments of cartilage and bone are seen in the synovial tissue.

At least two underlying mechanisms are believed to
be involved in the pathogenesis of neuropathic arthritis.
An abnormal autonomic nervous system is thought to
be responsible for the increased blood flow to the joint
and subsequent resorption of bone. Loss of bone, particularly in the diabetic foot, may be the initial manifestation. With the loss of deep pain, proprioception, and
protective neuromuscular reflexes, the joint is subjected
to repeated injuries including ligamental tears and bone
fractures. The mechanism of injury that occurs following
frequent intraarticular glucocorticoid injections is thought
to be due to the analgesic effect of glucocorticoids leading

TABLE 22-2

DISORDERS ASSOCIATED WITH NEUROPATHIC JOINT DISEASE	
Diabetes mellitus	Amyloidosis
Tabes dorsalis	Leprosy
Meningomyelocele	Congenital indifference to pain
Syringomyelia	Peroneal muscular atrophy

to overuse of an already damaged joint, which results in
accelerated cartilage damage. It is not understood why
only a few patients with neuropathies develop neuropathic arthritis.

Clinical Manifestations

Neuropathic joint disease usually begins in a single joint
and then progresses to involve other joints, depending
on the underlying neurologic disorder. The involved
joint progressively becomes enlarged from bony overgrowth and synovial effusion. Loose bodies may be palpated in the joint cavity. Joint instability, subluxation,
and crepitus occur as the disease progresses. Neuropathic
joints may develop rapidly, and a totally disorganized
joint with multiple bony fragments may evolve in a
patient within weeks or months. The amount of pain
experienced by the patient is less than would be anticipated based on the degree of joint involvement. Patients
may experience sudden joint pain from intraarticular
fractures of osteophytes or condyles.

Neuropathic arthritis is encountered most often in
patients with diabetes mellitus, with the incidence estimated in the range of 0.5%. The usual age of onset is
≥50 years following several years of diabetes, but exceptions
occur. The tarsal and tarsometatarsal joints are most often
affected, followed by the metatarsophalangeal and talotibial
joints. The knees and spine are occasionally involved. In
about 20%, neuropathic arthritis may be present in both
feet. Patients often attribute the onset of foot pain to
antecedent trauma such as twisting their foot. Neuropathic changes may develop rapidly following a foot fracture or dislocation. Swelling of the foot and ankle are
often present. Downward collapse of the tarsal bones leads
to convexity of the sole, referred to as a "rocker foot."
Large osteophytes may protrude from the top of the foot.
Calluses frequently form over the metatarsal heads and
may lead to infected ulcers and osteomyelitis. Radiographs may show resorption and tapering of the distal
metatarsal bones. The term *Lisfranc fracture-dislocation* is
sometimes used to describe the destructive changes at the
tarsometatarsal joints.

Diagnosis

The diagnosis of neuropathic arthritis is based on the
clinical features and characteristic radiographic findings
in a patient with an underlying sensory neuropathy.
The differential diagnosis of neuropathic arthritis includes
osteomyelitis, osteonecrosis, advanced osteoarthritis,
stress fractures, and CPPD. Radiographs in neuropathic
arthritis initially show changes of osteoarthritis with joint
space narrowing, subchondral bone sclerosis, osteophytes,
and joint effusions followed later by marked destructive
and hypertrophic changes. Soft-tissue swelling, bone
resorption, fractures, large osteophytes, extraarticular

bone fragments, and subluxation are present with advanced arthropathy. The radiographic findings of neuropathic arthritis may be difficult to differentiate from those of osteomyelitis, especially in the diabetic foot. The joint margins in a neuropathic joint tend to be distinct, while in osteomyelitis, they are blurred. Imaging studies and cultures of fluid and tissue from the joint are often required to exclude osteomyelitis. MRI is helpful in differentiating these disorders. Another useful study is a bone scan using indium 111–labeled white blood cells or indium 111–labeled immunoglobulin G, which will show an increased uptake in osteomyelitis but not in a neuropathic joint. A technetium bone scan will not distinguish osteomyelitis from neuropathic arthritis, as increased uptake is observed in both. The joint fluid in neuropathic arthritis is noninflammatory; may be xanthochromic or even bloody; and may contain fragments of synovium, cartilage, and bone. The finding of calcium pyrophosphate dihydrate crystals suggests the diagnosis of a crystal-associated neuropathic-like arthropathy. In the absence of such crystals, the presence of an increased number of leukocytes may indicate osteomyelitis.

℞ Treatment:
NEUROPATHIC JOINT DISEASE

The primary focus of treatment is to provide stabilization of the joint. Treatment of the underlying disorder, even if successful, does not usually alter the joint disease. Braces and splints are helpful. Their use requires close surveillance, since patients may be unable to appreciate pressure from a poorly adjusted brace. In the diabetic patient, early recognition and treatment of a Charcot's foot by prohibiting weight bearing of the foot for at least 8 weeks may possibly prevent severe disease from developing. Fusion of a very unstable joint may improve function, but nonunion is frequent, especially when immobilization of the joint is inadequate.

HYPERTROPHIC OSTEOARTHROPATHY AND CLUBBING

Hypertrophic osteoarthropathy (HOA) is characterized by clubbing of digits and, in more advanced stages, by periosteal new bone formation and synovial effusions. HOA occurs in primary or familial form and usually begins in childhood. The secondary form of HOA is associated with intrathoracic malignancies, suppurative lung disease, congenital heart disease, and a variety of other disorders and is more common in adults. Clubbing is almost always a feature of HOA but can occur as an isolated manifestation (Fig. 22-2). The presence of clubbing in isolation is generally considered to represent either an early stage or an element in the spectrum of

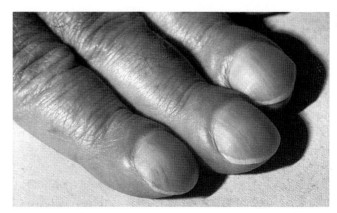

FIGURE 22-2
Clubbing of fingers. *(Reprinted from the Clinical Slide Collection on the Rheumatic Diseases, Copyright 1991, 1995. Used by permission of the American College of Rheumatology.)*

HOA. The presence of only clubbing in a patient usually has the same clinical significance as HOA.

Pathology and Pathophysiology

In HOA, the bone changes in the distal extremities begin as periostitis followed by new bone formation. At this stage, a radiolucent area may be observed between the new periosteal bone and subjacent cortex. As the process progresses, multiple layers of new bone are deposited, which become contiguous with the cortex and result in cortical thickening. The outer portion of bone is laminated in appearance, with an irregular surface. Initially, the process of periosteal new bone formation involves the proximal and distal diaphyses of the tibia, fibula, radius, and ulna and, less frequently, the femur, humerus, metacarpals, metatarsals, and phalanges. Occasionally, scapulae, clavicles, ribs, and pelvic bones are also affected. In long-standing disease, these changes extend to involve metaphyses and musculotendinous insertions. The adjacent interosseous membranes may become ossified. The distribution of the bone manifestations is usually bilateral and symmetric. The soft tissue overlying the distal third of the arms and legs may be thickened. Mononuclear cell infiltration may be present in the adjacent soft tissue. Proliferation of connective tissue occurs in the nail bed and volar pad of digits, giving the distal phalanges a clubbed appearance. Small blood vessels in the clubbed digits are dilated and have thickened walls. In addition, the number of arteriovenous anastomoses is increased. The synovia of involved joints show edema, varying degrees of synovial cell proliferation, thickening of the subsynovium, vascular congestion, vascular obliteration with thrombi, and small numbers of lymphocyte infiltrates.

Several theories have been suggested for the pathogenesis of HOA. Most have been disproved or have not explained the development in all clinical disorders associated with HOA. Previously proposed neurogenic and humoral theories are no longer considered likely explanations for HOA. The neurogenic theory was based on the observation that vagotomy resulted in symptomatic improvement in a small number of patients with lung tumors and HOA. It was postulated that vagal stimuli from the tumor site led via a neural reflex to efferent nerve impulses to the distal extremities, resulting in HOA. This theory, however, did not explain HOA in conditions where vagal stimulation did not occur, as in cyanotic congenital heart disease or arterial aneurysms. The humoral theory postulated that soluble substances that are normally inactivated or removed during passage through the lung reached the systemic circulation in an active form and stimulated the changes of HOA. Substances proposed included prostaglandins, ferritin, bradykinin, estrogen, and growth hormone. These substances seemed unlikely candidates, since their blood levels in HOA patients overlapped those in individuals without HOA. Furthermore, these substances did not explain the development of localized HOA associated with arterial aneurysms or infected arterial grafts.

Recent studies have suggested a role for platelets in the development of HOA. It has been observed that megakaryocytes and large platelet particles, present in venous circulation, were fragmented in their passage through normal lung. In patients with cyanotic congenital heart disease and in other disorders associated with right-to-left shunts, these large platelet particles bypass the lung and reach the distal extremities, where they can interact with endothelial cells. Platelet clumps have been demonstrated to form on an infected heart valve in bacterial endocarditis, in the wall of arterial aneurysms, and on infected arterial grafts. These platelet particles may also reach the distal extremities and interact with endothelial cells. Platelet-endothelial activation in the distal portion of extremities would then result in the release of platelet-derived growth factor (PDGF) and other factors leading to the proliferation of connective tissue and periosteum. Stimulation of fibroblasts by PDGF and transforming growth factor β results in cell growth and collagen synthesis. Elevated plasma levels of von Willebrand factor antigen have been found in patients with both primary and secondary forms of HOA, indicating endothelial activation or damage. Abnormalities of collagen synthesis have been demonstrated in the involved skin of patients with primary HOA. Fibroblasts from affected skin were shown to have increased collagen synthesis, increased $\alpha1(I)$ procollagen mRNA, and evidence for upregulation of collagen transcription. Other factors are undoubtedly involved in the pathogenesis of HOA, and further studies are needed to better understand this disorder.

Clinical Manifestations

Primary or familial HOA, also referred to as *pachydermoperiostosis* or *Touraine-Solente-Golé syndrome*, usually begins insidiously at puberty. In a smaller number of patients, the onset is in the first year of life. The disorder is inherited as an autosomal dominant trait with variable expression and is nine times more common in boys than in girls. Approximately one-third of patients have a family history of primary HOA.

Primary HOA is characterized by clubbing, periostitis, and unusual skin features. A small number of patients with this syndrome do not express clubbing. The skin changes and periostitis are prominent features of this syndrome. The skin becomes thickened and coarse. Deep nasolabial folds develop, and the forehead may become furrowed. Patients may have heavy-appearing eyelids and ptosis. The skin is often greasy, and there may be excessive sweating of the hands and feet. Patients may also experience acne vulgaris, seborrhea, and folliculitis. In a few patients, the skin over the scalp becomes very thick and corrugated, a feature that has been descriptively termed *cutis verticis gyrata*. The distal extremities, particularly the legs, become thickened owing to proliferation of new bone and soft tissue; when the process is extensive, the distal lower extremities resemble those of an elephant. The periostitis is usually not painful, as it may be in secondary HOA. Clubbing of the fingers may be extensive, producing large, bulbous deformities and clumsiness. Clubbing also affects the toes. Patients may experience articular and periarticular pain, especially in the ankles and knees, and joint motion may be mildly restricted owing to periarticular bone overgrowth. Non-inflammatory effusions occur in the wrists, knees, and ankles. Synovial hypertrophy is not found. Associated abnormalities observed in patients with primary HOA include hypertrophic gastropathy, bone marrow failure, female escutcheon, gynecomastia, and cranial suture defects. In patients with primary HOA, the symptoms disappear when adulthood is reached.

HOA secondary to an underlying disease occurs more frequently than primary HOA. It accompanies a variety of disorders and may precede clinical features of the associated disorder by months. Clubbing is more frequent than the full syndrome of HOA in patients with associated illnesses. Because clubbing evolves over months and is usually asymptomatic, it is often recognized first by the physician and not the patient. Patients may experience a burning sensation in their fingertips. Clubbing is characterized by widening of the fingertips, enlargement of the distal volar pad, convexity of the nail contour, and the loss of the normal 15° angle between the proximal nail and cuticle. The thickness of the digit at the base of the nail is greater than the thickness at the distal interphalangeal joint. An objective measurement of finger clubbing can be made by determining the diameter at the base of the nail and at the distal interphalangeal joint of all 10 digits. Clubbing is present when the sum of the individual digit ratios is >10. At the bedside, clubbing can be appreciated by having the patient place the dorsal surface of the distal phalanges of the fourth fingers together with the nails of the fourth fingers opposing each other. Normally, an open area is visible between the bases of the opposing fingernails; when clubbing is present, this open space is no longer visible. The base of the nail feels spongy when compressed, and the nail can be easily rocked on its bed. Marked periungual erythema is usually present. When clubbing is advanced, the finger may have a drumstick appearance, and the distal interphalangeal joint can be hyperextended. Periosteal involvement in the distal extremities may produce a burning or deep-seated aching pain. The pain can be quite incapacitating and is aggravated by dependency and relieved by elevation of the affected limbs. The overlying soft tissue may be swollen, and the skin slightly erythematous. Pressure applied over the distal forearms and legs may be quite painful.

Patients may also experience joint pain, most often in the ankles, wrists, and knees. Joint effusions may be present; usually they are small and noninflammatory. The small joints of the hands are rarely affected. Severe joint or bone pain may be the presenting symptom of an underlying lung malignancy and may precede the appearance of clubbing. In addition, the progression of HOA tends to be more rapid when associated with malignancies, most notably bronchogenic carcinoma. Unlike primary HOA, excessive sweating and oiliness of the skin and thickening of the facial skin are uncommon in secondary HOA.

HOA occurs in 5–10% of patients with intrathoracic malignancies, the most common being bronchogenic carcinoma and pleural tumors (Table 22-3). Lung metastases infrequently cause HOA. HOA is also seen in patients with intrathoracic infections, including lung abscesses, empyema, bronchiectasis, chronic obstructive lung disease, and, uncommonly, pulmonary tuberculosis. HOA may also accompany chronic interstitial pneumonitis, sarcoidosis, and cystic fibrosis. In the latter, clubbing is more common than the full syndrome of HOA. Other causes of clubbing include congenital heart disease with right-to-left shunts, bacterial endocarditis, Crohn's disease, ulcerative colitis, sprue, and neoplasms of the esophagus, liver, and small and large bowel. In patients with congenital heart disease with right-to-left shunts, clubbing alone occurs more often than the full syndrome of HOA.

Unilateral clubbing has been found in association with aneurysms of major extremity arteries, with infected arterial grafts, and with arteriovenous fistulas of brachial vessels. Clubbing of the toes but not fingers has been associated with an infected abdominal aortic aneurysm and patent ductus arteriosus. Clubbing of a single digit may follow trauma and has been reported in tophaceous gout and sarcoidosis. While clubbing occurs more commonly than the full syndrome in most diseases, periostitis in the absence of clubbing has been observed in the affected limb of patients with infected arterial grafts.

Hyperthyroidism (Graves' disease), treated or untreated, is occasionally associated with clubbing and periostitis of the bones of the hands and feet. This condition is referred to as *thyroid acropachy*. Periostitis is asymptomatic and occurs in the midshaft and diaphyseal portion of the metacarpal and phalangeal bones. The long bones of the extremities are seldom affected. Elevated levels of long-acting thyroid stimulator are found in the serum of these patients.

Laboratory Findings

The laboratory abnormalities reflect the underlying disorder. The synovial fluid of involved joints has <500 white cells per microliter, and the cells are predominantly mononuclear. Radiographs show a faint radiolucent line beneath the new periosteal bone along the shaft of long bones at their distal end. These changes are observed most frequently at the ankles, wrists, and knees. The ends of the distal phalanges may show osseous resorption. Radionuclide studies show pericortical linear uptake along the cortical margins of long bones that may be present before any radiographic changes.

TABLE 22-3

DISORDERS ASSOCIATED WITH HYPERTROPHIC OSTEOARTHROPATHY	
Pulmonary	Cardiovascular
Bronchogenic carcinoma and other neoplasms	Cyanotic congenital heart disease
Lung abscesses, empyema, bronchiectasis	Subacute bacterial endocarditis
Chronic interstitial pneumonitis	Infected arterial grafts[a]
Cystic fibrosis	Aortic aneurysm[b]
Chronic obstructive lung disease	Aneurysm of major extremity artery[a]
Sarcoidosis	Patent ductus arteriosus[b]
Gastrointestinal	Arteriovenous fistula of major extremity vessel[a]
Inflammatory bowel disease	
Sprue	Thyroid (thyroid acropachy)
Neoplasms: esophagus, liver, bowel	Hyperthyroidism (Graves' disease)

[a]Unilateral involvement.
[b]Bilateral lower extremity involvement.

℞ **Treatment:**
HYPERTROPHIC OSTEOARTHROPATHY

The treatment of HOA is to identify the associated disorder and treat it appropriately. The symptoms and signs of HOA may disappear completely with removal or effective chemotherapy of a tumor or with antibiotic therapy and drainage of a chronic pulmonary infection. Vagotomy or percutaneous block of the vagus nerve leads to symptomatic relief in some patients. Aspirin, NSAIDs, or analgesics may help control symptoms of HOA.

REFLEX SYMPATHETIC DYSTROPHY SYNDROME

The reflex sympathetic dystrophy syndrome is now referred to as *complex regional pain syndrome, type 1*, by the new Classification of the International Association for the Study of Pain. It is characterized by pain and swelling, usually of a distal extremity, accompanied by vasomotor instability, trophic skin changes, and the rapid development of bony demineralization. Further detail about reflex sympathetic dystrophy and its treatment can be found in *Harrison's Principles of Internal Medicine,* 17th edition, Chap. 371.

TIETZE SYNDROME AND COSTOCHONDRITIS

Tietze syndrome is manifested by painful swelling of one or more costochondral articulations. The age of onset is usually before 40, and both sexes are affected equally. In most patients only one joint is involved, usually the second or third costochondral joint. The onset of anterior chest pain may be sudden or gradual. The pain may radiate to the arms or shoulders and is aggravated by sneezing, coughing, deep inspirations, or twisting motions of the chest. The term *costochondritis* is often used interchangeably with *Tietze syndrome*, but some workers restrict the former term to pain of the costochondral articulations without swelling. Costochondritis is observed in patients over age 40; tends to affect the third, fourth, and fifth costochondral joints; and occurs more often in women. Both syndromes may mimic cardiac or upper abdominal causes of pain. Rheumatoid arthritis, ankylosing spondylitis, and Reiter's syndrome may involve costochondral joints but are distinguished easily by their other clinical features. Other skeletal causes of anterior chest wall pain are xiphoidalgia and the slipping rib syndrome, which usually involves the tenth rib. Malignancies such as breast cancer, prostate cancer, plasma cell cytoma, and sarcoma can invade the ribs, thoracic spine, or chest wall and produce symptoms suggesting Tietze syndrome. They should be easily distinguishable by radiographs and biopsy. Analgesics, anti-inflammatory drugs, and local glucocorticoid injections usually relieve symptoms.

MYOFASCIAL PAIN SYNDROME

Myofascial pain syndrome is characterized by localized musculoskeletal pain and tenderness in association with trigger points. The pain is deep and aching and may be accompanied by a burning sensation. Myofascial pain may follow trauma, overuse, or prolonged static contraction of a muscle or muscle group, which may occur when reading or writing at a desk or working at a computer. In addition, this syndrome may be associated with underlying osteoarthritis of the neck or low back. Trigger points are a diagnostic feature of this syndrome. Pain is referred from trigger points to defined areas distant from the original tender points. Palpation of the trigger point reproduces or accentuates the pain. The trigger points are usually located in the center of a muscle belly, but they can occur at other sites, such as costosternal junctions, the xiphoid process, ligamentous and tendinous insertions, fascia, and fatty areas. Trigger point sites in muscle have been described as feeling indurated and taut, and palpation may cause the muscle to twitch. These findings, however, have been shown not to be unique for myofascial pain syndrome, since in a controlled study they were also present in fibromyalgia patients and normal subjects. Myofascial pain most often involves the posterior neck, low back, shoulders, and chest. Chronic pain in the muscles of the posterior neck may involve referral of pain from the trigger point in the erector neck muscle or upper trapezius to the head, leading to persistent headaches, which may last for days. Trigger points in the paraspinal muscles of the low back may refer pain to the buttock. Pain may be referred down the leg from a trigger point in the gluteus medius and can mimic sciatica. A trigger point in the infraspinatus muscle may produce local and referred pain over the lateral deltoid and down the outside of the arm into the hand. Injection of a local anesthetic such as 1% lidocaine into the trigger point site often results in pain relief. Another useful technique is first to spray from the trigger point toward the area of referred pain with an agent such as ethyl chloride and then to stretch the muscle. This maneuver may need to be repeated several times. Massage and application of ultrasound to the affected area also may be beneficial. Patients should be instructed in methods to prevent muscle stresses related to work and recreation. Posture and resting positions are important in preventing muscle tension. The prognosis in most patients is good. In some patients, myofascial pain syndrome may evolve into fibromyalgia (Chap. 21). Patients at risk for developing fibromyalgia are thought to be those with anxiety, depression, nonrestorative sleep, and fatigue.

TUMORS OF JOINTS

Primary tumors and tumor-like disorders of synovium are uncommon but should be considered in the differential diagnosis of monarticular joint disease. In addition, metastases to bone and primary bone tumors adjacent to a joint may produce joint symptoms.

Pigmented villonodular synovitis is characterized by the slowly progressive, exuberant, benign proliferation of synovial tissue, usually involving a single joint. The most common age of onset is in the third decade, and women are affected slightly more often than men. The cause of this disorder is unknown.

The synovium has a brownish color and numerous large, finger-like villi that fuse to form pedunculated nodules. There is marked hyperplasia of synovial cells in the stroma of the villi. Hemosiderin granules and lipids are found in the cytoplasm of macrophages and in the interstitial tissue. Multinucleated giant cells may be present. The proliferative synovium grows into the subsynovial tissue and invades adjacent cartilage and bone.

The clinical picture of pigmented villonodular synovitis is characterized by the insidious onset of swelling and pain in one joint, most commonly the knee. Other joints affected include the hips, ankles, calcaneocuboid joints, elbows, and small joints of the fingers or toes. The disease may also involve the common flexor sheath of the hands or fingers. Less commonly, tendon sheaths in the wrist, ankle, or foot may be involved. Symptoms may be mild and intermittent and may be present for years before the patient seeks medical attention. Radiographs may show joint space narrowing, erosions, and subchondral cysts. The joint fluid contains blood and is dark red or almost black in color. Lipid-containing macrophages may be present in the fluid. The joint fluid may be clear if hemorrhages have not occurred.

The treatment of pigmented villonodular synovitis is complete synovectomy. With incomplete synovectomy, the villonodular synovitis recurs, and the rate of tissue growth may be faster than it was originally. Irradiation of the involved joint has been successful in some patients.

Synovial chondromatosis is a disorder characterized by multiple focal metaplastic growths of normal-appearing cartilage in the synovium or tendon sheath. Segments of cartilage break loose and continue to grow as loose bodies. When calcification and ossification of loose bodies occur, the disorder is referred to as *synovial osteochondromatosis*. The disorder is usually monarticular and affects young to middle-aged individuals. The knee is most often involved, followed by hip, elbow, and shoulder. Symptoms are pain, swelling, and decreased motion of the joint. Radiographs may show several rounded calcifications within the joint cavity. Treatment is synovectomy; however, the tumor may recur.

Hemangiomas occur in synovium and in tendon sheaths. The knee is affected most commonly. Recurrent episodes of joint swelling and pain usually begin in childhood. The joint fluid is bloody. Treatment is excision of the lesion. *Lipomas* occur most often in the knee, originating in the subsynovial fat on either side of the patellar tendon. Lipomas also appear in tendon sheaths of the hands, wrists, feet, and ankles. In some instances, surgical removal is necessary.

Synovial sarcoma is a malignant neoplasm often found near a large joint of both upper and lower extremities, being more common in the lower extremity. It seldom arises within the joint itself. Synovial sarcomas constitute 10% of soft-tissue sarcomas. The tumor is believed to arise from primitive mesenchymal tissue that differentiates into epithelial cells and/or spindle cells. Small foci of calcification may be present in the tumor mass. It occurs most often in young adults and is more common in men. The tumor presents as a slowly growing deep-seated mass near a joint, without much pain. The area of the knee is the most common site, followed by the foot, ankle, elbow, and shoulder. Other primary sites include the buttocks, abdominal wall, retroperitoneum, and mediastinum. The tumor spreads along tissue planes. The most common site of visceral metastasis is lung. The diagnosis is made by biopsy. Treatment is wide resection of the tumor including adjacent muscle and regional lymph nodes, followed by chemotherapy and radiation therapy. Currently used chemotherapeutic agents are doxorubicin, ifosfamide, and cisplatin. Amputation of the involved distal extremity may be required. Chemotherapy may be beneficial in some patients with metastatic disease. Isolated pulmonary metastasis can be surgically removed. The 5-year survival with treatment is variable depending on the staging of the tumor, ranging from approximately 25–60% or higher. Synovial sarcomas tend to recur locally and eventually metastasize to regional lymph nodes, lungs, and skeleton.

FURTHER READINGS

AGUILAR C et al: Bone and joint disease in sickle cell disease. Hematol Oncol Clin North Am 19:929, 2005

ALBAZAZ R et al: Complex regional pain syndrome: A review. Ann Vasc Surg 22:297, 2008

ARMAN MI et al: Brief report. Frequency and features of rheumatic findings in thalassaemia minor: A blind controlled study. Br J Rheumatol 31:197, 1992

CARELESS DJ, COHEN MG: Rheumatic manifestations of hyperlipidemia and antihyperlipidemia drug therapy. Semin Arthritis Rheum 23:90, 1993

CRONIN ME: Rheumatic aspects of endocrinopathies, in *Arthritis and Allied Conditions,* 15th ed, WJ Koopman (ed). Philadelphia, Lippincott Williams & Wilkins, 2005, pp 2559–2576

CUNNANE G: Hemochromatosis, in *Kelley's Textbook of Rheumatology,* 8th ed, GS Firestein et al (eds). Philadelphia, Saunders, 2009, pp 1809–1815

DIXON J: Tumors of bone, in *Rheumatology,* 4th ed, MC Hochberg et al (eds). Philadelphia, Mosby, 2008, pp 2043–2056

ELLMAN MH: Neuropathic joint disease (Charcot joints), in *Arthritis and Allied Conditions,* 15th ed, WJ Koopman (ed). Philadelphia, Lippincott Williams & Wilkins, 2005, pp 1911–1932

GORODKIN R, HERRICK AL: Reflex sympathetic dystrophy (complex regional pain syndrome type I), in *Rheumatology,* 4th ed, MC Hochberg et al (eds). Philadelphia, Mosby, 2008, pp 725–732

HECK LW JR: Arthritis associated with hematologic disorders, storage diseases, disorders of lipid metabolism, and dysproteinemias, in *Arthritis and Allied Conditions,* 15th ed, WJ Koopman (ed). Philadelphia, Lippincott Williams & Wilkins, 2005, pp 1969–1990

270 HUSNI EM, DONOHUE JP: Painful shoulder and reflex sympathetic dystrophy syndrome, in *Arthritis and Allied Conditions*, 15th ed, WJ Koopman (ed). Philadelphia, Lippincott Williams & Wilkins, 2005, pp 2133–2152

JANSEN NW et al: Understanding haemophilic arthropathy: An exploration of current open issues. Br J Haematol 143:632, 2008

JORDAN JM. Arthritis in hemochromatosis or iron storage disease. Curr Opin Rheumatol 16:62, 2004

KALUNIAN KC, SUN B: Rheumatic manifestations of hemoglobinopathies, in *Kelley's Textbook of Rheumatology*, 8th ed, GS Firestein et al (eds). Philadelphia, Saunders, 2009, pp 1827–1831

KASSIMOS DG, CREAMER P: Neuropathic arthropathy, in *Rheumatology*, 4th ed, MC Hochberg et al (eds). Philadelphia, Mosby, 2008, pp 1771–1776

MARTINEZ-LAVIN M, PINEDA C: Digital clubbing and hypertrophic osteoarthropathy, in *Rheumatology*, 4th ed, MC Hochberg et al (eds). Philadelphia, Mosby, 2008, pp 1683–1687

ROSENBERG EA: Tumors and tumor-like lesions of joints and related structures, in *Kelley's Textbook of Rheumatology*, 8th ed, GS Firestein et al (eds). Philadelphia, Saunders, 2009, pp 1883–1902

SPICKNALL KE et al: Clubbing: An update on diagnosis, differential diagnosis, pathophysiology, and clinical relevance. J Am Acad Dermatol 52:1020, 2005

TYLER WK et al: Pigmented villonodular synovitis. J Am Acad Orthop Surg 14(6):376, 2006

UPCHURCH KS, BRETTLER DB: Hemophilic arthropathy, in *Kelley's Textbook of Rheumatology*, 8th ed, GS Firestein et al (eds). Philadelphia, Saunders, 2009, pp 1817–1825

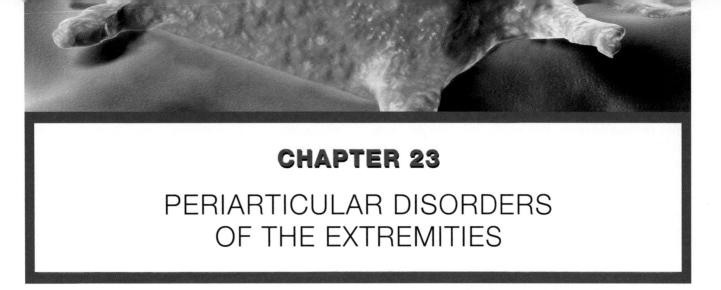

CHAPTER 23

PERIARTICULAR DISORDERS OF THE EXTREMITIES

Carol A. Langford ■ Bruce C. Gilliland†

A number of periarticular disorders have become increasingly common over the past two to three decades, due in part to greater participation in recreational sports by individuals of a wide range of ages. This chapter discusses some of the more common periarticular disorders of the extremities.

BURSITIS

Bursitis is inflammation of a bursa, which is a thin-walled sac lined with synovial tissue. The function of the bursa is to facilitate movement of tendons and muscles over bony prominences. Excessive frictional forces from overuse, trauma, systemic disease (e.g., rheumatoid arthritis, gout), or infection may cause bursitis. *Subacromial bursitis* (subdeltoid bursitis) is the most common form of bursitis. The subacromial bursa, which is contiguous with the subdeltoid bursa, is located between the undersurface of the acromion and the humeral head and is covered by the deltoid muscle. Bursitis is caused by repetitive overhead motion and often accompanies rotator cuff tendinitis. Another frequently encountered form is *trochanteric bursitis*, which involves the bursa around the insertion of the gluteus medius onto the greater trochanter of the femur. Patients experience pain over the lateral aspect of the hip and upper thigh and have tenderness over the posterior aspect of the greater trochanter. External rotation and resisted abduction of the hip elicit pain. *Olecranon bursitis* occurs over the posterior elbow, and when the area is acutely inflamed, infection or gout should be excluded by aspirating the bursa and performing a Gram stain and culture on the fluid as well as examining the fluid for urate crystals. *Achilles bursitis* involves the bursa located above the insertion of the tendon to the calcaneus and results from overuse and wearing tight shoes. *Retrocalcaneal bursitis* involves the bursa that is located between the calcaneus and posterior surface of the Achilles tendon. The pain is experienced at the back of the heel, and swelling appears on the medial and/or lateral side of the tendon. It occurs in association with spondyloarthropathies, rheumatoid arthritis, gout, or trauma. *Ischial bursitis* (weaver's bottom) affects the bursa separating the gluteus medius from the ischial tuberosity and develops from prolonged sitting and pivoting on hard surfaces. *Iliopsoas bursitis* affects the bursa that lies between the iliopsoas muscle and hip joint and is lateral to the femoral vessels. Pain is experienced over this area and is made worse by hip extension and flexion. *Anserine bursitis* is an inflammation of the sartorius bursa located over the medial side of the tibia just below the knee and under the conjoint

†Deceased. A contributor to *Harrison's Principles of Internal Medicine* since the 11th edition, Dr. Gilliland passed away on February 17, 2007.

tendon and is manifested by pain on climbing stairs. Tenderness is present over the insertion of the conjoint tendon of the sartorius, gracilis, and semitendinosus. *Prepatellar bursitis* (housemaid's knee) occurs in the bursa situated between the patella and overlying skin and is caused by kneeling on hard surfaces. Gout or infection may also occur at this site. Treatment of bursitis consists of prevention of the aggravating situation, rest of the involved part, administration of a nonsteroidal anti-inflammatory drug (NSAID) where appropriate for an individual patient, or local glucocorticoid injection.

ROTATOR CUFF TENDINITIS AND IMPINGEMENT SYNDROME

Tendinitis of the rotator cuff is the major cause of a painful shoulder and is currently thought to be caused by inflammation of the tendon(s). The rotator cuff consists of the tendons of the supraspinatus, infraspinatus, subscapularis, and teres minor muscles, and inserts on the humeral tuberosities. Of the tendons forming the rotator cuff, the supraspinatus tendon is the most often affected, probably because of its repeated impingement (*impingement syndrome*) between the humeral head and the undersurface of the anterior third of the acromion and coracoacromial ligament above, as well as the reduction in its blood supply that occurs with abduction of the arm (**Fig. 23-1**). The tendon of the infraspinatus and that of the long head of the biceps are less commonly involved. The process begins with edema and

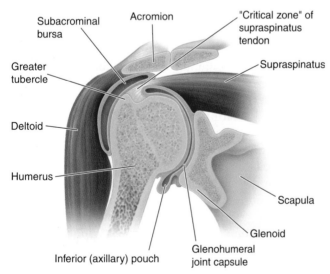

FIGURE 23-1

Coronal section of the shoulder illustrating the relationships of the glenohumeral joint, the joint capsule, the subacromial bursa, and the rotator cuff (supraspinatus tendon). *[From F Kozin, in Arthritis and Allied Conditions, 13th ed, WJ Koopman (ed). Baltimore, Williams & Wilkins, 1997; with permission.]*

hemorrhage of the rotator cuff, which evolves to fibrotic thickening and eventually to rotator cuff degeneration with tendon tears and bone spurs. Subacromial bursitis also accompanies this syndrome. Symptoms usually appear after injury or overuse, especially with activities involving elevation of the arm with some degree of forward flexion. Impingement syndrome occurs in persons participating in baseball, tennis, swimming, or occupations that require repeated elevation of the arm. Those over age 40 are particularly susceptible. Patients complain of a dull aching in the shoulder, which may interfere with sleep. Severe pain is experienced when the arm is actively abducted into an overhead position. The arc between 60° and 120° is especially painful. Tenderness is present over the lateral aspect of the humeral head just below the acromion. NSAIDs, local glucocorticoid injection, and physical therapy may relieve symptoms. Surgical decompression of the subacromial space may be necessary in patients refractory to conservative treatment.

Patients may tear the supraspinatus tendon acutely by falling on an outstretched arm or lifting a heavy object. Symptoms are pain along with weakness of abduction and external rotation of the shoulder. Atrophy of the supraspinatus muscles develops. The diagnosis is established by arthrogram, ultrasound, or MRI. Surgical repair may be necessary in patients who fail to respond to conservative measures. In patients with moderate to severe tears and functional loss, surgery is indicated.

CALCIFIC TENDINITIS

This condition is characterized by deposition of calcium salts, primarily hydroxyapatite, within a tendon. The exact mechanism of calcification is not known but may be initiated by ischemia or degeneration of the tendon. The supraspinatus tendon is most often affected because it is frequently impinged on and has a reduced blood supply when the arm is abducted. The condition usually develops after age 40. Calcification within the tendon may evoke acute inflammation, producing sudden and severe pain in the shoulder. However, it may be asymptomatic or not related to the patient's symptoms.

BICIPITAL TENDINITIS AND RUPTURE

Bicipital tendinitis, or tenosynovitis, is produced by friction on the tendon of the long head of the biceps as it passes through the bicipital groove. When the inflammation is acute, patients experience anterior shoulder pain that radiates down the biceps into the forearm. Abduction and external rotation of the arm are painful and limited. The bicipital groove is very tender to palpation. Pain may be elicited along the course of the tendon by resisting supination of the forearm with the elbow at 90°

(Yergason's supination sign). Acute rupture of the tendon may occur with vigorous exercise of the arm and is often painful. In a young patient, it should be repaired surgically. Rupture of the tendon in an older person may be associated with little or no pain and is recognized by the presence of persistent swelling of the biceps ("Popeye" muscle) produced by the retraction of the long head of the biceps. Surgery is usually not necessary in this setting.

DE QUERVAIN'S TENOSYNOVITIS

In this condition, inflammation involves the abductor pollicis longus and the extensor pollicis brevis as these tendons pass through a fibrous sheath at the radial styloid process. The usual cause is repetitive twisting of the wrist. It may occur in pregnancy, and it also occurs in mothers who hold their babies with the thumb outstretched. Patients experience pain on grasping with their thumb, such as with pinching. Swelling and tenderness are often present over the radial styloid process. The Finkelstein sign is positive, which is elicited by having the patient place the thumb in the palm and close the fingers over it. The wrist is then ulnarly deviated, resulting in pain over the involved tendon sheath in the area of the radial styloid. Treatment consists initially of splinting the wrist and an NSAID. When severe or refractory to conservative treatment, glucocorticoid injections can be very effective.

PATELLAR TENDINITIS (JUMPER'S KNEE)

Tendinitis involves the patellar tendon at its attachment to the lower pole of the patella. Patients may experience pain when jumping during basketball or volleyball, going up stairs, or doing deep knee squats. Tenderness is noted on examination over the lower pole of the patella. Treatment consists of rest, icing, and NSAIDs, followed by strengthening and increasing flexibility.

ADHESIVE CAPSULITIS

Often referred to as "frozen shoulder," adhesive capsulitis is characterized by pain and restricted movement of the shoulder, usually in the absence of intrinsic shoulder disease. Night pain is often present in the affected shoulder. Adhesive capsulitis, however, may follow bursitis or tendinitis of the shoulder or be associated with systemic disorders such as chronic pulmonary disease, myocardial infarction, and diabetes mellitus. Prolonged immobility of the arm contributes to the development of adhesive capsulitis, and reflex sympathetic dystrophy is thought to be a pathogenic factor. The capsule of the shoulder is thickened, and a mild chronic inflammatory infiltrate and fibrosis may be present.

Adhesive capsulitis occurs more commonly in women after age 50. Pain and stiffness usually develop gradually over several months to a year but progress rapidly in some patients. Pain may interfere with sleep. The shoulder is tender to palpation, and both active and passive movement is restricted. Radiographs of the shoulder show osteopenia. The diagnosis is confirmed by arthrography, in that only a limited amount of contrast material, usually <15 mL, can be injected under pressure into the shoulder joint.

In most patients, the condition improves spontaneously 1–3 years after onset. While pain usually improves, most patients are left with some limitation of shoulder motion. Early mobilization of the arm following an injury to the shoulder may prevent the development of this disease. Slow but forceful injection of contrast material into the joint may lyse adhesions and stretch the capsule, resulting in improvement of shoulder motion. Manipulation under anesthesia may be helpful in some patients. Once the disease is established, therapy may have little effect on its natural course. Local injections of glucocorticoids, NSAIDs, and physical therapy may provide relief of symptoms.

LATERAL EPICONDYLITIS (TENNIS ELBOW)

Lateral epicondylitis, or tennis elbow, is a painful condition involving the soft tissue over the lateral aspect of the elbow. The pain originates at or near the site of attachment of the common extensors to the lateral epicondyle and may radiate into the forearm and dorsum of the wrist. This painful condition is thought to be caused by small tears of the extensor aponeurosis resulting from repeated resisted contractions of the extensor muscles. The pain usually appears after work or recreational activities involving repeated motions of wrist extension and supination against resistance. Most patients with this disorder injure themselves in activities other than tennis, such as pulling weeds, carrying suitcases or briefcases, or using a screwdriver. The injury in tennis usually occurs when hitting a backhand with the elbow flexed. Shaking hands and opening doors can reproduce the pain. Striking the lateral elbow against a solid object may also induce pain.

The treatment is usually rest along with administration of an NSAID. Ultrasound, icing, and friction massage may also help relieve pain. When pain is severe, the elbow is placed in a sling or splinted at 90° of flexion. When the pain is acute and well localized, injection of a glucocorticoid using a small-gauge needle may be effective. Following injection, the patient should be advised to rest the arm for at least 1 month and avoid activities that would aggravate the elbow. Once symptoms have subsided, the patient should begin rehabilitation to strengthen and increase flexibility of the extensor muscles before resuming physical activity involving the arm. A fore-arm band placed 2.5–5.0 cm (1–2 in.) below the elbow may help to reduce tension on the extensor muscles at their attachment to the lateral epicondyle. The patient should be advised to restrict activities requiring forcible extension and supination of the wrist. Improvement may take several months. The patient may continue to experience mild pain but, with care, can usually avoid the return of debilitating pain. In an occasional patient, surgical release of the extensor aponeurosis may be necessary.

MEDIAL EPICONDYLITIS

Medial epicondylitis is an overuse syndrome resulting in pain over the medial side of the elbow with radiation into the forearm. The cause of this syndrome is considered to be repetitive resisted motions of wrist flexion and pronation, which lead to microtears and granulation tissue at the origin of the pronator teres and forearm flexors, particularly the flexor carpi radialis. This overuse syndrome is usually seen in patients >35 years and is much less common than lateral epicondylitis. It occurs most often in work-related repetitive activities but also occurs with recreational activities such as swinging a golf club (golfer's elbow) or throwing a baseball. On physical examination, there is tenderness just distal to the medial epicondyle over the origin of the forearm flexors. Pain can be reproduced by resisting wrist flexion and pronation with the elbow extended. Radiographs are usually normal. The differential diagnosis of patients with medial elbow symptoms includes tears of the pronator teres, acute medial collateral ligament tear, and medial collateral ligament instability. Ulnar neuritis has been found in 25–50% of patients with medial epicondylitis and is associated with tenderness over the ulnar nerve at the elbow as well as hypesthesia and paresthesia on the ulnar side of the hand.

The initial treatment of medial epicondylitis is conservative, involving rest, NSAIDs, friction massage, ultrasound, and icing. Some patients may require splinting. Injections of glucocorticoids at the painful site may also be effective. Patients should be instructed to rest at least 1 month. Also, patients should be started on physical therapy once the pain has subsided. In patients with chronic debilitating medial epicondylitis that remains unresponsive after at least a year of treatment, surgical release of the flexor muscle at its origin may be necessary and is often successful.

PLANTAR FASCIITIS

Plantar fasciitis is a common cause of foot pain in adults, with the peak incidence occurring in people between the ages of 40 and 60 years. It is also seen more frequently in a younger population consisting of runners, aerobic exercise dancers, and ballet dancers. The pain originates at or near the site of the plantar fascia attachment to the medial tuberosity of the calcaneus. The plantar fascia is a thick fibrous band that extends distally, dividing into five slips that insert into each metatarsal head. Its function is to tighten and elevate the longitudinal arch as well as to invert the hind foot during the push-off phase of gait. Plantar fasciitis is thought to be the result of repetitive microtrauma to the tissue. Pathology of involved fascia reveals degeneration of fibrous tissue with or without fibroblast proliferation and chronic inflammation. Several factors that increase the risk of developing plantar fasciitis include obesity, pes planus (excessive pronation of the foot), pes cavus (high-arched foot), limited dorsiflexion of the ankle, prolonged standing, walking on hard surfaces, and faulty shoes. In runners, excessive running and a change to a harder running surface may precipitate plantar fasciitis.

The diagnosis of plantar fasciitis can usually be made on the basis of history and physical examination alone. The onset of inferior heel pain of plantar fasciitis is typically gradual, but in some individuals it can be abrupt. Patients experience severe pain with the first steps on arising in the morning or following inactivity during the day. The pain usually lessens with weight-bearing activity during the day, only to worsen with continued activity. Pain is made worse on walking barefoot or up stairs. On examination, maximal tenderness is elicited on palpation over the inferior heel corresponding to the site of attachment of the plantar fascia.

Imaging studies may be indicated when the diagnosis is not clear. Plain radiographs may show heel spurs, which are of little diagnostic significance as they may be present in patients with or without plantar fasciitis. A calcaneal stress fracture may be detected on plain radiographs; however, a bone scan is more sensitive. Bone scan in plantar fasciitis demonstrates increased uptake at the attachment of the plantar fascia to the calcaneus. Ultrasonography in plantar fasciitis can demonstrate thickening of the fascia and diffuse hypoechogenicity, indicating edema at the attachment of the plantar fascia to the calcaneus. MRI is a sensitive method for detecting plantar fasciitis, but it is usually not required for establishing the diagnosis.

The differential diagnosis of inferior heel pain includes calcaneal stress fractures, the spondyloarthritides, rheumatoid arthritis, gout, neoplastic or infiltrative bone processes, and nerve compression/entrapment syndromes. The diagnosis of these disorders is made on clinical features, imaging studies, and laboratory findings, which distinguish them from plantar fasciitis.

Long-term studies have found that resolution of symptoms occurs within 12 months in more than 80% of patients with plantar fasciitis. Treatment should begin immediately with the diagnosis of plantar fasciitis. The patient is advised to reduce or discontinue activities that can exacerbate plantar fasciitis. Initial treatment consists of ice, heat, massage, and stretching. Stretching of the plantar fascia and calf muscles are commonly employed and can be beneficial. Orthotics provide medial arch support and can be effective in relieving symptoms. Foot strapping or taping is commonly performed, and some patients may benefit by wearing a night splint designed to keep the ankle in a neutral position. A short course of NSAIDs can be given to alleviate symptoms in patients where the benefits outweigh the risks. Local glucocorticoid injections have also been shown to be efficacious but may carry an increased risk for plantar fascia rupture. Plantar fasciotomy is reserved for those patients who have failed to improve after at least 6–12 months of conservative treatment.

FURTHER READINGS

BUCHBINDER R: Plantar fasciitis. N Engl J Med 350:2159, 2004

DALTON SE: The shoulder, in *Rheumatology*, 4th ed, MC Hochberg et al (eds). Philadelphia, Mosby, 2008, pp 619–634

FRIEMAN BG et al: Rotator cuff disease: A review of diagnosis, pathophysiology, and current trends in treatment. Arch Phys Med Rehabil 75:604, 1994

HUSNI EM, DONOHUE JP: Painful shoulder and reflex sympathetic dystrophy syndrome, in *Arthritis and Allied Conditions*, 15th ed, WJ Koopman (ed). Philadelphia, Lippincott Williams & Wilkins, 2005, pp 2133–2152

JACOBS JW: How to perform local soft-tissue glucocorticoid injections. Best Pract Res Clin Rheumatol 23:193, 2009

MARTIN SD, THORNHILL TS: Shoulder pain, in *Kelley's Textbook of Rheumatology*, 8th ed, GS Firestein et al (eds). Philadelphia, Saunders, 2009, pp 587–615

MATSEN FA 3RD: Clinical practice. Rotator-cuff failure. N Engl J Med 358:2138, 2008

NEER CS II: Impingement lesions. Clin Orthop 173:70, 1983

NEUFELD SK, CERRATO R: Plantar fasciitis: Evaluation and treatment. J Am Acad Orthop Surg 16:338, 2008

SHERIDAN MA, HANNAFIN JA: Upper extremity: Emphasis on frozen shoulder. Orthop Clin North Am 37:531, 2006

CHAPTER 23

Periarticular Disorders of the Extremities

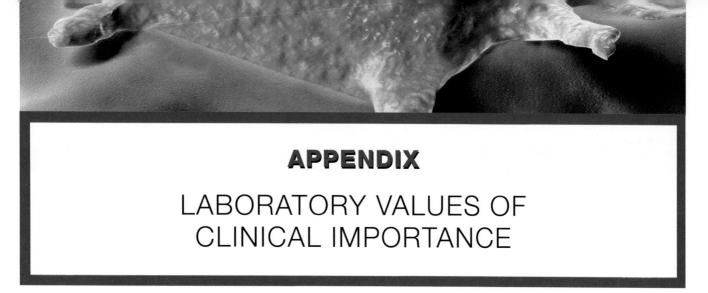

APPENDIX

LABORATORY VALUES OF CLINICAL IMPORTANCE

Alexander Kratz ■ Michael A. Pesce ■ Daniel J. Fink†

INTRODUCTORY COMMENTS

The following are tables of reference values for laboratory tests, special analytes, and special function tests. A variety of factors can influence reference values. Such variables include the population studied, the duration and means of specimen transport, laboratory methods and instrumentation, and even the type of container used for the collection of the specimen. The reference or "normal" ranges given in this appendix may therefore not be appropriate for all laboratories, and these values should only be used as general guidelines. Whenever possible, reference values provided by the laboratory performing the testing should be utilized in the interpretation of laboratory data. Values supplied in this Appendix reflect typical reference ranges in adults. Pediatric reference ranges may vary significantly from adult values.

In preparing the Appendix, the authors have taken into account the fact that the system of international units (SI, système international d'unités) is used in most countries and in some medical journals. However, clinical laboratories may continue to report values in "conventional" units. Therefore, both systems are provided in the Appendix. The dual system is also used in the text except for (1) those instances in which the numbers remain the same but only the terminology is changed (mmol/L for meq/L or IU/L for mIU/mL), when only the SI units are given; and (2) most pressure measurements (e.g., blood and cerebrospinal fluid pressures), when the conventional units (mmHg, mmH$_2$O) are used. In all other instances in the text the SI unit is followed by the traditional unit in parentheses.

---

†Deceased.

TABLE A-1

HEMATOLOGY AND COAGULATION

ANALYTE	SPECIMEN[a]	SI UNITS	CONVENTIONAL UNITS
Activated clotting time	WB	70–180 s	70–180 seconds
Activated protein C resistance (factor V Leiden)	P	Not applicable	Ratio > 2.1
Alpha$_2$ antiplasmin	P	0.87–1.55	87–155%
Antiphospholipid antibody panel			
PTT-LA (lupus anticoagulant screen)	P	Negative	Negative
Platelet neutralization procedure	P	Negative	Negative
Dilute viper venom screen	P	Negative	Negative
Anticardiolipin antibody	S		
IgG		0–15 arbitrary units	0–15 GPL
IgM		0–15 arbitrary units	0–15 MPL
Antithrombin III	P		
Antigenic		220–390 mg/L	22–39 mg/dL
Functional		0.7–1.30 U/L	70–130%
Anti-Xa assay (heparin assay)	P		
Unfractionated heparin		0.3–0.7 kIU/L	0.3–0.7 IU/mL
Low-molecular-weight heparin		0.5–1.0 kIU/L	0.5–1.0 IU/mL
Danaparoid (Orgaran)		0.5–0.8 kIU/L	0.5–0.8 IU/mL
Autohemolysis test	WB	0.004–0.045	0.4%–4.50%
Autohemolysis test with glucose	WB	0.003–0.007	0.3%–0.7%
Bleeding time (adult)		<7.1 min	<7.1 min
Bone marrow: see **Table A-8**			
Clot retraction	WB	0.50–1.00/2 h	50–100%/2 h
Cryofibrinogen	P	Negative	Negative
D-Dimer	P	0.22–0.74 µg/mL	0.22–0.74 µg/mL
Differential blood count	WB		
Neutrophils		0.40–0.70	40–70%
Bands		0.0–0.05	0–5%
Lymphocytes		0.20–0.50	20–50%
Monocytes		0.04–0.08	4–8%
Eosinophils		0.0–0.6	0–6%
Basophils		0.0–0.02	0–2%
Eosinophil count	WB	150–300/µL	150–300/mm^3
Erythrocyte count	WB		
Adult males		4.30–5.60 × 10^{12}/L	4.30–5.60 × 10^6/mm^3
Adult females		4.00–5.20 × 10^{12}/L	4.00–5.20 × 10^6/mm^3
Erythrocyte life span	WB		
Normal survival		120 days	120 days
Chromium labeled, half life ($t_{1/2}$)		25–35 days	25–35 days
Erythrocyte sedimentation rate	WB		
Females		0–20 mm/h	0–20 mm/h
Males		0–15 mm/h	0–15 mm/h
Euglobulin lysis time	P	7200–14400 s	120–240 min
Factor II, prothrombin	P	0.50–1.50	50–150%
Factor V	P	0.50–1.50	50–150%
Factor VII	P	0.50–1.50	50–150%
Factor VIII	P	0.50–1.50	50–150%
Factor IX	P	0.50–1.50	50–150%
Factor X	P	0.50–1.50	50–150%
Factor XI	P	0.50–1.50	50–150%
Factor XII	P	0.50–1.50	50–150%
Factor XIII screen	P	Not applicable	Present

(Continued)

HEMATOLOGY AND COAGULATION

ANALYTE	SPECIMEN[a]	SI UNITS	CONVENTIONAL UNITS
Factor inhibitor assay	P	<0.5 Bethesda Units	<0.5 Bethesda Units
Fibrin (ogen) degradation products	P	0–1 mg/L	0–1 µg/mL
Fibrinogen	P	2.33–4.96 g/L	233–496 mg/dL
Glucose-6-phosphate dehydrogenase (erythrocyte)	WB	<2400 s	<40 min
Ham's test (acid serum)	WB	Negative	Negative
Hematocrit	WB		
Adult males		0.388–0.464	38.8–46.4
Adult females		0.354–0.444	35.4–44.4
Hemoglobin			
Plasma	P	6–50 mg/L	0.6–5.0 mg/dL
Whole blood	WB		
Adult males		133–162 g/L	13.3–16.2 g/dL
Adult females		120–158 g/L	12.0–15.8 g/dL
Hemoglobin electrophoresis	WB		
Hemoglobin A		0.95–0.98	95–98%
Hemoglobin A_2		0.015–0.031	1.5–3.1%
Hemoglobin F		0–0.02	0–2.0%
Hemoglobins other than A, A_2, or F		Absent	Absent
Heparin-induced thrombocytopenia antibody	P	Negative	Negative
Joint fluid crystal	JF	Not applicable	No crystals seen
Joint fluid mucin	JF	Not applicable	Only type I mucin present
Leukocytes			
Alkaline phosphatase (LAP)	WB	0.2–1.6 µkat/L	13–100 µ/L
Count (WBC)	WB	3.54–9.06 × 10^9/L	3.54–9.06 × 10^3/mm³
Mean corpuscular hemoglobin (MCH)	WB	26.7–31.9 pg/cell	26.7–31.9 pg/cell
Mean corpuscular hemoglobin concentration (MCHC)	WB	323–359 g/L	32.3–35.9 g/dL
Mean corpuscular hemoglobin of reticulocytes (CH)	WB	24–36 pg	24–36 pg
Mean corpuscular volume (MCV)	WB	79–93.3 fL	79–93.3 µm³
Mean platelet volume (MPV)	WB	9.00–12.95 fL	9.00–12.95 µm³
Osmotic fragility of erythrocytes	WB		
Direct		0.0035–0.0045	0.35–0.45%
Index		0.0030–0.0065	0.30–0.65%
Partial thromboplastin time, activated	P	26.3–39.4 s	26.3–39.4 s
Plasminogen	P		
Antigen		84–140 mg/L	8.4–14.0 mg/dL
Functional		0.70–1.30	70–130%
Plasminogen activator inhibitor 1	P	4–43 µg/L	4–43 ng/mL
Platelet aggregation	PRP	Not applicable	>65% aggregation in response to adenosine diphosphate, epinephrine, collagen, ristocetin, and arachidonic acid
Platelet count	WB	165–415 × 10^9/L	165–415 × 10^3/mm³
Platelet, mean volume	WB	6.4–11 fL	6.4–11.0 µm³
Prekallikrein assay	P	0.50–1.5	50–150%
Prekallikrein screen	P		No deficiency detected
Protein C	P		
Total antigen		0.70–1.40	70–140%
Functional		0.70–1.30	70–130%
Protein S	P		
Total antigen		0.70–1.40	70–140%
Functional		0.65–1.40	65–140%
Free antigen		0.70–1.40	70–140%
Prothrombin gene mutation G20210A	WB	Not applicable	Not present

(Continued)

TABLE A-1 (*CONTINUED*)

HEMATOLOGY AND COAGULATION

ANALYTE	SPECIMEN[a]	SI UNITS	CONVENTIONAL UNITS
Prothrombin time	P	12.7–15.4 s	12.7–15.4 s
Protoporphyrin, free erythrocyte	WB	0.28–0.64 μmol/L of red blood cells	16–36 μg/dL of red blood cells
Red cell distribution width	WB	<0.145	<14.5%
Reptilase time	P	16–23.6 s	16–23.6 s
Reticulocyte count	WB		
Adult males		0.008–0.023 red cells	0.8–2.3% red cells
Adult females		0.008–0.020 red cells	0.8–2.0% red cells
Reticulocyte hemoglobin content	WB	>26 pg/cell	>26 pg/cell
Ristocetin cofactor (functional von Willebrand factor)	P		
Blood group O		0.75 mean of normal	75% mean of normal
Blood group A		1.05 mean of normal	105% mean of normal
Blood group B		1.15 mean of normal	115% mean of normal
Blood group AB		1.25 mean of normal	125% mean of normal
Sickle cell test	WB	Negative	Negative
Sucrose hemolysis	WB	<0.1	<10% hemolysis
Thrombin time	P	15.3–18.5 s	15.3–18.5 s
Total eosinophils	WB	150–300 × 10⁶/L	150–300/mm³
Transferrin receptor	S, P	9.6–29.6 nmol/L	9.6–29.6 nmol/L
Viscosity			
Plasma	P	1.7–2.1	1.7–2.1
Serum	S	1.4–1.8	1.4–1.8
Von Willebrand factor (vWF) antigen (factor VIII:R antigen)	P		
Blood group O		0.75 mean of normal	75% mean of normal
Blood group A		1.05 mean of normal	105% mean of normal
Blood group B		1.15 mean of normal	115% mean of normal
Blood group AB		1.25 mean of normal	125% mean of normal
Von Willebrand factor multimers	P	Normal distribution	Normal distribution
White blood cells: see "leukocytes"			

[a]P, plasma; JF, joint fluid; PRP, platelet-rich plasma; S, serum; WB, whole blood.

TABLE A-2

CLINICAL CHEMISTRY AND IMMUNOLOGY

ANALYTE	SPECIMEN[a]	SI UNITS	CONVENTIONAL UNITS
Acetoacetate	P	20–99 μmol/L	0.2–1.0 mg/dL
Adrenocorticotropin (ACTH)	P	1.3–16.7 pmol/L	6.0–76.0 pg/mL
Alanine aminotransferase (AST, SGPT)	S	0.12–0.70 μkat/L	7–41 U/L
Albumin	S		
Female		41–53 g/L	4.1–5.3 g/dL
Male		40–50 g/L	4.0–5.0 g/L
Aldolase	S	26–138 nkat/L	1.5–8.1 U/L
Aldosterone (adult)			
Supine, normal sodium diet	S, P	55–250 pmol/L	2–9 ng/dL
Upright, normal sodium diet	S, P		2–5-fold increase over supine value
Supine, low-sodium diet	S, P		2–5-fold increase over normal sodium diet level
	U	6.38–58.25 nmol/d	2.3–21.0 μg/24 h
Alpha fetoprotein (adult)	S	0–8.5 μg/L	0–8.5 ng/mL
Alpha₁ antitrypsin	S	1.0–2.0 g/L	100–200 mg/dL
Ammonia, as NH₃	P	11–35 μmol/L	19–60 μg/dL

CLINICAL CHEMISTRY AND IMMUNOLOGY

ANALYTE	SPECIMEN[a]	SI UNITS	CONVENTIONAL UNITS
Amylase (method dependent)	S	0.34–1.6 μkat/L	20–96 U/L
Androstenedione (adult)	S	1.75–8.73 nmol/L	50–250 ng/dL
Angiotensin-converting enzyme (ACE)	S	0.15–1.1 μkat/L	9–67 U/L
Anion gap	S	7–16 mmol/L	7–16 mmol/L
Apo B/Apo A-1 ratio		0.35–0.98	0.35–0.98
Apolipoprotein A-1	S	1.19–2.40 g/L	119–240 mg/dL
Apolipoprotein B	S	0.52–1.63 g/L	52–163 mg/dL
Arterial blood gases			
$[HCO_3^-]$		22–30 mmol/L	22–30 meq/L
P_{CO_2}		4.3–6.0 kPa	32–45 mmHg
pH		7.35–7.45	7.35–7.45
P_{O_2}		9.6–13.8 kPa	72–104 mmHg
Aspartate aminotransferase (AST, SGOT)	S	0.20–0.65 μkat/L	12–38 U/L
Autoantibodies			
Anti-adrenal antibody	S	Not applicable	Negative at 1:10 dilution
Anti–double-strand (native) DNA	S	Not applicable	Negative at 1:10 dilution
Anti–glomerular basement membrane antibodies	S		
Qualitative		Negative	Negative
Quantitative		<5 kU/L	<5 U/mL
Anti-granulocyte antibody	S	Not applicable	Negative
Anti–Jo-1 antibody	S	Not applicable	Negative
Anti-La antibody	S	Not applicable	Negative
Anti-mitochondrial antibody	S	Not applicable	Negative
Antineutrophil cytoplasmic autoantibodies, cytoplasmic (C-ANCA)	S		
Qualitative		Negative	Negative
Quantitative (antibodies to proteinase 3)		<2.8 kU/L	<2.8 U/mL
Antineutrophil cytoplasmic autoantibodies, perinuclear (P-ANCA)	S		
Qualitative		Negative	Negative
Quantitative (antibodies to myeloperoxidase)		<1.4 kU/L	<1.4 U/mL
Antinuclear antibody	S	Not applicable	Negative at 1:40
Anti–parietal cell antibody	S	Not applicable	Negative at 1:20
Anti-Ro antibody	S	Not applicable	Negative
Anti-platelet antibody	S	Not applicable	Negative
Anti-RNP antibody	S	Not applicable	Negative
Anti-Scl 70 antibody	S	Not applicable	Negative
Anti-Smith antibody	S	Not applicable	Negative
Anti–smooth-muscle antibody	S	Not applicable	Negative at 1:20
Anti-thyroglobulin	S	Not applicable	Negative
Anti-thyroid antibody	S	<0.3 kIU/L	<0.3 IU/mL
B type natriuretic peptide (BNP)	P	Age and gender specific: <167 ng/L	Age and gender specific: <167 pg/mL
Bence Jones protein, serum	S	Not applicable	None detected
Bence Jones protein, urine, qualitative	U	Not applicable	None detected in 50× concentrated urine
Bence Jones Protein, urine, quantitative	U		
Kappa		<25 mg/L	<2.5 mg/dL
Lambda		<50 mg/L	<5.0 mg/dL
β_2-Microglobulin			
	S	<2.7 mg/L	<0.27 mg/dL
	U	<120 μg/d	<120 μg/day
Bilirubin	S		
Total		5.1–22 μmol/L	0.3–1.3 mg/dL
Direct		1.7–6.8 μmol/L	0.1–0.4 mg/dL
Indirect		3.4–15.2 μmol/L	0.2–0.9 mg/dL

(Continued)

TABLE A-2 (*CONTINUED*)

CLINICAL CHEMISTRY AND IMMUNOLOGY

ANALYTE	SPECIMEN[a]	SI UNITS	CONVENTIONAL UNITS
C peptide (adult)	S, P	0.17–0.66 nmol/L	0.5–2.0 ng/mL
C1-esterase-inhibitor protein	S		
Antigenic		124–250 mg/L	12.4–24.5 mg/dL
Functional		Present	Present
CA 125	S	0–35 kU/L	0–35 U/mL
CA 19-9	S	0–37 kU/L	0–37 U/mL
CA 15-3	S	0–34 kU/L	0–34 U/mL
CA 27-29	S	0–40 kU/L	0–40 U/mL
Calcitonin	S		
Male		3–26 ng/L	3–26 pg/mL
Female		2–17 ng/L	2–17 pg/mL
Calcium	S	2.2–2.6 mmol/L	8.7–10.2 mg/dL
Calcium, ionized	WB	1.12–1.32 mmol/L	4.5–5.3 mg/dL
Carbon dioxide content (TCO_2)	P (sea level)	22–30 mmol/L	22–30 meq/L
Carboxyhemoglobin (carbon monoxide content)	WB		
Nonsmokers		0–0.04	0–4%
Smokers		0.04–0.09	4–9%
Onset of symptoms		0.15–0.20	15–20%
Loss of consciousness and death		>0.50	>50%
Carcinoembryonic antigen (CEA)	S		
Nonsmokers		0.0–3.0 µg/L	0.0–3.0 ng/mL
Smokers	S	0.0–5.0 µg/L	0.0–5.0 ng/mL
Ceruloplasmin	S	250–630 mg/L	25–63 mg/dL
Chloride	S	102–109 mmol/L	102–109 meq/L
Cholesterol: see **Table A-5**			
Cholinesterase	S	5–12 kU/L	5–12 U/mL
Complement			
C3	S	0.83–1.77 g/L	83–177 mg/dL
C4	S	0.16–0.47 g/L	16–47 mg/dL
Total hemolytic complement (CH50)	S	50–150%	50–150%
Factor B	S	0.17–0.42 g/L	17–42 mg/dL
Coproporphyrins (types I and III)	U	150–470 µmol/d	100–300 µg/d
Cortisol			
Fasting, 8 A.M.–12 noon	S	138–690 nmol/L	5–25 µg/dL
12 noon–8 P.M.		138–414 nmol/L	5–15 µg/dL
8 P.M.–8 A.M.		0–276 nmol/L	0–10 µg/dL
Cortisol, free	U	55–193 nmol/24 h	20–70 µg/24 h
C-reactive protein	S	0.2–3.0 mg/L	0.2–3.0 mg/L
Creatine kinase (total)	S		
Females		0.66–4.0 µkat/L	39–238 U/L
Males		0.87–5.0 µkat/L	51–294 U/L
Creatine kinase-MB	S		
Mass		0.0–5.5 µg/L	0.0–5.5 ng/mL
Fraction of total activity (by electrophoresis)		0–0.04	0–4.0%
Creatinine	S		
Female		44–80 µmol/L	0.5–0.9 ng/mL
Male		53–106 µmol/L	0.6–1.2 ng/mL
Cryoproteins	S	Not applicable	None detected
Dehydroepiandrosterone (DHEA) (adult)			
Male	S	6.2–43.4 nmol/L	180–1250 ng/dL
Female		4.5–34.0 nmol/L	130–980 ng/dL
Dehydroepiandrosterone (DHEA) sulfate	S		
Male (adult)		100–6190 µg/L	10–619 µg/dL
Female (adult, premenopausal)		120–5350 µg/L	12–535 µg/dL
Female (adult, postmenopausal)		300–2600 µg/L	30–260 µg/dL
Deoxycorticosterone (DOC) (adult)	S	61–576 nmol/L	2–19 ng/dL
11-Deoxycortisol (adult) (compound S) (8:00 A.M.)	S	0.34–4.56 nmol/L	12–158 ng/dL

(Continued)

CLINICAL CHEMISTRY AND IMMUNOLOGY

ANALYTE	SPECIMEN[a]	SI UNITS	CONVENTIONAL UNITS
Dihydrotestosterone			
Male	S, P	1.03–2.92 nmol/L	30–85 ng/dL
Female		0.14–0.76 nmol/L	4–22 ng/dL
Dopamine	P	<475 pmol/L	<87 pg/mL
Dopamine	U	425–2610 nmol/d	65–400 µg/d
Epinephrine	P		
Supine (30 min)		<273 pmol/L	<50 pg/mL
Sitting		<328 pmol/L	<60 pg/mL
Standing (30 min)		<491 pmol/L	<90 pg/mL
Epinephrine	U	0–109 nmol/d	0–20 µg/d
Erythropoietin	S	4–27 U/L	4–27 U/L
Estradiol	S, P		
Female			
Menstruating:			
Follicular phase		74–532 pmol/L	<20–145 pg/mL
Mid-cycle peak		411–1626 pmol/L	112–443 pg/mL
Luteal phase		74–885 pmol/L	<20–241 pg/mL
Postmenopausal		217 pmol/L	<59 pg/mL
Male		74 pmol/L	<20 pg/mL
Estrone	S, P		
Female			
Menstruating:			
Follicular phase		55–555 pmol/L	15–150 pg/mL
Luteal phase		55–740 pmol/L	15–200 pg/mL
Postmenopausal		55–204 pmol/L	15–55 pg/mL
Male		55–240 pmol/L	15–65 pg/mL
Fatty acids, free (nonesterified)	P	<0.28–0.89 mmol/L	<8–25 mg/dL
Ferritin	S		
Female		10–150 µg/L	10–150 ng/mL
Male		29–248 µg/L	29–248 ng/mL
Follicle stimulating hormone (FSH)	S, P		
Female			
Menstruating:			
Follicular phase		3.0–20.0 IU/L	3.0–20.0 mIU/mL
Ovulatory phase		9.0–26.0 IU/L	9.0–26.0 mIU/mL
Luteal phase		1.0–12.0 IU/L	1.0–12.0 mIU/mL
Postmenopausal		18.0–153.0 IU/L	18.0–153.0 mIU/mL
Male		1.0–12.0 IU/L	1.0–12.0 mIU/mL
Free testosterone, adult			
Female	S	2.1–23.6 pmol/L	0.6–6.8 pg/mL
Male		163–847 pmol/L	47–244 pg/mL
Fructosamine	S	<285 µmol/L	<285 µmol/L
Gamma glutamyltransferase	S	0.15–0.99 µkat/L	9–58 U/L
Gastrin	S	<100 ng/L	<100 pg/mL
Glucagon	P	20–100 ng/L	20–100 pg/mL
Glucose (fasting)	P		
Normal		4.2–6.1 mmol/L	75–110 mg/dL
Impaired glucose tolerance		6.2–6.9 mmol/L	111–125 mg/dL
Diabetes mellitus		>7.0 mmol/L	>125 mg/dL
Glucose, 2 h postprandial	P	3.9–6.7 mmol/L	70–120 mg/dL
Growth hormone (resting)	S	0.5–17.0 µg/L	0.5–17.0 ng/mL
Hemoglobin A_{1c}	WB	0.04–0.06 Hb fraction	4.0–6.0%
High-density lipoprotein (HDL) (see **Table A-5**)			
Homocysteine	P	4.4–10.8 µmol/L	4.4–10.8 µmol/L
Human chorionic gonadotropin (hCG)	S		
Non-pregnant female		<5 IU/L	<5 mIU/mL
1–2 weeks postconception		9–130 IU/L	9–130 mIU/mL

(Continued)

TABLE A-2 (*CONTINUED*)

CLINICAL CHEMISTRY AND IMMUNOLOGY

ANALYTE	SPECIMEN[a]	SI UNITS	CONVENTIONAL UNITS
2–3 weeks postconception		75–2600 IU/L	75–2600 mIU/mL
3–4 weeks postconception		850–20,800 IU/L	850–20,800 mIU/mL
4–5 weeks postconception		4000–100,200 IU/L	4000–100,200 mIU/mL
5–10 weeks postconception		11,500–289,000 IU/L	11,500–289,000 mIU/mL
10–14 weeks postconception		18,300–137,000 IU/L	18,300–137,000 mIU/mL
Second trimester		1400–53,000 IU/L	1400–53,000 mIU/mL
Third trimester		940–60,000 IU/L	940–60,000 mIU/mL
β-Hydroxybutyrate	P	0–290 µmol/L	0–3 mg/dL
5-Hydroindoleacetic acid (5-HIAA)	U	10.5–36.6 µmol/d	2–7 mg/d
17-Hydroxyprogesterone (adult)	S		
Male		0.15–7.5 nmol/L	5–250 ng/dL
Female			
Follicular phase		0.6–3.0 nmol/L	20–100 ng/dL
Midcycle peak		3–7.5 nmol/L	100–250 ng/dL
Luteal phase		3–15 nmol/L	100–500 ng/dL
Postmenopausal		≤ 2.1 nmol/L	≤ 70 ng/dL
Hydroxyproline	U, 24 hour	38–500 µmol/d	38–500 µmol/d
Immunofixation	S	Not applicable	No bands detected
Immunoglobulin, quantitation (adult)			
IgA	S	0.70–3.50 g/L	70–350 mg/dL
IgD	S	0–140 mg/L	0–14 mg/dL
IgE	S	24–430 µg/L	10–179 IU/mL
IgG	S	7.0–17.0 g/L	700–1700 mg/dL
IgG_1	S	2.7–17.4 g/L	270–1740 mg/dL
IgG_2	S	0.3–6.3 g/L	30–630 mg/dL
IgG_3	S	0.13–3.2 g/L	13–320 mg/dL
IgG_4	S	0.11–6.2 g/L	11–620 mg/dL
IgM	S	0.50–3.0 g/L	50–300 mg/dL
Insulin	S, P	14.35–143.5 pmol/L	2–20 µU/mL
Iron	S	7–25 µmol/L	41–141 µg/dL
Iron-binding capacity	S	45–73 µmol/L	251–406 µg/dL
Iron-binding capacity saturation	S	0.16–0.35	16–35%
Joint fluid crystal	JF	Not applicable	No crystals seen
Joint fluid mucin	JF	Not applicable	Only type I mucin present
Ketone (acetone)	S, U	Negative	Negative
17 Ketosteroids	U	0.003–0.012 g/d	3–12 mg/d
Lactate	P, arterial	0.5–1.6 mmol/L	4.5–14.4 mg/dL
	P, venous	0.5–2.2 mmol/L	4.5–19.8 mg/dL
Lactate dehydrogenase	S	2.0–3.8 µkat/L	115–221 U/L
Lactate dehydrogenase isoenzymes	S		
Fraction 1 (of total)		0.14–0.26	14–26%
Fraction 2		0.29–0.39	29–39%
Fraction 3		0.20–0.25	20–25%
Fraction 4		0.08–0.16	8–16%
Fraction 5		0.06–0.16	6–16%
Lipase (method dependent)	S	0.51–0.73 µkat/L	3–43 U/L
Lipids: see **Table A-5**			
Lipoprotein (a)	S	0–300 mg/L	0–30 mg/dL
Low-density lipoprotein (LDL) (see **Table A-5**)			
Luteinizing hormone (LH)	S, P		
Female			
Menstruating:			
Follicular phase		2.0–15.0 U/L	2.0–15.0 U/L
Ovulatory phase		22.0–105.0 U/L	22.0–105.0 U/L
Luteal phase		0.6–19.0 U/L	0.6–19.0 U/L
Postmenopausal		16.0–64.0 U/L	16.0–64.0 U/L
Male		2.0–12.0 U/L	2.0–12.0 U/L

(Continued)

CLINICAL CHEMISTRY AND IMMUNOLOGY

ANALYTE	SPECIMEN[a]	SI UNITS	CONVENTIONAL UNITS
Magnesium	S	0.62–0.95 mmol/L	1.5–2.3 mg/dL
Metanephrine	P	<0.5 nmol/L	<100 pg/mL
Metanephrine	U	30–211 mmol/mol creatinine	53–367 μg/g creatinine
Methemoglobin	WB	0.0–0.01	0–1%
Microalbumin urine	U		
24-h urine		0.0–0.03 g/d	0–30 mg/24 h
Spot urine		0.0–0.03 g/g creatinine	0–30 μg/mg creatinine
Myoglobin	S		
Male		19–92 μg/L	19–92 μg/L
Female		12–76 μg/L	12–76 μg/L
Norepinephrine	U	89–473 nmol/d	15–80 μg/d
Norepinephrine	P		
Supine (30 min)		650–2423 pmol/L	110–410 pg/mL
Sitting		709–4019 pmol/L	120–680 pg/mL
Standing (30 min)		739–4137 pmol/L	125–700 pg/mL
N-telopeptide (cross linked), NTx	S		
Female, premenopausal		6.2–19.0 nmol BCE	6.2–19.0 nmol BCE
Male		5.4–24.2 nmol BCE	5.4–24.2 nmol BCE
Bone collagen equivalent (BCE)			
N-telopeptide (cross linked), NTx	U		
Female, premenopausal		17–94 nmol BCE/mmol creatinine	17–94 nmol BCE/mmol creatinine
Female, postmenopausal		26–124 nmol BCE/mmol creatinine	26–124 nmol BCE/mmol creatinine
Male		21–83 nmol BCE/mmol creatinine	21–83 nmol BCE/mmol creatinine
Bone collagen equivalent (BCE)			
5′ Nucleotidase	S	0.02–0.19 μkat/L	0–11 U/L
Osmolality	P	275–295 mosmol/kg serum water	275–295 mosmol/kg serum water
	U	500–800 mosmol/kg water	500–800 mosmol/kg water
Osteocalcin	S	11–50 μg/L	11–50 ng/mL
Oxygen content	WB		
Arterial (sea level)		17–21	17–21 vol%
Venous (sea level)		10–16	10–16 vol%
Oxygen percent saturation (sea level)	WB		
Arterial		0.97	94–100%
Venous, arm		0.60–0.85	60–85%
Parathyroid hormone (intact)	S	8–51 ng/L	8–51 pg/mL
Phosphatase, alkaline	S	0.56–1.63 μkat/L	33–96 U/L
Phosphorus, inorganic	S	0.81–1.4 mmol/L	2.5–4.3 mg/dL
Porphobilinogen	U	None	None
Potassium	S	3.5–5.0 mmol/L	3.5–5.0 meq/L
Prealbumin	S	170–340 mg/L	17–34 mg/dL
Progesterone	S, P		
Female			
Follicular		<3.18 nmol/L	<1.0 ng/mL
Midluteal		9.54–63.6 nmol/L	3–20 ng/mL
Male		<3.18 nmol/L	<1.0 ng/mL
Prolactin	S	0–20 μg/L	0–20 ng/mL
Prostate-specific antigen (PSA)	S		
Male			
<40 years		0.0–2.0 μg/L	0.0–2.0 ng/mL
>40 years		0.0–4.0 μg/L	0.0–4.0 ng/mL

(Continued)

TABLE A-2 (CONTINUED)

CLINICAL CHEMISTRY AND IMMUNOLOGY

ANALYTE	SPECIMEN[a]	SI UNITS	CONVENTIONAL UNITS
PSA, free; in males 45–75 years, with PSA values between 4 and 20 μg/mL	S	>0.25 associated with benign prostatic hyperplasia	>25% associated with benign prostatic hyperplasia
Protein fractions	S		
Albumin		35–55 g/L	3.5–5.5 g/dL (50–60%)
Globulin		20–35 g/L	2.0–3.5 g/dL (40–50%)
Alpha$_1$		2–4 g/L	0.2–0.4 g/dL (4.2–7.2%)
Alpha$_2$		5–9 g/L	0.5–0.9 g/dL (6.8–12%)
Beta		6–11 g/L	0.6–1.1 g/dL (9.3–15%)
Gamma		7–17 g/L	0.7–1.7 g/dL (13–23%)
Protein, total	S	67–86 g/L	6.7–8.6 g/dL
Pyruvate	P, arterial	40–130 μmol/L	0.35–1.14 mg/dL
	P, venous	40–130 μmol/L	0.35–1.14 mg/dL
Rheumatoid factor	S, JF	<30 kIU/L	<30 IU/mL
Serotonin	WB	0.28–1.14 μmol/L	50–200 ng/mL
Serum protein electrophoresis	S	Not applicable	Normal pattern
Sex hormone binding globulin (adult)	S		
Male		13–71 nmol/L	13–71 nmol/L
Female		18–114 nmol/L	18–114 nmol/L
Sodium	S	136–146 mmol/L	136–146 meq/L
Somatomedin-C (IGF-1) (adult)	S		
16–24 years		182–780 μg/L	182–780 ng/mL
25–39 years		114–492 μg/L	114–492 ng/mL
40–54 years		90–360 μg/L	90–360 ng/mL
>54 years		71–290 μg/L	71–290 ng/mL
Somatostatin	P	<25 ng/L	<25 pg/mL
Testosterone, total, morning sample	S		
Female		0.21–2.98 nmol/L	6–86 ng/dL
Male		9.36–37.10 nmol/L	270–1070 ng/dL
Thyroglobulin	S	0.5–53 μg/L	0.5–53 ng/mL
Thyroid-binding globulin	S	13–30 mg/L	1.3–3.0 mg/dL
Thyroid-stimulating hormone	S	0.34–4.25 mIU/L	0.34–4.25 μIU/mL
Thyroxine, free (fT$_4$)	S	10.3–21.9 pmol/L	0.8–1.7 ng/dL
Thyroxine, total (T$_4$)	S	70–151 nmol/L	5.4–11.7 μg/dL
(Free) thyroxine index	S	6.7–10.9	6.7–10.9
Transferrin	S	2.0–4.0 g/L	200–400 mg/dL
Triglycerides (see **Table A-5**)	S	0.34–2.26 mmol/L	30–200 mg/dL
Triiodothyronine, free (fT$_3$)	S	3.7–6.5 pmol/L	2.4–4.2 pg/mL
Triiodothyronine, total (T$_3$)	S	1.2–2.1 nmol/L	77–135 ng/dL
Troponin I	S		
Normal population, 99 %tile		0–0.08 μg/L	0–0.08 ng/mL
Cut-off for MI		>0.4 μg/L	>0.4 ng/mL
Troponin T	S		
Normal population, 99 %tile		0–0.1 μg/L	0–0.01 ng/mL
Cut-off for MI		0–0.1 μg/L	0–0.1 ng/mL
Urea nitrogen	S	2.5–7.1 mmol/L	7–20 mg/dL
Uric acid	S		
Females		0.15–0.33 μmol/L	2.5–5.6 mg/dL
Males		0.18–0.41 μmol/L	3.1–7.0 mg/dL
Urobilinogen	U	0.09–4.2 μmol/d	0.05–25 mg/24 h
Vanillylmandelic acid (VMA)	U, 24h	<30 μmol/d	<6 mg/d
Vasoactive intestinal polypeptide	P	0–60 ng/L	0–60 pg/mL

[a]P, plasma; S, serum; U, urine; WB, whole blood; JF, joint fluid.

TOXICOLOGY AND THERAPEUTIC DRUG MONITORING

DRUG	THERAPEUTIC RANGE		TOXIC LEVEL	
	SI UNITS	CONVENTIONAL UNITS	SI UNITS	CONVENTIONAL UNITS
Acetaminophen	66–199 µmol/L	10–30 µg/mL	>1320 µmol/L	>200 µg/mL
Amikacin				
Peak	34–51 µmol/L	20–30 µg/mL	>60 µmol/L	>35 µg/mL
Trough	0–17 µmol/L	0–10 µg/mL	>17 µmol/L	>10 µg/mL
Amitriptyline/nortriptyline (total drug)	430–900 nmol/L	120–250 ng/mL	>1800 nmol/L	>500 ng/mL
Amphetamine	150–220 nmol/L	20–30 ng/mL	>1500 nmol/L	>200 ng/mL
Bromide	1.3–6.3 mmol/L	Sedation: 10–50 mg/dL	6.4–18.8 mmol/L	51–150 mg/dL: mild toxicity
	9.4–18.8 mmol/L		>18.8 mmol/L	
		Epilepsy: 75–150 mg/dL	>37.5 mmol/L	>150 mg/dL: severe toxicity
				>300 mg/dL: lethal
Carbamazepine	17–42 µmol/L	4–10 µg/mL	85 µmol/L	>20 µg/mL
Chloramphenicol				
Peak	31–62 µmol/L	10–20 µg/mL	>77 µmol/L	>25 µg/mL
Trough	15–31 µmol/L	5–10 µg/mL	>46 µmol/L	>15 µg/mL
Chlordiazepoxide	1.7–10 µmol/L	0.5–3.0 µg/mL	>17 µmol/L	>5.0 µg/mL
Clonazepam	32–240 nmol/L	10–75 ng/mL	>320 nmol/L	>100 ng/mL
Clozapine	0.6–2.1 µmol/L	200–700 ng/mL	>3.7 µmol/L	>1200 ng/mL
Cocaine			>3.3 µmol/L	>1.0 µg/mL
Codeine	43–110 nmol/mL	13–33 ng/mL	>3700 nmol/mL	>1100 ng/mL (lethal)
Cyclosporine				
Renal transplant				
0–6 months	208–312 nmol/L	250–375 ng/mL	>312 nmol/L	>375 ng/mL
6–12 months after transplant	166–250 nmol/L	200–300 ng/mL	>250 nmol/L	>300 ng/mL
>12 months	83–125 nmol/L	100–150 ng/mL	>125 nmol/L	>150 ng/mL
Cardiac transplant				
0–6 months	208–291 nmol/L	250–350 ng/mL	>291 nmol/L	>350 ng/mL
6–12 months after transplant	125–208 nmol/L	150–250 ng/mL	>208 nmol/L	>250 ng/mL
>12 months	83–125 nmol/L	100–150 ng/mL	>125 nmol/L	150 ng/mL
Lung transplant				
0–6 months	250–374 nmol/L	300–450 ng/mL	>374 nmol/L	>450 ng/mL
Liver transplant				
0–7 days	249–333 nmol/L	300–400 ng/mL	>333 nmol/L	>400 ng/mL
2–4 weeks	208–291 nmol/L	250–350 ng/mL	>291 nmol/L	>350 ng/mL
5–8 weeks	166–249 nmol/L	200–300 ng/mL	>249 nmol/L	>300 ng/mL
9–52 weeks	125–208 nmol/L	150–250 ng/mL	>208 nmol/L	>250 ng/mL
>1 year	83–166 nmol/L	100–200 ng/mL	>166 nmol/L	>200 ng/mL
Desipramine	375–1130 nmol/L	100–300 ng/mL	>1880 nmol/L	>500 ng/mL
Diazepam (and metabolite)				
Diazepam	0.7–3.5 µmol/L	0.2–1.0 µg/mL	>7.0 µmol/L	>2.0 µg/mL
Nordazepam	0.4–6.6 µmol/L	0.1–1.8 µg/mL	>9.2 µmol/L	>2.5 µg/mL
Digoxin	0.64–2.6 nmol/L	0.5–2.0 ng/mL	>3.1 nmol/L	>2.4 ng/mL
Disopyramide	>7.4 µmol/L	2.5 µg/mL	20.6 µmol/L	>7 µg/mL
Doxepin and nordoxepin				
Doxepin	0.36–0.98 µmol/L	101–274 ng/mL	>1.8 µmol/L	>503 ng/mL
Nordoxepin	0.38–1.04 µmol/L	106–291 ng/mL	>1.9 µmol/L	>531 ng/mL
Ethanol				
Behavioral changes			>4.3 mmol/L	>20 mg/dL
Legal limit			≥17 mmol/L	≥80 mg/dL
Critical with acute exposure			>54 mmol/L	>250 mg/dL

(Continued)

TOXICOLOGY AND THERAPEUTIC DRUG MONITORING

DRUG	THERAPEUTIC RANGE		TOXIC LEVEL	
	SI UNITS	CONVENTIONAL UNITS	SI UNITS	CONVENTIONAL UNITS
Ethylene glycol				
Toxic			>2 mmol/L	>12 mg/dL
Lethal			>20 mmol/L	>120 mg/dL
Ethosuxamide	280–700 µmol/L	40–100 µg/mL	>700 µmol/L	>100 µg/mL
Flecainide	0.5–2.4 µmol/L	0.2–1.0 µg/mL	>3.6 µmol/L	>1.5 µg/mL
Gentamicin				
Peak	10–21 µmol/mL	5–10 µg/mL	> 25 µmol/mL	>12 µg/mL
Trough	0–4.2 µmol/mL	0–2 µg/mL	> 4.2 µmol/mL	>2 µg/mL
Heroin (diacetyl morphine)			>700 µmol/L	>200 ng/mL (as morphine)
Ibuprofen	49–243 µmol/L	10–50 µg/mL	>97 µmol/L	>200 µg/mL
Imipramine (and metabolite)				
Desimipramine	375–1130 nmol/L	100–300 ng/mL	>1880 nmol/L	>500 ng/mL
Total imipramine + desimipramine	563–1130 nmol/L	150–300 ng/mL	>1880 nmol/L	>500 ng/mL
Lidocaine	5.1–21.3 µmol/L	1.2–5.0 µg/mL	>38.4 µmol/L	>9.0 µg/mL
Lithium	0.5–1.3 meq/L	0.5–1.3 meq/L	>2 mmol/L	>2 meq/L
Methadone	1.3–3.2 µmol/L	0.4–1.0 µg/mL	>6.5 µmol/L	>2 µg/mL
Methamphetamine		20–30 ng/mL		0.1–1.0 µg/mL
Methanol			>6 mmol/L	>20 mg/dL
			>16 mmol/L	>50 mg/dL, severe toxicity
			>28 mmol/L	>89 mg/dL, lethal
Methotrexate				
Low-dose	0.01–0.1 µmol/L	0.01–0.1 µmol/L	>0.1 mmol/L	>0.1 mmol/L
High-dose (24h)	<5.0 µmol/L	<5.0 µmol/L	>5.0 µmol/L	>5.0 µmol/L
High-dose (48h)	<0.50 µmol/L	<0.50 µmol/L	>0.5 µmol/L	>0.5 µmol/L
High-dose (72h)	<0.10 µmol/L	<0.10 µmol/L	>0.1 µmol/L	>0.1 µmol/L
Morphine	35–250 µmol/L	10–70 ng/mL	180–14000 µmol/L	50–4000 ng/mL
Nitroprusside (as thiocyanate)	103–499 µmol/L	6–29 µg/mL	860 µmol/L	>50 µg/mL
Nortriptyline	190–569 nmol/L	50–150 ng/mL	>1900 nmol/L	>500 ng/mL
Phenobarbital	65–172 µmol/L	15–40 µg/mL	>215 µmol/L	>50 µg/mL
Phenytoin	40–79 µmol/L	10–20 µg/mL	>118 µmol/L	>30 µg/mL
Phenytoin, free	4.0–7.9 µg/mL	1–2 µg/mL	>13.9 µg/mL	>3.5 µg/mL
% Free	0.08–0.14	8–14%		
Primidone and metabolite				
Primidone	23–55 µmol/L	5–12 µg/mL	>69 µmol/L	>15 µg/mL
Phenobarbital	65–172 µmol/L	15–40 µg/mL	>215 µmol/L	>50 µg/mL
Procainamide				
Procainamide	17–42 µmol/L	4–10 µg/mL	>51 µmol/L	>12 µg/mL
NAPA (N-acetylpro-cainamide)	22–72 µmol/L	6–20 µg/mL	>126 µmol/L	>35 µg/mL
Quinidine	>6.2–5.4 µmol/L	2.0–5.0 µg/mL	>31 µmol/L	>10 µg/mL
Salicylates	145–2100 µmol/L	2–29 mg/dL	>2172 µmol/L	>30 mg/dL
Sirolimus (trough level)				
Kidney transplant	4.4–13.1 nmol/L	4–12 ng/mL	>16 nmol/L	>15 ng/mL

(Continued)

TOXICOLOGY AND THERAPEUTIC DRUG MONITORING

DRUG	THERAPEUTIC RANGE		TOXIC LEVEL	
	SI UNITS	CONVENTIONAL UNITS	SI UNITS	CONVENTIONAL UNITS
Tacrolimus (FK506) (trough)				
Kidney and liver				
0–2 months post transplant	12–19 nmol/L	10–15 ng/mL	>25 nmol/L	>20 ng/mL
>2 months post transplant	6–12 nmol/L	5–10 ng/mL		
Heart				
0–2 months post transplant	19–25 nmol/L	15–20 ng/mL	>25 nmol/L	>20 ng/mL
3–6 months post transplant	12–19 nmol/L	10–15 ng/mL		
>6 months post transplant	10–12 nmol/L	8–10 ng/mL		
Theophylline	56–111 µg/mL	10–20 µg/mL	>140 µg/mL	>25 µg/mL
Thiocyanate				
After nitroprusside infusion	103–499 µmol/L	6–29 µg/mL	860 µmol/L	>50 µg/mL
Nonsmoker	17–69 µmol/L	1–4 µg/mL		
Smoker	52–206 µmol/L	3–12 µg/mL		
Tobramycin				
Peak	11–22 µg/L	5–10 µg/mL	>26 µg/L	>12 µg/mL
Trough	0–4.3 µg/L	0–2 µg/mL	>4.3 µg/L	>2 µg/mL
Valproic acid	350–700 µmol/L	50–100 µg/mL	>1000 µmol/L	>150 µg/mL
Vancomycin				
Peak	14–28 µmol/L	20–40 µg/mL	>55 µmol/L	>80 µg/mL
Trough	3.5–10.4 µmol/L	5–15 µg/mL	>14 µmol/L	>20 µg/mL

APPENDIX

Laboratory Values of Clinical Importance

TABLE A-4

VITAMINS AND SELECTED TRACE MINERALS

SPECIMEN	ANALYTE[a]	REFERENCE RANGE	
		SI UNITS	CONVENTIONAL UNITS
Aluminum	S	<0.2 μmol/L	<5.41 μg/L
	U, random	0.19–1.11 μmol/L	5–30 μg/L
Arsenic	WB	0.03–0.31 μmol/L	2–23 μg/L
	U, 24 h	0.07–0.67 μmol/d	5–50 μg/d
Cadmium	WB	<44.5 nmol/L	<5.0 μg/L
Coenzyme Q10 (ubiquinone)	P	433–1532 μg/L	433–1532 μg/L
B carotene	S	0.07–1.43 μmol/L	4–77 μg/dL
Copper			
	S	11–22 μmol/L	70–140 μg/dL
	U, 24 h	<0.95 μmol/d	<60 μg/d
Folic acid	RC	340–1020 nmol/L cells	150–450 ng/mL cells
Folic acid	S	12.2–40.8 nmol/L	5.4–18.0 ng/mL
Lead (adult)	S	<0.5 μmol/L	<10 μg/dL
Mercury			
	WB	3.0–294 nmol/L	0.6–59 μg/L
	U, 24 h	<99.8 nmol/L	<20 μg/L
Selenium	S	0.8–2.0 μmol/L	63–160 μg/L
Vitamin A	S	0.7–3.5 μmol/L	20–100 μg/dL
Vitamin B$_1$ (thiamine)	S	0–75 nmol/L	0–2 μg/dL
Vitamin B$_2$ (riboflavin)	S	106–638 nmol/L	4–24 μg/dL
Vitamin B$_6$	P	20–121 nmol/L	5–30 ng/mL
Vitamin B$_{12}$	S	206–735 pmol/L	279–996 pg/mL
Vitamin C (ascorbic acid)	S	23–57 μmol/L	0.4–1.0 mg/dL
Vitamin D$_3$, 1,25-dihydroxy	S	60–108 pmol/L	25–45 pg/mL
Vitamin D$_3$, 25-hydroxy	P		
Summer		37.4–200 nmol/L	15–80 ng/mL
Winter		34.9–105 nmol/L	14–42 ng/mL
Vitamin E	S	12–42 μmol/L	5–18 μg/mL
Vitamin K	S	0.29–2.64 nmol/L	0.13–1.19 ng/mL
Zinc	S	11.5–18.4 μmol/L	75–120 μg/dL

[a]P, plasma; RC, red cells; S, serum; WB, whole blood; U, urine.

TABLE A-5

CLASSIFICATION OF LDL, TOTAL, AND HDL CHOLESTEROL

LDL Cholesterol, mg/dL (mmol/L)

<70 (<1.81)	Therapeutic option for very high risk patients
<100 (<2.59)	Optimal
100–129 (2.59–3.34)	Near optimal/above optimal
130–159 (3.36–4.11)	Borderline high
160–189 (4.14–4.89)	High
≥190 (≥4.91)	Very high

Total Cholesterol, mg/dL (mmol/L)

<200 (<5.17)	Desirable
200–239 (5.17–6.18)	Borderline high
≥240 (≥6.21)	High

HDL Cholesterol, mg/dL (mmol/L)

<40 (<1.03)	Low
≥60 (≥1.55)	High

Note: LDL, low-density lipoprotein; HDL, high-density lipoprotein
Source: Executive summary of the third report of the National Cholesterol Education Program (NCEP) expert panel on detection, evaluation, and treatment of high blood cholesterol in adults (adult treatment panel III). JAMA 285:2486, 2001; and Implications of recent clinical trials for the National Cholesterol Education Program Adult Treatment Panel III Guidelines: SM Grundy et al for the Coordinating Committee of the National Cholesterol Education Program. Circulation 110:227, 2004.

TABLE A-6

CEREBROSPINAL FLUID (CSF)[a]

CONSTITUENT	REFERENCE RANGE	
	SI UNITS	CONVENTIONAL UNITS
Osmolarity	292–297 mmol/kg water	292–297 mosmol/L
Electrolytes		
Sodium	137–145 mmol/L	137–145 meq/L
Potassium	2.7–3.9 mmol/L	2.7–3.9 meq/L
Calcium	1.0–1.5 mmol/L	2.1–3.0 meq/L
Magnesium	1.0–1.2 mmol/L	2.0–2.5 meq/L
Chloride	116–122 mmol/L	116–122 meq/L
CO_2 content	20–24 mmol/L	20–24 meq/L
P_{CO_2}	6–7 kPa	45–49 mmHg
pH	7.31–7.34	
Glucose	2.22–3.89 mmol/L	40–70 mg/dL
Lactate	1–2 mmol/L	10–20 mg/dL
Total protein		
Lumbar	0.15–0.5 g/L	15–50 mg/dL
Cisternal	0.15–0.25 g/L	15–25 mg/dL
Ventricular	0.06–0.15 g/L	6–15 mg/dL
Albumin	0.066–0.442 g/L	6.6–44.2 mg/dL
IgG	0.009–0.057 g/L	0.9–5.7 mg/dL
IgG index[b]	0.29–0.59	
Oligoclonal bands	<2 bands not present in matched serum sample	
Ammonia	15–47 µmol/L	25–80 µg/dL
Creatinine	44–168 µmol/L	0.5–1.9 mg/dL
Myelin basic protein	<4 µg/L	
CSF pressure		50–180 mmH$_2$O
CSF volume (adult)	~150 mL	
Red blood cells	0	0
Leukocytes		
Total	0–5 mononuclear cells per µL	0–5 mononuclear cells per mm³
Differential		
Lymphocytes	60–70%	
Monocytes	30–50%	
Neutrophils	None	

[a]Since cerebrospinal fluid concentrations are equilibrium values, measurements of the same parameters in blood plasma obtained at the same time are recommended. However, there is a time lag in attainment of equilibrium, and cerebrospinal levels of plasma constituents that can fluctuate rapidly (such as plasma glucose) may not achieve stable values until after a significant lag phase.

[b]IgG index = CSF IgG(mg/dL) $\times$ serum albumin(g/dL)/Serum IgG(g/dL) $\times$ CSF albumin(mg/dL).

TABLE A-7

URINE ANALYSIS

	REFERENCE RANGE	
	SI UNITS	CONVENTIONAL UNITS
Acidity, titratable	20–40 mmol/d	20–40 meq/d
Ammonia	30–50 mmol/d	30–50 meq/d
Amylase		4–400 U/L
Amylase/creatinine clearance ratio [(Cl_{am}/Cl_{cr}) × 100]	1–5	1–5
Calcium (10 meq/d or 200 mg/d dietary calcium)	<7.5 mmol/d	<300 mg/d
Creatine, as creatinine		
Female	<760 µmol/d	<100 mg/d
Male	<380 µmol/d	<50 mg/d
Creatinine	8.8–14 mmol/d	1.0–1.6 g/d
Eosinophils	<100,000 eosinophils/L	<100 eosinophils/mL
Glucose (glucose oxidase method)	0.3–1.7 mmol/d	50–300 mg/d
5-Hydroxyindoleacetic acid (5-HIAA)	10–47 µmol/d	2–9 mg/d
Iodine, spot urine		
WHO classification of iodine deficiency		
Not iodine deficient	>100 µg/L	>100 µg/L
Mild iodine deficiency	50–100 µg/L	50–100 µg/L
Moderate iodine deficiency	20–49 µg/L	20–49 µg/L
Severe iodine deficiency	<20 µg/L	<20 µg/L
Microalbumin		
Normal	0.0–0.03 g/d	0–30 mg/d
Microalbuminuria	0.03–0.30 g/d	30–300 mg/d
Clinical albuminuria	>0.3 g/d	>300 mg/d
Microalbumin/creatinine ratio		
Normal	0–3.4 g/mol creatinine	0–30 µg/mg creatinine
Microalbuminuria	3.4–34 g/mol creatinine	30–300 µg/mg creatinine
Clinical albuminuria	>34 g/mol creatinine	>300 µg/mg creatinine
Oxalate		
Male	80–500 µmol/d	7–44 mg/d
Female	45–350 µmol/d	4–31 mg/d
pH	5.0–9.0	5.0–9.0
Phosphate (phosphorus) (varies with intake)	12.9–42.0 mmol/d	400–1300 mg/d
Potassium (varies with intake)	25–100 mmol/d	25–100 meq/d
Protein	<0.15 g/d	<150 mg/d
Sediment		
Red blood cells	0–2/high power field	
White blood cells	0–2/high power field	
Bacteria	None	
Crystals	None	
Bladder cells	None	
Squamous cells	None	
Tubular cells	None	
Broad casts	None	
Epithelial cell casts	None	
Granular casts	None	
Hyaline casts	0–5/low power field	
Red blood cell casts	None	
Waxy casts	None	
White cell casts	None	
Sodium (varies with intake)	100–260 mmol/d	100–260 meq/d
Specific gravity	1.001–1.035	1.001–1.035
Urea nitrogen	214–607 mmol/d	6–17 g/d
Uric acid (normal diet)	1.49–4.76 mmol/d	250–800 mg/d

Note: WHO, World Health Organization.

TABLE A-8

DIFFERENTIAL NUCLEATED CELL COUNTS OF BONE MARROW ASPIRATES[a]

	OBSERVED RANGE, %	95% CONFIDENCE INTERVALS, %	MEAN, %
Blast cells	0–3.2	0–3.0	1.4
Promyelocytes	3.6–13.2	3.2–12.4	7.8
Neutrophil myelocytes	4–21.4	3.7–10.0	7.6
Eosinophil myelocytes	0–5.0	0–2.8	1.3
Metamyelocytes	1–7.0	2.3–5.9	4.1
Neutrophils			
Males	21.0–45.6	21.9–42.3	32.1
Females	29.6–46.6	28.8–45.9	37.4
Eosinophils	0.4–4.2	0.3–4.2	2.2
Eosinophils plus eosinophil myelocytes	0.9–7.4	0.7–6.3	3.5
Basophils	0–0.8	0–0.4	0.1
Erythroblasts			
Male	18.0–39.4	16.2–40.1	28.1
Females	14.0–31.8	13.0–32.0	22.5
Lymphocytes	4.6–22.6	6.0–20.0	13.1
Plasma cells	0–1.4	0–1.2	0.6
Monocytes	0–3.2	0–2.6	1.3
Macrophages	0–1.8	0–1.3	0.4
M:E ratio			
Males	1.1–4.0	1.1–4.1	2.1
Females	1.6–5.4	1.6–5.2	2.8

[a]Based on bone marrow aspirate from 50 healthy volunteers (30 men, 20 women).
Source: From BJ Bain: The bone marrow aspirate of healthy subjects. Br J Haematol 94(1):206, 1996.

TABLE A-9

STOOL ANALYSIS

	REFERENCE RANGE	
	SI UNITS	CONVENTIONAL UNITS
Amount	0.1–0.2 kg/d	100–200 g/24 h
Coproporphyrin	611–1832 nmol/d	400–1200 µg/24 h
Fat		
Adult		<7 g/d
Adult on fat-free diet		<4 g/d
Fatty acids	0–21 mmol/d	0–6 g/24 h
Leukocytes	None	None
Nitrogen	<178 mmol/d	<2.5 g/24 h
pH	7.0–7.5	
Occult blood	Negative	Negative
Trypsin		20–95 U/g
Urobilinogen	85–510 µmol/d	50–300 mg/24 h
Uroporphyrins	12–48 nmol/d	10–40 µg/24 h
Water	<0.75	<75%

Source: Modified from FT Fishbach, MB Dunning III: *A Manual of Laboratory and Diagnostic Tests,* 7th ed., Lippincott Williams & Wilkins, Philadelphia, 2004.

SPECIAL FUNCTION TESTS

TABLE A-10

RENAL FUNCTION TESTS

	REFERENCE RANGE	
	SI UNITS	**CONVENTIONAL UNITS**
Clearances (corrected to 1.72 m^2 body surface area)		
Measures of glomerular filtration rate		
Inulin clearance (CI)		
Males (mean ± 1 SD)	2.1 ± 0.4 mL/s	124 ± 25.8 mL/min
Females (mean ± 1 SD)	2.0 ± 0.2 mL/s	119 ± 12.8 mL/min
Endogenous creatinine clearance	1.5–2.2 mL/s	91–130 mL/min
Measures of effective renal plasma flow and tubular function		
p-Aminohippuric acid clearance (CI$_{PAH}$)		
Males (mean ± 1 SD)	10.9 ± 2.7 mL/s	654 ± 163 mL/min
Females (mean ± 1 SD)	9.9 ± 1.7 mL/s	594 ± 102 mL/min
Concentration and dilution test		
Specific gravity of urine		
After 12-h fluid restriction	>1.025	>1.025
After 12-h deliberate water intake	≤1.003	≤1.003
Protein excretion, urine	<0.15 g/d	<150 mg/d
Specific gravity, maximal range	1.002–1.028	1.002–1.028
Tubular reabsorption, phosphorus	0.79–0.94 of filtered load	79–94% of filtered load

TABLE A-11

CIRCULATORY FUNCTION TESTS

	RESULTS: REFERENCE RANGE	
TEST	**SI UNITS (RANGE)**	**CONVENTIONAL UNITS (RANGE)**
Arteriovenous oxygen difference	30–50 mL/L	30–50 mL/L
Cardiac output (Fick)	2.5–3.6 L/m^2 of body surface area per min	2.5–3.6 L/m^2 of body surface area per min
Contractility indexes		
Max. left ventricular dp/dt (dp/dt)/DP when DP = 5.3 kPa (40 mmHg) (DP, diastolic pressure)	220 kPa/s (176–250 kPa/s) (37.6 ± 12.2)/s	1650 mmHg/s (1320–1880 mmHg/s) (37.6 ± 12.2)/s
Mean normalized systolic ejection rate (angiography)	3.32 ± 0.84 end-diastolic volumes per second	3.32 ± 0.84 end-diastolic volumes per second
Mean velocity of circumferential fiber shortening (angiography)	1.83 ± 0.56 circumferences per second	1.83 ± 0.56 circumferences per second
Ejection fraction: stroke volume/end-diastolic volume (SV/EDV)	0.67 ± 0.08 (0.55–0.78)	0.67 ± 0.08 (0.55–0.78)
End-diastolic volume	70 ± 20.0 mL/m^2 (60–88 mL/m^2)	70 ± 20.0 mL/m^2 (60–88 mL/m^2)
End-systolic volume	25 ± 5.0 mL/m^2 (20–33 mL/m^2)	25 ± 5.0 mL/m^2 (20–33 mL/m^2)
Left ventricular work		
Stroke work index	50 ± 20.0 (g·m)/m^2 (30–110)	50 ± 20.0 (g·m)/m^2 (30–110)
Left ventricular minute work index	1.8–6.6 [(kg·m)/m^2]/min	1.8–6.6 [(kg·m)/m^2]/min
Oxygen consumption index	110–150 mL	110–150 mL
Maximum oxygen uptake	35 mL/min (20–60 mL/min)	35 mL/min (20–60 mL/min)
Pulmonary vascular resistance	2–12 (kPa·s)/L	20–130 (dyn·s)/cm^5
Systemic vascular resistance	77–150 (kPa·s)/L	770–1600 (dyn·s)/cm^5

Source: E Braunwald et al: *Heart Disease*, 6th ed, Philadelphia, Saunders, 2001.

TABLE A-12

GASTROINTESTINAL TESTS

| | RESULTS | |
TEST	SI UNITS	CONVENTIONAL UNITS
Absorption tests		
D-Xylose: after overnight fast, 25 g xylose given in oral aqueous solution		
Urine, collected for following 5 h	25% of ingested dose	25% of ingested dose
Serum, 2 h after dose	2.0–3.5 mmol/L	30–52 mg/dL
Vitamin A: a fasting blood specimen is obtained and 200,000 units of vitamin A in oil is given orally	Serum level should rise to twice fasting level in 3–5 h	Serum level should rise to twice fasting level in 3–5 h
Bentiromide test (pancreatic function): 500 mg bentiromide (chymex) orally; *p*-aminobenzoic acid (PABA) measured		
Plasma		>3.6 (±1.1) µg/mL at 90 min
Urine	>50% recovered in 6 h	>50% recovered in 6 h
Gastric juice		
Volume		
24 h	2–3 L	2–3 L
Nocturnal	600–700 mL	600–700 mL
Basal, fasting	30–70 mL/h	30–70 mL/h
Reaction		
pH	1.6–1.8	1.6–1.8
Titratable acidity of fasting juice	4–9 µmol/s	15–35 meq/h
Acid output		
Basal		
Females (mean ± 1 SD)	0.6 ± 0.5 µmol/s	2.0 ± 1.8 meq/h
Males (mean ± 1 SD)	0.8 ± 0.6 µmol/s	3.0 ± 2.0 meq/h
Maximal (after SC histamine acid phosphate, 0.004 mg/kg body weight, and preceded by 50 mg promethazine, or after betazole, 1.7 mg/kg body weight, or pentagastrin, 6 µg/kg body weight)		
Females (mean ± 1 SD)	4.4 ± 1.4 µmol/s	16 ± 5 meq/h
Males (mean ± 1 SD)	6.4 ± 1.4 µmol/s	23 ± 5 meq/h
Basal acid output/maximal acid output ratio	≤0.6	≤0.6
Gastrin, serum	0–200 µg/L	0–200 pg/mL
Secretin test (pancreatic exocrine function): 1 unit/kg body weight, IV		
Volume (pancreatic juice) in 80 min	>2.0 mL/kg	>2.0 mL/kg
Bicarbonate concentration	>80 mmol/L	>80 meq/L
Bicarbonate output in 30 min	>10 mmol	>10 meq

TABLE A-13

NORMAL VALUES OF DOPPLER ECHOCARDIOGRAPHIC MEASUREMENTS IN ADULTS

	RANGE	MEAN
RVD (cm), measured at the base in apical 4-chamber view	2.6–4.3	3.5 ± 0.4
LVID (cm), measured in the parasternal long axis view	3.6–5.4	4.7 ± 0.4
Posterior LV wall thickness (cm)	0.6–1.1	0.9 ± 0.4
IVS wall thickness (cm)	0.6–1.1	0.9 ± 0.4
Left atrial dimension (cm), antero-posterior dimension	2.3–3.8	3.0 ± 0.3
Aortic root dimension (cm)	2.0–3.5	2.4 ± 0.4
Aortic cusps separation (cm)	1.5–2.6	1.9 ± 0.4
Percentage of fractional shortening	34–44%	36%
Mitral flow (m/s)	0.6–1.3	0.9
Tricuspid flow (m/s)	0.3–0.7	0.5
Pulmonary artery (m/s)	0.6–0.9	0.75
Aorta (m/s)	1.0–1.7	1.35

Note: RVD, right ventricular dimension; LVID, left ventricular internal dimension; LV, left ventricle; IVS, interventricular septum.

Source: From A Weyman: *Principles and Practice of Echocardiography*, 2d ed., Philadelphia, Lea & Febiger, 1994.

APPENDIX

Laboratory Values of Clinical Importance

TABLE A-14

SUMMARY OF VALUES USEFUL IN PULMONARY PHYSIOLOGY

	SYMBOL	TYPICAL VALUES	
		MAN, AGE 40, 75 kg, 175-cm TALL	WOMAN, AGE 40, 60 kg, 160-cm TALL
Pulmonary Mechanics			
Spirometry—volume-time curves			
Forced vital capacity	FVC	5.1 L	3.6 L
Forced expiratory volume in 1 s	FEV_1	4.1 L	2.9 L
FEV_1/FVC	$FEV_1\%$	80%	82%
Maximal mid-expiratory flow	MMF (FEF 25–27)	4.8 L/s	3.6 L/s
Maximal expiratory flow rate	MEFR (FEF 200–1200)	9.4 L/s	6.1 L/s
Spirometry—flow-volume curves			
Maximal expiratory flow at 50% of expired vital capacity	V_{max} 50 (FEF 50%)	6.1 L/s	4.6 L/s
Maximal expiratory flow at 75% of expired vital capacity	V_{max} 75 (FEF 75%)	3.1 L/s	2.5 L/s
Resistance to airflow			
Pulmonary resistance	RL (R_L)	<3.0 (cmH_2O/s)/L	
Airway resistance	Raw	<2.5 (cmH_2O/s)/L	
Specific conductance	SGaw	>0.13 cmH_2O/s	
Pulmonary compliance			
Static recoil pressure at total lung capacity	Pst TLC	25 ± 5 cmH_2O	
Compliance of lungs (static)	CL	0.2 L cmH_2O	
Compliance of lungs and thorax	C(L + T)	0.1 L cmH_2O	
Dynamic compliance of 20 breaths per minute	C dyn 20	0.25 ± 0.05 L/cmH_2O	
Maximal static respiratory pressures			
Maximal inspiratory pressure	MIP	>90 cmH_2O	>50 cmH_2O
Maximal expiratory pressure	MEP	>150 cmH_2O	>120 cmH_2O
Lung Volumes			
Total lung capacity	TLC	6.7 L	4.9 L
Functional residual capacity	FRC	3.7 L	2.8 L
Residual volume	RV	2.0 L	1.6 L
Inspiratory capacity	IC	3.3 L	2.3 L
Expiratory reserve volume	ERV	1.7 L	1.1 L
Vital capacity	VC	5.0 L	3.4 L
Gas Exchange (Sea Level)			
Arterial O_2 tension	Pa_{O_2}	12.7 ± 0.7 kPa (95 ± 5 mmHg)	
Arterial CO_2 tension	Pa_{CO_2}	5.3 ± 0.3 kPa (40 ± 2 mmHg)	
Arterial O_2 saturation	Sa_{O_2}	0.97 ± 0.02 (97 ± 2%)	
Arterial blood pH	pH	7.40 ± 0.02	
Arterial bicarbonate	HCO_3^-	24 + 2 meq/L	
Base excess	BE	0 ± 2 meq/L	
Diffusing capacity for carbon monoxide (single breath)	DL_{CO}	0.42 mL CO/s per mmHg (25 mL CO/min per mmHg)	
Dead space volume	V_D	2 mL/kg body wt	
Physiologic dead space; dead space-tidal volume ratio	V_D/V_T		
Rest		≤35% V_T	
Exercise		≤20% V_T	
Alveolar-arterial difference for O_2	$P(A - a)_{O_2}$	≤2.7 kPa ≤20 kPa (≤20 mmHg)	

TABLE A-15

BODY FLUIDS AND OTHER MASS DATA

	REFERENCE RANGE	
	SI UNITS	**CONVENTIONAL UNITS**
Ascitic fluid		
Body fluid		
Total volume (lean) of body weight	50% (in obese) to 70%	
Intracellular	0.3–0.4 of body weight	
Extracellular	0.2–0.3 of body weight	
Blood		
Total volume		
Males	69 mL per kg body weight	
Females	65 mL per kg body weight	
Plasma volume		
Males	39 mL per kg body weight	
Females	40 mL per kg body weight	
Red blood cell volume		
Males	30 mL per kg body weight	1.15–1.21 L/m^2 of body surface area
Females	25 mL per kg body weight	0.95–1.00 L/m^2 of body surface area
Body mass index	18.5–24.9 kg/m^2	18.5–24.9 kg/m^2

TABLE A-16

RADIATION-DERIVED UNITS

QUANTITY	OLD UNIT	SI UNIT	NAME FOR SI UNIT (AND ABBREVIATION)	CONVERSION
Activity	curie (Ci)	Disintegrations per second (dps)	becquerel (Bq)	1 Ci = 3.7×10^{10} Bq 1 mCi = 37 mBq 1 μCi = 0.037 MBq or 37 GBq 1 Bq = 2.703×10^{-11} Ci
Absorbed dose	rad	joule per kilogram (J/kg)	gray (Gy)	1 Gy = 100 rad 1 rad = 0.01 Gy 1 mrad = 10^{-3} cGy
Exposure	roentgen (R)	coulomb per kilogram (C/kg)	—	1 C/kg = 3876 R 1 R = 2.58×10^{-4} C/kg 1 mR = 258 pC/kg
Dose equivalent	rem	joule per kilogram (J/kg)	sievert (Sv)	1 Sv = 100 rem 1 rem = 0.01 Sv 1 mrem = 10 μSv

ACKNOWLEDGMENT

The authors acknowledge the contributions of Dr. Patrick M. Sluss, Dr. James L. Januzzi, and Dr. Kent B. Lewandrowski to this chapter in previous editions of Harrison's Principles of Internal Medicine.

FURTHER READINGS

KRATZ A et al: Case records of the Massachusetts General Hospital. Weekly clinicopathological exercises. Laboratory reference values. N Engl J Med 351(15):1548, 2004

LEHMAN HP, HENRY JB: SI units, in *Henry's Clinical Diagnosis and Management by Laboratory Methods*, 21st ed, RC McPherson, MR Pincus (eds). Philadelphia, Elsevier Saunders, 2007, pp 1404–1418

PESCE MA: Reference ranges for laboratory tests and procedures, in *Nelson's Textbook of Pediatrics*, 18th ed, RM Klegman et al (eds). Philadelphia, Elsevier Saunders, 2007, pp 2943–2949

SOLBERG HE: Establishment and use of reference values, in *Tietz Textbook of Clinical Chemistry and Molecular Diagnostics*, 4th ed, CA Burtis et al (eds). Philadelphia, Elsevier Saunders, 2006, pp 425–448

REVIEW AND SELF-ASSESSMENT*

Charles Wiener ▪ **Gerald Bloomfield** ▪ **Cynthia D. Brown**
▪ **Joshua Schiffer** ▪ **Adam Spivak**

QUESTIONS

DIRECTIONS: Choose the **one best** response to each question.

1. A 73-year-old woman with a medical history of obesity and diabetes mellitus presents to your clinic complaining of right knee pain that has been progressive and is worse with walking or standing. She has taken over-the-counter nonsteroidal anti-inflammatory drugs without relief. She wants to know what is wrong with her knee and what may have caused it. X-rays are performed and reveal cartilage loss and osteophyte formation. Which of the following represents the most potent risk factor for the development of osteoarthritis?

   A. Age
   B. Gender
   C. Genetic susceptibility
   D. Obesity
   E. Previous joint injury

2. A 54-year-old man is admitted for persistent lower abdominal and groin pain that began 7 months previously. Two months before his present admission, he required exploratory laparoscopy for acute abdominal pain and presumed cholecystitis. This revealed necrotic omental tissue and pericholecystitis necessitating omentectomy and cholecystectomy. However, the pain continued unchanged. He currently describes it as periumbilical and radiating into his groin and legs. It becomes worse with eating. The patient has also had episodic severe testicular pain, bowel urgency, nausea, vomiting, and diuresis. He has lost ~22.7 kg over the preceding 6 months. His past medical history is significant of hypertension that has recently become difficult to control.

   Medications on admission include aspirin, hydrochlorothiazide, hydromorphone, lansoprazole, metoprolol, and quinapril. On physical examination, the patient appears comfortable. His blood pressure is

2. *(Continued)*
   170/100 mmHg, his heart rate is 88 beats/min, and he is afebrile. He has normal first and second heart sounds without murmurs, and an S_4 is present. There are no carotid, renal, abdominal, or femoral bruits.

   His lungs are clear to auscultation. Bowel sounds are normal. Abdominal palpation demonstrates minimal diffuse tenderness without rebound or guarding. No masses are present, and the stool is negative for occult blood. During the examination, the patient develops Raynaud's phenomenon in his right hand that persists for several minutes. His neurologic examination is intact. Admission laboratory studies reveal an erythrocyte sedimentation rate of 72 mm/h, a BUN of 17 mg/dL, and a creatinine of 0.8 mg/dL. The patient has no proteinuria or hematuria. Tests for antinuclear antibodies, anti–double-stranded-DNA antibodies, and antineutrophil cytoplasmic antibodies are negative. Liver function tests are abnormal with an AST of 89 IU/L and an ALT of 112 IU/L. Hepatitis B surface antigen and e antigen are positive. Mesenteric angiography demonstrates small beaded aneurysms of the superior and inferior mesenteric veins. What is the most likely diagnosis?

   A. Hepatocellular carcinoma
   B. Ischemic colitis
   C. Microscopic polyangiitis
   D. Mixed cryoglobulinemia
   E. Polyarteritis nodosa

3. A 64-year-old African-American male is evaluated in the hospital for congestive heart failure, renal failure, and polyneuropathy. Physical examination on admission was notable for these findings and raised waxy papules in the axilla and inguinal region. Admission laboratories showed a BUN of 90 mg/dL

---

*Questions and answers were taken from Wiener C et al (eds): *Harrison's Principles of Internal Medicine Self-Assessment and Board Review*, 17th ed. New York, McGraw-Hill, 2008.

3. *(Continued)*

and a creatinine of 6.3 mg/dL. Total protein was 9.0 g/dL, with an albumin of 3.2 g/dL. Hematocrit was 24%, and white blood cell and platelet counts were normal. Urinalysis was remarkable for 3+ proteinuria but no cellular casts. Further evaluation included an echocardiogram with a thickened left ventricle and preserved systolic function. Which of the following tests is most likely to diagnose the underlying condition?

A. Bone marrow biopsy
B. Electromyogram (EMG) with nerve conduction studies
C. Fat pad biopsy
D. Right heart catheterization
E. Renal ultrasound

4. A 31-year-old woman presents to your clinic complaining of painful arthritis that is worse in the mornings when she wakes up. She was recently evaluated by an ophthalmologist for uveitis in her right eye. A recent laboratory report shows an erythrocyte sedimentation rate of 48 mm/h. Which of the following will be helpful in distinguishing relapsing polychondritis from rheumatoid arthritis (RA)?

A. Arthritis associated with RA is nonerosive.
B. Eye inflammation is absent in relapsing polychondritis.
C. Relapsing polychondritis will not present with vasculitis.
D. Relapsing polychondritis will present with high-titer rheumatoid factor.
E. The arthritis of relapsing polychondritis is asymmetric.

5. A 66-year-old woman with a history of rheumatoid arthritis and frequent pseudogout attacks in her left knee presents with night sweats and a 2-day history of left knee pain. On physical examination, her temperature is 38.6°C, heart rate is 110 beats/min, blood pressure is 104/78 mmHg, and oxygen saturation is 97% on room air. Her left knee is swollen, red, painful, and warm. With 5° of flexion or extension, she develops extreme pain. She has evidence of chronic joint deformity in her hands, knees, and spine. Peripheral white blood cell (WBC) count is 16,700 cells/μL with 95% neutrophils. A diagnostic tap of her left knee reveals 168,300 WBCs per microliter, 99% neutrophils, and diffuse needle-shaped birefringent crystals present. Gram stain shows rare gram-positive cocci in clusters. Management includes all of the following *except*

A. blood cultures
B. glucocorticoids
C. needle aspiration of joint fluid
D. orthopedic surgery consult
E. vancomycin

6. A 58-year-old female presents complaining of right shoulder pain. She does not recall any prior injury but notes that she feels that the shoulder has been getting progressively stiffer over the last several months. She previously had several episodes of bursitis of the right shoulder that were treated successfully with NSAIDs and steroid injections. The patient's past medical history is also significant for diabetes mellitus, for which she takes metformin and glyburide. On physical examination, the right shoulder is not warm or red but is tender to touch. Passive and active range of motion is limited in flexion, extension, and abduction. A right shoulder radiogram shows osteopenia without evidence of joint erosion or osteophytes. What is the most likely diagnosis?

A. Adhesive capsulitis
B. Avascular necrosis
C. Bicipital tendinitis
D. Osteoarthritis
E. Rotator cuff tear

7. A 44-year-old woman presents for evaluation of dry eyes and mouth. She first noticed these symptoms >5 years ago and the symptoms have worsened over time. She describes her eyes as gritty-feeling, as if there were sand in her eyes. Sometimes her eyes burn, and she states that it is difficult to be outside in bright sunlight. In addition, her mouth is quite dry. In her job, she is frequently asked to give business presentations and finds it increasingly difficult to complete a 30- to 60-minute presentation. She usually has water with her at all times. Although she reports good dental hygiene without any recent changes, her dentist has had to place fillings twice in the past 3 years for dental caries. Her only other past medical history is treated tuberculosis that she contracted while in the Peace Corps in Southeast Asia when in her twenties. She takes no medication regularly and does not smoke. Ocular examination reveals punctuate corneal ulcerations on rose Bengal stain, and the Schirmer test shows <5 mm of wetness after 5 min. Her oral mucosa is dry with thick mucous secretions, and the parotid glands are enlarged bilaterally. Laboratory examination reveals positive antibodies to Ro and La (SS-A and SS-B). In addition, her chemistries reveal sodium of 142 mEq/L, potassium 2.6 mEq/L, chloride 115 mEq/L, and bicarbonate of 15 mEq/L. What is the most likely cause of the hypokalemia and acidemia in this patient?

A. Diarrhea
B. Distal (type I) renal tubular acidosis
C. Hypoaldosteronism
D. Purging with underlying anorexia nervosa
E. Renal compensation for chronic respiratory alkalosis

8. A patient with end-stage renal disease on hemodialysis presents to your office with hand pain and you diagnose carpal tunnel syndrome. A serum thyroid-stimulating hormone level is normal. You also note bilateral knee effusions, which the patient states have been there for many months. Suspecting an amyloid deposition disease, you perform a fat pad biopsy. Which protein do you expect to find on immunohistochemical staining?

A. β_2-Microglobulin
B. Fibrinogen α-chain
C. Immunoglobulin light chain
D. Serum amyloid A
E. Transthyretin

9. A 41-year-old female presents to your clinic with 3 weeks of weakness, lethargy, and depressed mood. She notes increasing difficulty with climbing steps, rising from a chair, and combing her hair. She has no difficulty buttoning her blouse or writing. The patient also notes some dyspnea on exertion and orthopnea. She denies rash, joint aches, or constitutional symptoms. She is on no medications, and the past medical history is otherwise uninformative. The family history is notable only for coronary artery disease. The physical examination is notable for an elevated jugular venous pressure, an S_3, and some bibasilar crackles. The neurologic examination shows some marked proximal muscle weakness in the deltoids and biceps and the hip flexors. Distal muscle strength is normal. Sensory examination and reflexes are normal. Laboratories are unremarkable except for a negative antinuclear antibody screen and a creatinine kinase of 3200 IU/L. You suspect a diagnosis of polymyositis. All the following clinical conditions may occur in polymyositis *except*

A. an increased incidence of malignancy
B. interstitial lung disease
C. dilated cardiomyopathy
D. dysphagia
E. Raynaud's phenomenon

10. A 64-year-old man with congestive heart failure presents to the emergency room complaining of acute onset of severe pain in his right foot. The pain began during the night and awoke him from a deep sleep. He reports the pain to be so severe that he could not wear a shoe or sock to the hospital. His current medications are furosemide, 40 mg twice daily; carvedilol, 6.25 mg twice daily; candesartan, 8 mg once daily; and aspirin, 325 mg once daily. On examination, he is febrile to 38.5°C. The first toe of the right foot is erythematous and exquisitely tender to touch. There is significant swelling and effusion of

10. *(Continued)*
the first metatarsophalangeal joint on the right. No other joints are affected. Which of the following findings would be expected on arthrocentesis?

A. Glucose level of <25 mg/dL
B. Positive Gram stain
C. Presence of strongly negatively birefringent needle-shaped crystals under polarized light microscopy
D. Presence of weakly positively birefringent rhomboidal crystals under polarized light microscopy
E. White blood cell (WBC) count >100,000/µL

11. A 32-year-old African-American woman presents to her primary care doctor complaining of fatigue, joint stiffness and pain, mouth ulcers, and hair loss. She first noticed fatigue about 6 months ago, and at that time, a complete blood count and thyroid function tests were normal. Since then, she feels like her symptoms are getting progressively worse. She now states that she sleeps ≥10 h but continues to feel fatigued. She has also developed joint stiffness and pain in her hands, wrists, and knees that is present for about 1 h upon awakening. For the past month, she has had an area of hair loss on her scalp associated with a raised scaly rash. During this time, she intermittently developed painful mouth ulcerations that would spontaneously resolve. She also reports a severe "sunburn" on her face, upper neck, and back that occurred after <1 h of sun exposure and which was unusual for her. Her past medical history is positive for two spontaneous vaginal deliveries that were uncomplicated. She has not had any prior miscarriages. She is taking oral contraceptive pills and has no allergies. On physical examination, the vital signs are as follows: temperature 36.6°C, blood pressure 136/82 mmHg, heart rate 88 beats/min, respiratory rate 12 breaths/min, SaO$_2$ 98% on room air. She has a circular raised area on her right parietal area that is 3 cm in diameter. This area has an atrophic center with hair loss and is erythematous with a hyperpigmented rim. Her conjunctiva are pink and no scleral icterus is present. The oropharynx shows a single 2-mm aphthous ulceration on the buccal mucosa. Both wrists show some slight tenderness with palpation and pain with range of motion. The patient is incapable of closing her hands tightly. In addition, there is warmth and a possible effusion in the right knee and tenderness with range of motion in the left knee. Cardiovascular, pulmonary, abdominal, and neurologic examinations are normal. Laboratory studies show the following:

White blood cell count	2300/µL
Hemoglobin	8.9 g/dL
Hematocrit	26.7%
Mean corpuscular volume	88 fL

11. *(Continued)*

Mean corpuscular hemoglobin count   32 g/dL
Platelet   98,000/mL

The differential is 80% polymorphonuclear cells, 12% lymphocytes, 7% monocytes, 1% eosinophils, and 1% basophils. An antinuclear antibody (ANA) is positive at a titer of 1:640. Antibodies to double-stranded DNA are negative, and anti-Smith antibodies are positive at a titer of 1:160. The rheumatoid factor level is 37 IU/L. What is the most likely diagnosis?

A. Behçet's disease
B. Discoid lupus erythematosus
C. Rheumatoid arthritis
D. Sarcoidosis
E. Systemic lupus erythematosus

12. In this patient, which test should be performed next?

A. Chest radiograph
B. Echocardiogram
C. Electrocardiogram
D. Skin biopsy
E. Urinalysis

13. A 45-year-old obese man presents to the clinic several weeks after starting a jogging regimen. He describes right-sided heel pain that has worsened over this time. The pain is worse in the morning and when the patient is barefoot. On examination, pain can be elicited with palpation of the inferior medial right heel. Which of the following is required to make a definitive diagnosis of plantar fasciitis?

A. Compatible history and provocative testing
B. History and physical examination alone
C. History, physical examination, and nuclear medicine bone scan
D. History, physical examination, and heel ultrasound showing thickening of the fascia
E. History, physical examination, and plain radiograph demonstrating heel spur

14. Which of the following findings on joint aspiration is most likely to be associated with calcium pyrophosphate deposition disease (pseudogout)?

A. Fluid, clear and viscous; white blood cell count, 400/μL; crystals, rhomboidal and weakly positively birefringent
B. Fluid, cloudy and watery; white blood cell count, 8000/μL; no crystals
C. Fluid, dark brown and viscous; white blood cell count, 1200/μL; crystals, needle-like and strongly negatively birefringent

14. *(Continued)*

D. Fluid, cloudy and watery; white blood cell count, 12,000/μL; crystals, needle-like and strongly negatively birefringent
E. Fluid, cloudy and watery; white blood cell count, 4800/μL; crystals, rhomboidal and weakly positively birefringent

15. A 45-year-old woman presents to the emergency room for evaluation of fatigue, fever, and acute onset of joint pain and swelling of the right knee, left ankle, and right second toe. She reports that she was ill with a diarrheal illness about 2 weeks ago. She did not seek evaluation as the symptoms resolved spontaneously over 48 h. She did lose about 2.3 kg, which she has been unable to regain. Three days ago, she developed a feeling of malaise with fevers and pain in her right second toe. Additional joints have become inflamed over the ensuing 72 h. She denies any prior similar episodes. She is not currently sexually active and estimates her last sexual activity to be 8 months prior to presentation. She has a history of seasonal rhinitis, but is taking no medications currently. On examination, she is febrile at 38.4°C. Her left eye has evidence of conjunctival injection. There is a superficial ulcer on the inside of her lower lip that is not painful. The right knee is warm to the touch with an effusion. Passive movement results in pain. The left ankle is similarly warm and painful. The right second great toe has the appearance of a "sausage digit." There is also pain with palpation at the tendinous insertion of both Achilles tendons. There are no genital ulcers or discharge. No rash is present. Arthrocentesis is performed and is consistent with inflammatory arthritis without crystals or organisms seen on Gram stain. Cervical probes for *Neisseria gonorrhoeae* and *Chlamydia trachomatis* are negative. Reactive arthritis following *Campylobacter* infection is suspected with positive serum antibodies to *C. jejuni*. Which of the following statements is true regarding this diagnosis?

A. Chronic joint symptoms affect 15% of individuals, and recurrences of the acute syndrome may occur.
B. Presence of HLA-B27 antigen predicts individuals who are likely to have a better prognosis.
C. Reactive arthritis is self-limited and should be expected to resolve spontaneously over the next 2 weeks.
D. The causative organism has no effect on long-term outcomes following an initial episode of reactive arthritis.

16. A 54-year-old female with rheumatoid arthritis is treated with infliximab for refractory disease. All the following are potential side effects of this treatment *except*

A. demyelinating disorders
B. disseminated tuberculosis

16. *(Continued)*

    C. exacerbation of congestive heart failure

    D. pancytopenia

    E. pulmonary fibrosis

17. A 26-year-old man presents with severe bilateral pain in his hands, ankles, knees, and elbows. He is recovering from a sore throat and has had recent fevers to 38.9°C. Social history is notable for recent unprotected receptive oral intercourse with a man ~1 week ago. Physical examination reveals a well-developed man in moderate discomfort. He is afebrile. His pharynx is erythematous with pustular exudates on his tonsils. He has tender anterior cervical lymphadenopathy. His cardiac examination is notable for a normal S_1 and S_2 and a soft ejection murmur. His lungs are clear. Abdomen is benign with no organomegaly. He has no rash, and genital examination is normal. His bilateral proximal interphalangeal joints, metacarpophalangeal joints, wrists, ankles, and metatarsophalangeal joints are red, warm, and boggy with tenderness noted with both passive and active movement. A complete metabolic panel and complete blood count are all within normal limits. His erythrocyte sedimentation rate is 85 mm/h and C-reactive protein is 11 mg/dL. What is the most likely diagnosis?

    A. Acute HIV infection

    B. Acute rheumatic fever

    C. Lyme disease

    D. *Neisseria gonorrhoeae* infection

    E. Poststreptococcal reactive arthritis

18. A 27-year-old female with SLE is in remission; current treatment consists of azathioprine 75 mg/d and prednisone 5 mg/d. Last year she had a life-threatening exacerbation of her disease. She now strongly desires to become pregnant. Which of the following is the least appropriate action to take?

    A. Advise her that the risk of spontaneous abortion is high.

    B. Warn her that exacerbations can occur in the first trimester and in the postpartum period.

    C. Tell her it is unlikely that a newborn will have lupus.

    D. Advise her that fetal loss rates are higher if anticardiolipin antibodies are detected in her serum.

    E. Stop the prednisone just before she attempts to become pregnant.

19. A 48-year-old male has a long-standing history of ankylosing spondylitis. His most recent spinal film shows straightening of the lumbar spine, loss of lordosis, and "squaring" of the vertebral bodies. He currently is limited by pain with ambulation that is not improved with nonsteroidal anti-inflammatory

19. *(Continued)*

medications. Which of the following treatments has been shown to improve symptoms the best at this stage of the illness?

    A. Celecoxib

    B. Etanercept

    C. Prednisone

    D. Sulfasalazine

    E. Thalidomide

20. A 72-year-old woman presents to the emergency room for an episode of vision loss in her right eye. The vision loss came on abruptly and is described as a curtain falling across her visual field. She immediately called her daughter and upon arrival to the emergency room 40 min later, her vision had returned to normal. Recently she also has been experiencing dull throbbing headaches for which she is taking acetaminophen, with limited relief. She has a past medical history of hypercholesterolemia and coronary artery disease, undergoing angioplasty and stenting of the right coronary artery 8 years previously. She does not smoke currently but has a 40-pack-year history of tobacco, quitting only after her diagnosis of coronary artery disease. On review of systems, the patient recalls pain in her scalp with combing her hair, particularly on the right side, and occasional pain with chewing food. She has also recently noticed stiffness and pain in her hips, making it difficult to stand from seated position. On examination, she has 20/30 visual acuity in the left eye, and 20/100 visual acuity in the right eye. Funduscopic examination suggests anterior ischemic optic neuropathy. There are no carotid bruits present, but palpation of the temporal artery is painful. The neurologic examination is otherwise normal. The erythrocyte sedimentation rate (ESR) is 102 mm/h. The hemoglobin is 7.9 g/dL, and hematocrit is 25.5%. A head CT shows no acute ischemic event. Which of the following is the next most important step in the management of this patient?

    A. Initiate treatment with indomethacin, 75 mg twice daily.

    B. Initiate treatment with prednisone, 60 mg daily.

    C. Initiate treatment with unfractionated heparin adjusted based on activated partial thromboplastin time to obtain full anticoagulation.

    D. Perform magnetic resonance angiography of the brain.

    E. Perform a temporal artery biopsy.

21. A 64-year-old man with coronary artery disease and atrial fibrillation is referred for evaluation of fevers, arthralgias, pleuritis, and malar rash. The symptoms have developed over the past 6 months. The pleuritis

21. *(Continued)*

has responded to steroid therapy, but prednisone has been unable to be tapered off due to recurrence of symptoms at daily steroid doses <15 mg of prednisone. His medications include aspirin, procainamide, lovastatin, prednisone, and carvedilol. You suspect drug-induced lupus due to procainamide. Antibodies directed against which of the following proteins is most likely to be positive?

A. Cardiolipin
B. Double-stranded DNA
C. Histone
D. Ribonucleoprotein (RNP)
E. Ribosomal P

22. A 34-year-old man is admitted to the hospital for evaluation and treatment of renal failure and an abnormal CT of the chest. For the past 2 months, he has had fatigue, malaise, and intermittent fevers to as high as 38.2°C. About 3 weeks ago, he sought treatment from his primary provider for sinus pain and congestion with a purulent and bloody nasal discharge. He was treated for 2 weeks with ampicillinsulbactam, but his symptoms have only minimally improved. When he returned to his physician, a basic metabolic panel was performed which showed a creatinine of 2.8 mg/dL. A urinalysis showed 1+ protein with 25 red blood cells per high-power field. Red blood cell casts were present. His chest CT is shown below. Which of the following tests would be most likely to be positive in this individual?

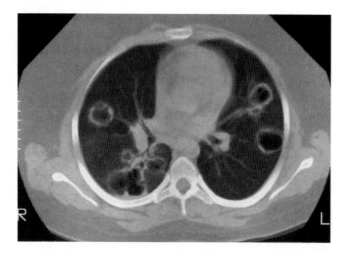

A. Antiglomerular basement membrane antibodies
B. Antiproteinase-3 antibodies
C. High titers of antibodies to antistreptolysin O
D. Perinuclear antineutrophil cytoplasmic antibodies
E. Positive blood cultures for *Staphylococcus aureus*

23. An 18-year-old man is admitted to the hospital with acute onset of crushing substernal chest pain that began abruptly 30 min ago. He reports the pain radiating to his neck and right arm. He has otherwise been in good health. He currently plays trumpet in his high school marching band but does not participate regularly in aerobic activities. On physical examination, he is diaphoretic and tachypneic. His blood pressure is 100/48 mmHg and heart rate is 110 beats/min. His cardiovascular examination has a regular rhythm but is tachycardic. A II/VI holosystolic murmur is heard best at the apex and radiates to the axilla. His lungs have bilateral rales at the bases. The electrocardiogram demonstrates 4 mm of ST elevation in the anterior leads. On further questioning regarding his past medical history, he recalls having been told that he was hospitalized for some problem with his heart when he was 2 years old. His mother, who accompanies him, reports that he received aspirin and γ globulin as treatment. Since that time, he has required intermittent follow-up with echocardiography. What is the most likely cause of this patient's acute coronary syndrome?

A. Dissection of the aortic root and left coronary ostia
B. Presence of a myocardial bridge overlying the left anterior descending artery
C. Stenosis of a coronary artery aneurysm
D. Vasospasm following cocaine ingestion
E. Vasculitis involving the left anterior descending artery

24. A 29-year-old male with episodic abdominal pain and stress-induced edema of the lips, the tongue, and occasionally the larynx is likely to have low functional or absolute levels of which of the following proteins?

A. C5A (complement cascade)
B. IgE
C. T-cell receptor, α chain
D. Cyclooxygenase
E. C1 esterase inhibitor

25. Which of the following joints are typically spared in osteoarthritis (OA)?

A. Ankle
B. Cervical spine
C. Distal interphalangeal joint
D. Hip
E. Knee

26. A 62-year-old woman is admitted to the hospital with pneumococcal bacteremia. Her past medical history is notable for a history of pneumonia due to

26. *(Continued)*

Haemophilus influenzae type B2 years ago and hypertension. On review of systems, she reports easy bruising, peripheral paresthesias, and symptoms of carpal tunnel syndrome. On physical examination, she has ecchymoses on her face and arms. Her nails are dystrophic and she has alopecia. Her tongue has indentations on both sides. Abdominal examination shows only hepatomegaly. She takes no medications or supplements and has no significant family history. A complete blood count shows a white blood cell count of 17,000/μL, hematocrit of 30%, and platelets of 300,000/μL. Differential shows 75% neutrophils, 20% lymphocytes. Serum albumin is 3.3 mg/dL, calcium 8.0 mg/dL, total protein 8.2 mg/dL, AST 32 U/L, ALT 32 U/L, total bilirubin 1.3 mg/dL, alkaline phosphatase 120 U/L. What is the most likely etiology of the patient's current infection?

A. Cyclical neutropenia
B. Functional asplenism
C. HIV infection
D. Sickle cell anemia
E. X-linked agammaglobulinemia

27. Which of the following statements regarding rheumatoid arthritis is true?

A. There is an association with the class II major histocompatibility complex allele HLA-B27.
B. The earliest lesion in rheumatoid arthritis is an increase in the number of synovial lining cells with microvascular injury.
C. Females are affected three times more often than are males, and this difference is maintained throughout life.
D. Africans and African Americans most commonly have the class II major histocompatibility complex allele HLA-DR4.
E. Titers of rheumatoid factor are not predictive of the severity of rheumatoid arthritis or its extraarticular manifestations.

28. Which of the following definitions best fits the term *enthesitis*?

A. Alteration of joint alignment so that articulating surfaces incompletely approximate each other
B. Inflammation at the site of tendinous or ligamentous insertion into bone
C. Inflammation of the periarticular membrane lining the joint capsule
D. Inflammation of a saclike cavity near a joint that decreases friction
E. A palpable vibratory or crackling sensation elicited with joint motion

29. A 35-year-old female presents to her primary care doctor complaining of diffuse body and joint pain. When asked to describe which of her joints are most affected, she answers, "All of them." There is no associated stiffness, redness, or swelling of the joints. No Raynaud's phenomenon has been appreciated. Occasionally she notes numbness in the fingers and toes. The patient complains of chronic pain and poor sleep quality that she feels is due to her pain. She previously was seen in the clinic for chronic headaches that were felt to be tension related. She has tried taking over-the-counter ibuprofen twice daily without relief of pain. She has no other medical problems. On physical examination, the patient appears comfortable. Her joints exhibit full range of motion without evidence of inflammatory arthritis. She does have pain with palpation at bilateral suboccipital muscle insertions, at C5, at the lateral epicondyle, in the upper outer quadrant of the buttock, at the medial fat pad of the knee proximal to the joint line, and unilaterally on the second right rib. The erythrocyte sedimentation rate is 12 s. Antinuclear antibodies are positive at a titer of 1:40 in a speckled pattern. The patient is HLA-B27 positive. Rheumatoid factor is negative. Radiograms of the cervical spine, hips, and elbows are normal. What is the most likely diagnosis?

A. Ankylosing spondylitis
B. Disseminated gonococcal infection
C. Fibromyalgia
D. Rheumatoid arthritis
E. Systemic lupus erythematosus

30. A 42-year-old woman comes to your clinic 1 week after her primary doctor diagnosed her with fibromyalgia. She describes years of fatigue, chronic pain, poor sleep, and irritability and is unable to work due to her symptoms. A review of her physical examination confirms the presence of pain on digital palpation at 14 of 18 characteristic sites. While relieved at finally having a diagnosis, she is concerned about what treatments are available. Which of the following should be your first treatment step?

A. Improve sleep and consider tricyclics
B. Initiation of a pain diary and frequent, brief clinic visits
C. Low-dose narcotics and a long-acting benzodiazepine
D. Referral for psychotherapy with a psychologist
E. Treatment of depression with a selective serotonin reuptake inhibitor (SSRI)

31. An 18-year-old man with ankylosing spondylitis (AS) is concerned about the development of disability due to his disease. Which of the following statements is

31. *(Continued)*
    true regarding the development and treatment of disability in AS?

    A. Anti–TNF-α (tumor necrosis factor α) inhibitors are now first-line therapy and have been shown to limit disability while being safe for long-term therapy.
    B. Despite the development of ankylosis of the spine, spinal fracture is a rare complication, affecting <10% of individuals with AS.
    C. Maintenance of an exercise program to maintain posture and range of motion is important in limiting disability.
    D. Nonsteroidal anti-inflammatory drugs (NSAIDs) decrease pain but have no effect on the development of disability in AS.

32. A 23-year-old woman was diagnosed with systemic lupus erythematosus based upon the presence of polyarthritis, malar rash with photosensitivity, and oral ulcerations. Antibodies to double-stranded DNA, Smith protein, and antinuclear antibodies were present in high titers. A urinalysis is normal. The patient is requesting treatment for the joint symptoms as she feels they limit her activities of daily living. What is the best choice for initial therapy in this individual?

    A. Hydroxychloroquine, 200–400 mg daily
    B. Methotrexate, 15 mg weekly
    C. Physical therapy only
    D. Prednisone, 1 mg/kg daily
    E. Quinacrine, 100 mg three times daily

33. A 43-year-old male presents to your office complaining of weakness in the right hand for 2 days. He reports that he had been in excellent health until 2 months ago, when he was diagnosed with hypertension. Since that diagnosis, he has lost 20 lb unintentionally and complains of frequent headaches and abdominal pain that is worse after eating. He previously was an injection drug user but now is maintained on methadone. His only medications are hydrochlorothiazide 25 mg/d, methadone 70 mg/d, and lisinopril 5 mg/d. On physical examination, the patient appears well developed and without distress. Blood pressure is 148/94. He is not tachycardic. The examination is otherwise notable only for the inability to extend the right wrist and fingers against gravity. Laboratory studies show an erythrocyte sedimentation rate (ESR) of 88 mm/h, an aspartate aminotransferase (AST) of 154 IU/L, and an alanine aminotransferase (ALT) of 176 IU/L.

33. *(Continued)*
    Which of the following tests is most useful in establishing a diagnosis?

    A. Hepatitis B surface antigen
    B. Hepatitis C viral load
    C. Anticytoplasmic neutrophil antibodies
    D Mesenteric angiography
    E. Radial nerve biopsy

34. A 45-year-old male has been hospitalized for several weeks in the intensive care unit for postsurgical complications after gastrojejunal bypass surgery. He is noted to have persistent fevers and on examination is found to have erythema, fluctuance, and tenderness over the posterior surface of the left elbow. Initial management of this disorder should include all the following *except*

    A. incision and drainage
    B. empirical antibiotics for gram-positive organisms
    C. aspiration of the collection for Gram stain and culture
    D. microscopic evaluation of aspirate for crystals
    E. pressure-relieving devices

35. A 42-year-old woman is being treated with cyclophosphamide, 2 mg/kg daily, for Wegener's granulomatosis manifested as glomerulonephritis, tracheal stenosis, and cavitary lung disease. All of the following are potential side effects of cyclophosphamide at this dose *except*

    A. neurotoxicity
    B. bone marrow suppression
    C. hemorrhagic cystitis
    D. infertility
    E. myelodysplasia

36. Which of the following statements best describes the function of proteins encoded by the human major histocompatibility complex (MHC) I and II genes?

    A. Activation of the complement system
    B. Binding to cell surface receptors on granulocytes and macrophages to initiate phagocytosis
    C. Nonspecific binding of antigen for presentation to T cells
    D. Specific antigen binding in response to B cell activation to promote neutralization and precipitation

37. A 32-year-old pregnant woman presents to the clinic with right thumb and wrist pain that has worsened over several weeks. She has pain when she pinches her thumb against her other fingers. On physical examination she has mild swelling and tenderness

37. *(Continued)*

over the radial styloid process, and pain is elicited when she places her thumb in her palm and grasps it with her fingers. A Phalen maneuver is negative. Which condition is most likely?

A. Carpal tunnel syndrome
B. De Quervain's tenosynovitis
C. Gouty arthritis of the first metacarpophalangeal joint
D. Palmar fasciitis
E. Rheumatoid arthritis

38. A 63-year-old white female is admitted to the hospital complaining of hemoptysis and shortness of breath. She had been well until 3 months ago, when she noted vague symptoms of fatigue and a 10-lb unintentional weight loss. Past medical history is notable only for osteoporosis. Her current symptoms began on the day of presentation with the expectoration of >200 mL of red blood in the emergency department. On physical examination, the patient is in marked respiratory distress with a respiratory rate of 44 breaths/min. Oxygen saturation is 78% on room air and 88% on nonrebreather mask. Pulse is 120 beats/min, with a blood pressure of 170/110. There are diffuse crackles throughout both lung fields, and the cardiac examination is significant only for a regular tachycardia. There are no rashes or joint swellings. Laboratory studies reveal a hemoglobin of 10.2 mg/dL with a mean corpuscular volume (MCV) of 88 μm^3 (fL). The white blood cell count is 9760/mm^3. Blood urea nitrogen (BUN) is 78 mg/dL, and creatinine is 3.2 mg/dL. The urinalysis shows 1+ proteinuria, moderate hemoglobin, 25 to 35 red blood cells (RBC) per high-power field, and occasional RBC casts. Chest computed tomography (CT) shows diffuse alveolar infiltrates consistent with alveolar hemorrhage. The antimyeloperoxidase titer is positive at 126 U/mL (normal <1.4 U/mL). What is the most likely diagnosis?

A. Goodpasture's disease
B. Wegener's granulomatosis
C. Microscopic polyangiitis
D. Polyarteritis nodosa
E. Cryoglobulinemia

39. A 62-year-old white male presents with a chief complaint of right knee pain and swelling. Past medical history is significant for obesity with a body mass index (BMI) of 34 kg/m^2, diet-controlled Type 2 diabetes mellitus, and hypertension. His medications include hydrochlorothiazide and acetaminophen as needed for pain. Physical examination is remarkable for a moderate-size effusion of the right knee, with

39. *(Continued)*

range of motion limited to 90° of flexion and 160° of extension. There is minimal warmth and no redness. He has crepitus with range of motion. With weight bearing, he has outward bowing of the legs bilaterally. A radiogram of the right knee shows osteophytes and joint space narrowing. Which of the following is the most likely finding on joint fluid examination?

A. A Gram stain showing gram-positive cocci in clusters
B. A white blood cell count of 1110/mm^3
C. A white blood cell count of 22,000/mm^3
D. Positively birefringent crystals on polarizing light microscopy
E. Negatively birefringent crystals on polarizing light microscopy

40. A 25-year-old female presents with a complaint of painful mouth ulcerations. She describes these lesions as shallow ulcers that last for 1 or 2 weeks. The ulcers have been appearing for the last 6 months. For the last 2 days, the patient has had a painful red eye. She has had no genital ulcerations, arthritis, skin rashes, or photosensitivity. On physical examination, the patient appears well developed and in no distress. She has a temperature of 37.6°C (99.7°F), heart rate of 86, blood pressure of 126/72, and respiratory rate of 16. Examination of the oral mucosa reveals two shallow ulcers with a yellow base on the buccal mucosa. The ophthalmologic examination is consistent with anterior uveitis. The cardiopulmonary examination is normal. She has no arthritis, but medially on the right thigh there is a palpable cord in the saphenous vein. Laboratory studies reveal an erythrocyte sedimentation rate of 68 s. White blood cell count is 10,230/mm^3 with a differential of 68% polymorphonuclear cells, 28% lymphocytes, and 4% monocytes. The antinuclear antibody and anti-dsDNA antibody are negative. C3 is 89 mg/dL, and C4 is 24 mg/dL. What is the most likely diagnosis?

A. Behçet's syndrome
B. Systemic lupus erythematosus
C. Discoid lupus erythematosus
D. Sjögren's syndrome
E. Cicatricial pemphigoid

41. What is the best initial treatment for this patient?

A. Topical glucocorticoids including ophthalmic prednisolone
B. Systemic glucocorticoids and azathioprine
C. Thalidomide
D. Colchicine
E. Intralesional interferon α

42. A 42-year-old man presents to your clinic complaining of left shoulder soreness that has been bothering him for 8 months. He experiences intermittent pain that is worse at night. Active abduction of his left arm over his head causes extreme pain. He describes his pain as a dull ache in his shoulder. He cannot identify a specific trauma that led to his pain but notes that he lifts weights and plays sports on a regular basis. On physical examination, he has tenderness over the lateral aspect of the humeral head and pain with arm abduction. Which of the following is the most likely cause of his symptoms?

A. Acromioclavicular arthritis
B. Bicipital tendonitis
C. Inflammation of the infraspinatus tendon
D. Inflammation of the supraspinatus tendon
E. Subluxation of the left humeral head

43. A 42-year-old male presents with complaints of a rash and joint pain. He first noticed the rash 6 months ago. It is primarily on the hands (see figure below), the extensor surfaces of the elbows, and the knees, low back, and scalp. Although he complains of the appearance of these lesions, they do not itch or hurt. The patient has not been previously evaluated for them and has recently noticed changes in the nail beds. For the last 2 weeks, the patient has had increasingly severe pain in the distal joints of the hands and feet. His hands are so painful that he is having trouble writing and holding utensils. The patient denies fevers, weight loss, fatigue, cough, shortness of breath, or changes in bowel or bladder habits. Which of the following is the most likely diagnosis?

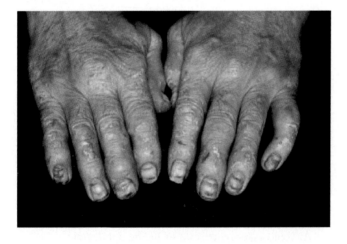

A. Arthritis associated with inflammatory bowel disease
B. Gout
C. Osteoarthritis
D. Psoriatic arthritis
E. Rheumatoid arthritis

44. Which of the following is the most common clinical manifestation of relapsing polychondritis?

A. Aortic regurgitation
B. Arthritis of weight-bearing joints
C. Auricular chondritis
D. Reduced hearing
E. Saddle nose deformity

45. A 60-year-old woman with a history of Sjögren's syndrome diagnosed 20 years ago presents to her primary care doctor complaining of facial swelling. Her xerostomia dry eye symptoms have not changed. She is known to be positive for rheumatoid factor in addition to Ro and La antibodies but is not thought to have rheumatoid arthritis. She previously had cutaneous vasculitis requiring treatment with prednisone, but she has been off steroids for 5 years without evidence of recurrence. She is currently using artificial tears and cevimeline, 30 mg three times daily. On physical examination, her right parotid gland is enlarged. It is not tender, but it is firm and hard to the touch. It is noted that the right parotid gland was similarly enlarged on a visit 3 months ago. She denies systemic illness or any new symptoms. What is the most likely diagnosis?

A. Adenoid cystic carcinoma
B. B-cell lymphoma
C. Impacted sialolith
D. Mumps
E. Recurrent vasculitis

46. A 42-year-old Turkish man presents to his physician complaining of recurring ulcers in the mouth and on his penis. He states that the ulcers are painful and last for about 2 weeks before spontaneously resolving. In addition, he intermittently gets skin lesions that he describes as painful nodules on his lower extremities. You suspect that he has Behçet's syndrome. A pathergy test is performed. What response would you expect after injecting 0.3 mL of sterile saline under the skin?

A. Development of 10 mm of induration with overlying erythema after 72 h
B. Development of a 2- to 3-mm papule at the site of insertion in 2–3 days
C. Development of granulomatous inflammation 4–6 weeks after the injection
D. Development of an urticarial reaction within 15 min
E. No reaction

47. A 45-year-old African-American woman with systemic lupus erythematosus (SLE) presents to the emergency room with complaints of headache and fatigue. Her prior manifestations of SLE have been arthralgias, hemolytic anemia, malar rash, and mouth ulcers, and

are commonly in the 10,000–30,000/µL range. The bacteria of septic arthritis usually enter the joint via hematogenous spread through synovial capillaries. Patients with rheumatoid arthritis are at high risk of a septic arthritis due to *Staphylococcus aureus* because of chronic inflammation and glucocorticoid therapy. The concurrent presence of pseudogout does not preclude the diagnosis of septic arthritis. In adults, the most common bacterial pathogens are *Neisseria gonorrhoeae* and *S. aureus*. Antibiotics, prompt surgical evaluation of possible arthroscopic drainage, and blood cultures to rule out bacteremia are all indicated. Prompt local and systemic treatment of infection can prevent destruction of cartilage, joint instability, or deformity. Direct instillation of antibiotics into the joint fluid is not necessary. If the smear shows no organisms, a third-generation cephalosporin is reasonable empirical therapy. In the presence of Gram-positive cocci in clusters, antistaphylococcal therapy should be instituted based on community prevalence of methicillin resistance or recent hospitalization (which would favor empirical vancomycin). Typically acute flairs of pseudogout can be addressed with glucocorticoids. However, this could portend a higher risk in the context of infection. Nonsteroidal anti-inflammatory agents might be a possibility depending on the patient's renal function and gastrointestinal history.

6. The answer is A.
(Chap. 23) Adhesive capsulitis is characterized by pain and restricted motion of the shoulder. Usually this occurs in the absence of intrinsic shoulder disease, including osteoarthritis and avascular necrosis. It is, however, more common in patients who have had bursitis or tendinitis previously as well as patients with other systemic illnesses, such as chronic pulmonary disease, ischemic heart disease, and diabetes mellitus. The etiology is not clear, but adhesive capsulitis appears to develop in the setting of prolonged immobility. Reflex sympathetic dystrophy may also occur in the setting of adhesive capsulitis. Clinically, this disorder is more commonly seen in females over age 50. Pain and stiffness develop over the course of months to years. On physical examination, the affected joint is tender to palpation, with a restricted range of motion. The gold standard for diagnosis is arthrography with limitation of the amount of injectable contrast to less than 15 mL. In most patients, adhesive capsulitis will regress spontaneously within 1 to 3 years. NSAIDs, glucocorticoid injections, physical therapy, and early mobilization of the arm are useful therapies.

7. The answer is B.
(Chap. 8) The patient in this vignette is presenting with severe dry eyes and mouth in the presence of autoantibodies to Ro and La (SS-A and SS-B, extractable nuclear and cytoplasmic antigens) consistent with the diagnosis of Sjögren's syndrome. This autoimmune disorder is associated with lymphocytic infiltration of exocrine glands that results

in decreased tear and saliva production as the most prominent symptom. Sjögren's syndrome affects women nine times more frequently than men and usually presents in middle age. Other autoimmune diseases often have associated xerostomia and dry eyes (secondary Sjögren's syndrome). High titers of antibodies to Ro and La are associated with longer disease duration, salivary gland enlargement, and the development of extra-glandular involvement, especially cutaneous vasculitis and demyelinating syndromes. One-third of patients with Sjögren's syndrome have extraglandular involvement of the disease, most commonly in the lungs and kidneys. In this patient with acidemia and hypokalemia, the possibility of renal disease due to Sjögren's syndrome should be considered. Interstitial nephritis is a common manifestation of Sjögren's syndrome in the kidneys. Distal (type I) renal tubular acidosis is also frequent, occurring in 25% of individuals with Sjögren's syndrome. Diagnosis could be confirmed by obtaining urine electrolytes to demonstrate a positive urine anion gap. Renal biopsy is not necessary. Treatment does not require immunosuppression as the acidemia can be treated with bicarbonate replacement. Diarrhea could cause similar electrolyte abnormalities with a non–anion gap acidosis, but the patient would be symptomatic. Furthermore, gastrointestinal symptoms do not commonly occur in Sjögren's syndrome. Hypoaldosteronism is associated with a type IV renal tubular acidosis that results in hyperkalemia and a non–anion gap acidosis. Renal compensation for respiratory alkalosis should not result in hypokalemia. Purging in anorexia nervosa could result in hypokalemia and increased risk of dental caries, but it would be associated with metabolic alkalosis rather than acidosis.

8. The answer is A.
(Chap. 15) Patients on hemodialysis are at risk for a particular type of amyloidosis due to deposition of β_2-microglobulin (Aβ_2M). The protein is above the molecular weight cut-off for clearance by the dialysis membrane and is becoming less common with the advent of newer dialysis techniques. The clinical syndrome is a rheumatologic one, with joint effusions, arthropathy, and cystic bone lesions predominating. The β_2-microglobulin can be found in joint synovium, and the joint fluid is usually noninflammatory. Serum amyloid A (secondary amyloid) is associated with chronic infections or inflammatory conditions. AL (immunoglobulin light chain deposition) is the most common type of amyloidosis and is due to a clonal population of B cells. Deposition of the fibrinogen α-chain (AFib) is a familial condition associated with a systemic amyloidosis. Transthyretin is associated with a familial form of amyloidosis that is transmitted in an autosomal dominant fashion. These usually manifest in midlife with neuropathy and cardiomyopathy. One variant of transthyretin amyloid has a carrier frequency of up to 4% in African Americans and is associated with a late-onset cardiomyopathy.

9. **The answer is A.**

(Chap. 16) Polymyositis is an inflammatory myopathy that presents as symmetric, progressive muscle weakness. The patient reports difficulty with everyday tasks requiring the use of proximal muscles, such as getting up from a chair and climbing steps. Distal muscle strength is usually preserved until late in the course. In addition to the musculoskeletal findings, there are numerous extramuscular manifestations. This patient may have systemic symptoms of fever, malaise, weight loss, and Raynaud's phenomenon. There may be "overlap" features with other autoimmune diseases, such as systemic lupus erythematosus (SLE) and scleroderma. Involvement of the striated muscles and the upper esophagus may lead to dysphagia. Conduction defects, arrhythmia, and dilated cardiomyopathy may occur. Interstitial lung disease may precede myopathy or occur early in the disease, often in association with the presence of antibodies to t-RNA synthetases. Although dermatomyositis is linked with an increased incidence of cancer, polymyositis does not seem to be associated with an increased incidence.

10. **The answer is C.**

(Chap. 19) Acute gouty arthritis is frequently seen in individuals on diuretic therapy. Diuretics result in hyperuricemia through enhanced urate reabsorption in the proximal tubule of the kidney in the setting of volume depletion. Hyperuricemia remains asymptomatic in many individuals but may manifest as acute gout. Acute gout is an intensely inflammatory arthritis that frequently begins at night. While any joint may be affected, the initial presentation of gout is often in the great toe at the metatarsophalangeal joint. There is associated joint swelling, effusion, erythema, and exquisite tenderness. A typical patient will complain that the pain is so great that they are unable to wear socks or allow sheets or blankets to cover the toes. Arthrocentesis will reveal an inflammatory cloudy-appearing fluid. The diagnosis of gout is confirmed by the demonstration of monosodium urate crystals seen both extracellularly and intracellularly within neutrophils. Monosodium urate crystals appear strongly negatively birefringent under polarized light microscopy and have a typical needle- and rod-shaped appearance. The WBC count is usually <50,000/μL with values >100,000/μL being more likely to be associated with a septic arthritis. Likewise, very low glucose levels and a positive Gram stain are not manifestations of acute gout but are common in septic arthritis. Calcium pyrophosphate dihydrate crystals appear as weakly positively birefringent rhomboidal crystals and are seen in pseudogout.

11. **and 12. The answers are E and E.**

(Chap. 4) This patient is presenting with symptoms that are consistent with systemic lupus erythematosus (SLE). SLE can present with a wide variety of complaints affecting every organ system. The most common complaints with SLE are fatigue (95%), arthralgias (95%), photosensitivity (70%), anemia (70%), leukopenia (65%), and nonerosive polyarthritis (60%)—all of which are present in this patient. In addition, this patient has mouth ulcers, which are seen in 40% of patients. The scalp lesion is consistent with discoid lupus erythematosus, which can be a benign condition if presenting as an isolated condition. Only 5% of individuals with isolated discoid lesions develop SLE; however, up to 20% of those with SLE will have discoid lesions. The presence of a positive ANA is sensitive, but not specific, for SLE as 98% of individuals with SLE will have a positive ANA during the course of the disease. Alternatively, persistent negative ANA results can rule out SLE. Antibodies to double-stranded DNA and to the Smith protein (nuclear U1 RNA) are both specific for SLE in high titers. Some 70% of individuals with SLE will have positive antibodies for ds-DNA, and 25% will have antibodies to the Smith protein. Individuals with anti-Sm antibodies often also have antibodies to ribonucleoprotein as well. The level of rheumatoid factor in this patient falls within the equivocal range and is not diagnostic of rheumatoid arthritis. Further, the patient's discoid rash and photosensitivity as well as positive serologies would further eliminate rheumatoid arthritis from the differential diagnosis. Behçet's disease presents with oral and genital ulcerations, and 50% will also have nonerosive arthritis. However, the skin lesions for Behçet's disease do not usually appear as discoid lesions, and Behçet's is inconsistent with the serology studies. Finally, sarcoidosis can mimic the arthritic disease of SLE. The rash associated with sarcoidosis is papular lesions along the nasolabial folds (lupus pernio) and erythema nodosum.

Nephritis is the most serious manifestation of SLE and, with infection, is the leading cause of death in the first decade following diagnosis. However, in most individuals, nephritis is clinically silent until the disease is advanced. For this reason, it is recommended that all patients suspected of having SLE undergo a urinalysis. In the presence of nephritis, the expected findings would include microscopic hematuria and proteinuria in early disease. In more severe disease, red cell casts and nephrotic range proteinuria may be seen. A skin biopsy of the discoid lesion would show hyperkeratosis and follicular plugging. A mononuclear cell infiltrate is often seen near the dermal-epidermal junction. While a biopsy would be diagnostic for discoid lupus, it would not alter management. An electrocardiogram would be indicated if the patient were complaining of pain consistent with pericarditis. Likewise, the presence of a murmur on examination may prompt an echocardiogram to assess for Libmann-Sachs valvular disease in a patient with SLE. However, these tests are not indicated in an asymptomatic patient. If sarcoidosis were being considered, chest radiography would be appropriate to assess for hilar lymphadenopathy and interstitial lung disease, but they are not indicated in this case.

13. The answer is B.

(Chap. 23) The plantar fascia is a thick fibrous band that extends from the medial tuberosity of the calcaneus to insert on each of the five metatarsal heads. Plantar fasciitis is thought to be the result of repeated microtrauma to the tissue. It is a common disorder leading to foot pain and can be diagnosed on the basis of history and physical examination alone. All of the imaging modalities listed above can support the diagnosis, but by themselves are neither sufficient nor necessary for diagnosis. Management includes stretching and orthotics in addition to reducing activities that elicit pain. Local glucocorticoid injections have also been shown effective but may have a risk of plantar fascia rupture. The differential diagnosis includes calcaneal stress fracture, spondyloarthropathy, rheumatoid arthritis, gout, neoplastic or infiltrative bone processes, and nerve entrapment/compression syndromes.

14. The answer is E.

(Chaps. 17 and 20; Baker, N Engl J Med 329:1013–1020, 1993.) The analysis of synovial fluid begins at the bedside. When fluid is withdrawn from a joint into a syringe, its clarity and color should be assessed. Cloudiness or turbidity is caused by the scattering of light as it is reflected off particles in the fluid; these particles are usually white blood cells, although crystals may also be present. The viscosity of synovial fluid is due to its hyaluronate content. In patients with inflammatory joint disease, synovial fluid contains enzymes that break down hyaluronate and reduce fluid viscosity. In contrast, synovial fluid taken from a joint in a person with a degenerative joint disease, a noninflammatory condition, would be expected to be clear and have good viscosity. The color of the fluid can indicate recent or old hemorrhage into the joint space. Pigmented villonodular synovitis is associated with noninflammatory fluid that is dark brown in color ("crankcase oil") as a result of repeated hemorrhage into the joint. Gout and calcium pyrophosphate deposition disease produce inflammatory synovial effusions, which are cloudy and watery. In addition, these disorders may be diagnosed by identification of crystals in the fluid: Sodium urate crystals of gout are needle-like and strongly negatively birefringent, whereas calcium pyrophosphate crystals are rhomboidal and weakly positively birefringent.

15. The answer is A.

(Chap. 9) Reactive arthritis is an acute inflammatory arthritis that occurs in the context of an infection elsewhere in the body. The most common causes of reactive arthritis are diarrhea and urethritis. Individuals with reactive arthritis typically present with asymmetric polyarthritis with associated fever, fatigue, and weight loss. Most often these symptoms begin 1–4 weeks after an antecedent illness. The arthritis usually begins with a single joint affected, but additional joints become inflamed over the next 1–2 weeks. The arthritis is painful with frequent effusions present. The

most commonly affected joints are those of the lower extremities. Dactylitis presenting as a "sausage digit" with diffuse swelling of a single toe or finger may occur. Pain at tendinous insertion, known as *enthesitis*, is also a feature of reactive arthritis. Extraarticular manifestations of reactive arthritis include urethritis, prostatitis, uveitis, and oral ulcers. In rare instances, life-threatening systemic manifestations can occur including cardiac conduction defects, aortic insufficiency, pulmonary infiltrates, and central nervous system disease. The arthritis typically persists for 3–5 months and can be present for up to a year. Fifteen percent of individuals will develop chronic joint symptoms, and relapses with recurrence of acute arthritis may occur. Risk factors for a worse outcome include presence of HLA-B27 antigen and epidemic shigellosis.

16. The answer is E.

(Chap. 5) Anti–TNF-α therapy for rheumatoid arthritis has been used since 2000. Two agents are currently used: infliximab is a chimeric human-mouse anti–TNF-α monoclonal antibody, and etanercept is a soluble p75 TNF-α monoclonal antibody. These agents are potent immunosuppressants, and six types of common side effects have been described. Serious infections are most frequently seen, with a marked increase in disseminated tuberculosis. Other side effects include pancytopenia, demyelinating disorders, exacerbations of congestive heart failure, hypersensitivity to the infusion or injection, and the development of drug-induced systemic lupus erythematosus. An increased incidence of malignancy is of theoretical concern, but this has not been borne out in the limited follow-up of patients treated with these drugs. Pulmonary fibrosis has not been reported.

17. The answer is E.

(Chap. 6) This patient has a small-joint, symmetric polyarthritis in the setting of a very recent sore throat. Although acute HIV commonly presents with a sore throat, other common features, such as rash, are missing. Moreover, the incubation period between this patient's high-risk sexual encounter and clinical syndrome would be too short for acute HIV infection. Certainly, this patient should be screened for HIV infection. The patient meets clinical criteria for group A *Streptococcus* throat infection given his recent fever, pustular exudates on examination, tender cervical lymph nodes, and lack of cough. His syndrome is consistent with a reactive arthritis, given the symmetric small-joint involvement and very short incubation period. Acute rheumatic fever is also seen with streptococcal throat infections but is very uncommon in the developed world. One would expect to see a latency period ranging between 1 and 5 weeks between resolution of sore throat and arthritis; asymmetric large-joint involvement; and possibly evidence of carditis, chorea, erythema marginatum, or subcutaneous nodules to suspect a diagnosis of acute rheumatic fever.

Gonococcal infection can cause pharyngitis but is more commonly associated with single large-joint infection or enthesopathy, but not small-joint polyarthritis. Lyme disease is a clinical diagnosis contingent upon tick exposure, a classic target lesion rash, and, if present, a migratory large-joint arthritis.

18. The answer is E.

(Chap. 4) Although most clinicians believe that females with SLE should not become pregnant if they have active disease or advanced renal or cardiac disease, the presence of SLE itself is not an absolute contraindication to pregnancy. The outcome of pregnancy is best for females who are in remission at the time of conception. Even in females with quiescent disease, exacerbations may occur (usually in the first trimester and the immediate postpartum period), and 25–40% of these pregnancies end in spontaneous abortion. Fetal loss rates are higher in patients with lupus anticoagulant or anticardiolipin antibodies. Flare-ups should be anticipated and vigorously treated with steroids. Steroids given throughout pregnancy also usually have no adverse effects on the child. In this case, the fact that the female had a life-threatening bout of disease a year ago would argue against stopping her drugs at this time. Neonatal lupus, which is manifested by thrombocytopenia, rash, and heart block, is rare but can occur when mothers have anti-Ro antibodies.

19. The answer is B.

(Chap. 9) Before the introduction of anti–tumor necrosis factor (TNF) α therapy, the mainstay of treatment for ankylosing spondylitis was nonsteroidal anti-inflammatory drugs (NSAIDs) and exercise therapy. In 2000, infliximab and etanercept were introduced and since that time have been shown to confer a rapid, profound, and sustained reduction in all clinical and laboratory measures of disease activity. Even patients with long-standing disease and ankylosis show significant improvement in spinal mobility and pain relief. MRI findings in patients treated with these agents also show marked improvement in marrow edema, enthesitis, and joint effusions. The long-term effects of these agents are not known.

Other treatments for AS can be used, including NSAIDs and COX-2 inhibitors, to decrease pain, especially in mild cases. An ongoing exercise program is encouraged to maintain posture and range of motion. In patients with more severe pain, sulfasalazine or methotrexate may be added with modest benefit, especially in those with peripheral arthritis. Diverse other agents have been tried, including thalidomide, bisphosphonates, and radium-224. Glucocorticoids have no role in the treatment of this disease.

20. The answer is B.

(Chap. 10) This patient is presenting with amaurosis fugax with evidence of decreased visual acuity and anterior

ischemic optic neuropathy in the setting of a compatible clinical history of giant cell arteritis (temporal arteritis). In an individual >50 years, this clinical history should prompt immediate initiation of glucocorticoids in order to prevent the development of monocular blindness. Giant cell arteritis is exquisitely sensitive to steroid therapy, and initiation of prednisone, 40–60 mg daily, is usually effective at managing the symptoms. If ocular symptoms recur, prednisone may be increased further. Once symptoms are controlled, gradual tapering of the steroid dose should occur. Most patients do require prolonged courses of steroid, usually for >2 years. The elevation in ESR can be a useful marker of disease activity during a steroid taper. Aspirin is often used in combination with glucocorticoids as it has been shown to decrease ischemic complications of giant cell arteritis. Indomethacin is not frequently used and should not be used alone in a patient presenting with symptoms of ischemic optic neuropathy. There is no role for anticoagulation in the treatment of giant cell arteritis. Definitive diagnosis of giant cell arteritis is confirmed by temporal artery biopsy, which should be performed in this patient. However, treatment should not be withheld for performance of the biopsy as sudden and irreversible blindness may occur. Ultrasonography of the temporal artery may also be a suggestive. While the patient's age and history of coronary artery disease raise the suspicion of a transient ischemic attack, the patient's other symptoms in this case make giant cell arteritis more likely. These symptoms are chronic, occurring over several weeks to months prior to presentation. The symptoms include new-onset headache, jaw claudication, scalp pain, and symptoms of polymyalgia rheumatica. In this clinical setting, performance of magnetic resonance angiography would not be indicated.

21. The answer is C.

(Chap. 4) Drug-induced lupus can occur with a variety of medications and should be considered when individuals present atypically. Individuals with drug-induced lupus are more likely to be male and of Caucasian race. Drug-induced lupus usually presents with fever, malaise, intense arthralgias/myalgias, serositis, and rash. The brain and kidneys are rarely involved. Discontinuation of the medication usually leads to resolution of the symptoms over a period of weeks, although anti-inflammatory medications may need to be utilized to control symptoms until the inflammation subsides. Common drugs that cause lupus include procainamide, propafenone, hydralazine, propylthiouracil, lithium, phenytoin, carbamazepine, sulfasalazine, and minocycline. Beta blockers, angiotensin-converting enzyme inhibitors, lovastatin, and simvastatin have also been reported to cause drug-induced lupus. Antibody testing usually reveals a positive antinuclear antibody and antihistone antibodies. Antibodies to ds-DNA are rare. Anticardiolipin antibodies are seen in antiphospholipid antibody syndrome, which would present with arterial

and venous thromboembolic disease. Anti-RNP antibodies are seen with mixed connective tissue disease that usually presents with features of lupus, rheumatoid arthritis, and/or scleroderma. Anti-ribosomal P antibodies are associated with depression and psychosis with central nervous system involvement of SLE.

22. The answer is B.
(Chap. 10) The presenting symptoms of this patient include rapidly progressive renal failure, sinusitis, and cavitary lung disease. These symptoms are consistent with the diagnosis of Wegener's granulomatosis (WG). WG is characterized by granulomatous vasculitis of small vessels that primarily manifests in the airways and kidneys. An uncommon disease, WG has an estimated prevalence of three per 100,000 population. The male-to-female ratio is equal. The upper airway is involved in 95% of patients and, in this setting, the disease often presents as chronic sinusitis unresponsive to antibiotic therapy. Facial pain and bloody nasal discharge are commonly present. Untreated disease can progress to complete cartilaginous destruction with nasal septal perforation and saddle nose deformity. The lungs are the second most commonly affected organ in about 85% of individuals with WG. The spectrum of lung disease may vary widely from asymptomatic pulmonary infiltrates to massive hemoptysis. In this patient, there are characteristic cavitary lung lesions that help to differentiate WG from microscopic polyangiitis, as no cavitary disease is seen in microscopic polyangiitis. Rapidly progressive glomerulonephritis is present in 77% of patients and is responsible for the majority of deaths in WG. Nonspecific symptoms are also present when the disease is active including fatigue, weight loss, and fevers. Diagnosis of WG is made by demonstration of necrotizing vasculitis on tissue biopsy of an affected organ. Serologic testing can offer supporting evidence for the diagnosis of WG. Ninety percent of individuals with WG will demonstrate antibodies to cytoplasmic antineutrophil cytoplasmic antibodies (cANCA). The specific cANCA target in WG is proteinase-3. Rapid initiation of therapy is important. Prior to the use of cyclophosphamide, WG was almost universally fatal within 5 years, even with the use of glucocorticoids. With the combined use of glucocorticoids and cyclophosphamide, survival is now 75–80% at 5 years. Perinuclear antineutrophil cytoplasmic antibodies (pANCA) are usually directed against myeloperoxidase. The pANCA are seen in a minority of patients with WG but are more commonly present in microscopic polyangiitis. Antistreptolysin O antibodies are seen with poststreptococcal glomerulonephritis. This patient's prior upper respiratory symptoms were primarily sinusitis and not associated with pharyngitis, and the CT scan of the chest would not be expected to be abnormal.

Antiglomerular basement membrane (anti-GBM) antibodies are present in Goodpasture's syndrome. This pulmonary-renal syndrome frequently presents with rapidly progressive glomerulonephritis and respiratory failure. Diffuse alveolar hemorrhage is common. The CT of the chest in Goodpasture's syndrome would not be expected to show cavitary lung lesions. Endocarditis due to *S. aureus* may cause a similar CT appearance with multiple septic emboli causing cavitary lung disease. However, the constellation of findings with sinusitis and glomerulonephritis would not be expected.

23. The answer is C.
(Chap. 10; JW Newberger et al: Circulation 110:2747, 2004.) The most likely cause of the acute coronary syndrome in this patient is thrombosis of a coronary artery aneurysm in an individual with a past history of Kawasaki disease. Kawasaki disease is an acute multisystem disease that primarily presents in children <5 years of age. The clinical manifestations in childhood are nonsuppurative cervical lymphadenitis; desquamation of the fingertips; and erythema of the oral cavity, lips, and palms. Approximately 25% of cases are associated with coronary artery aneurysms that occur late in illness in the convalescent stage. Early treatment (within 7–10 days of onset) with IV immunoglobulin and high-dose aspirin decreases the risk of developing coronary aneurysms to about 5%. Even if coronary artery aneurysms develop, most regress over the course of the first year if the size is <6 mm. Aneurysms >8 mm, however, are unlikely to regress. Complications of persistent coronary artery aneurysms include rupture, thrombosis and recanalization, and stenosis at the outflow area. Dissection of the aortic root and coronary ostia is a common cause of death in Marfan's syndrome and can also be seen with aortitis due to Takayasu's arteritis. In this patient, there is no history of hypertension, limb ischemia, or systemic symptoms that would suggest an active vasculitis. In addition, there are no other ischemic symptoms that would be expected in Takayasu's arteritis. Myocardial bridging overlying a coronary artery is seen frequently at autopsy but is an unusual cause of ischemia. The possibility of cocaine use as a cause of myocardial ischemia in a young individual must be considered, but given the clinical history, it is a less likely cause of ischemia in this case.

24. The answer is E.
(Chap. 1; Frank, N Engl J Med 316:1525–1530, 1987.) Complement activity, which results from the sequential interaction of a large number of plasma and cell-membrane proteins, plays an important role in the inflammatory response. The classic pathway of complement activation is initiated by an antibody-antigen interaction. The first complement component (C1, a complex composed of three proteins) binds to immune complexes with activation mediated by C1q. Active C1 then initiates the cleavage and concomitant activation of components C4 and C2. The activated C1 is destroyed by a plasma protease inhibitor termed *C1 esterase inhibitor*. This molecule also regulates clotting factor XI and kallikrein. Patients with a

deficiency of C1 esterase inhibitor may develop angioedema, sometimes leading to death by asphyxia. Attacks may be precipitated by stress or trauma. In addition to low antigenic or functional levels of C1 esterase inhibitor, patients with this autosomal dominant condition may have normal levels of C1 and C3 but low levels of C4 and C2. Danazol therapy produces a striking increase in the level of this important inhibitor and alleviates the symptoms in many patients. An acquired form of angioedema caused by a deficiency of C1 esterase inhibitor has been described in patients with autoimmune or malignant disease.

25. The answer is A.
(Chap. 18) OA is the most common type of arthritis. Roughly 12% of the U.S. population above the age of 60 has evidence of OA of the knee. OA in the hands may affect 10% of the elderly. Commonly affected sites include the cervical and lumbosacral spine, hip, and the knee. In the hands, both the proximal and distal interphalangeal joints are frequently affected. The wrist, elbow, and ankle are typically spared. The ankle joint's articular cartilage may be the reason it is less susceptible to OA, but this remains unclear. There is a notable difference between affected joints in osteoarthritis in comparison to rheumatoid arthritis (RA); the lumbar spine and distal interphalangeal joints are rarely affected in RA, and the wrist joints are almost always involved.

26. The answer is B.
(Chap. 15) Recurrent infections due to encapsulated organisms strongly suggests asplenism. Functional asplenism along with easy bruising, neuropathy, and macroglossia suggests amyloidosis. Other findings that argue for amyloidosis are alopecia, dystrophic nails, and the elevated globulin fraction. The functional asplenism of amyloidosis is due to direct involvement of the spleen, although hypersplenism may be present. HIV-infected patients are more likely to have recurrent infections but without splenomegaly, and they are not more susceptible to encapsulated organisms than other patients. A new diagnosis of sickle cell anemia is unlikely given the patient's demographic. Cyclical neutropenia usually occurs in children, although there are also adult forms. The cycle of cyclical neutropenia is usually 3 weeks. X-linked agammaglobulinemia is a rare congenital disorder of males whose B cells do not mature. Patients with this disorder do not make immunoglobulins and develop severe upper respiratory infections, often with encapsulated organisms.

27. The answer is B.
(Chap. 5) The prevalence of rheumatoid arthritis (RA) is 0.8%, and females are three times more likely to be affected than are males. However, as the population ages, the prevalence increases and the sex difference diminishes. RA is found throughout the world and affects people of all races. Age of onset is most commonly 35 to 50 years. Family studies show a clear genetic predisposition. First-degree relatives have approximately four times the expected rate of RA. Other risk factors for RA include the class II major histocompatibility antigen HLA-DR4. Approximately 70% of patients with RA have HLA-DR4. However, this association is not true in Africans or African Americans, among whom 75% do not show this allele. The role of this allele in the pathogenesis of RA remains unknown because the cause of RA is unknown. The earliest lesion in RA is microvascular injury with an increase in the number of synovial lining cells. Increased numbers of mononuclear cells are seen in the synovial lining, and this is thought to be under the control of CD4+ T lymphocytes. As the inflammation continues, the articular matrix is degraded by collagenases and cathepsins produced by the inflammatory cells. Other cytokines produced by the inflammatory cells include IL-1 and TNF-α. Over time, bone and cartilage are destroyed, leading to the end-stage clinical manifestations. Rheumatoid factor (RF) is an IgM molecule directed against the Fc portion of IgG and is found in two-thirds of patients with RA. However, this molecule is found in approximately 5% of healthy persons and more than 10% of persons older than age 60. It is not known to have a role in the pathogenesis of the disease, but titers of RF are shown to be predictive of the severity of clinical manifestations or the presence of extraarticular manifestations.

28. The answer is B.
(Chap. 9) Enthesopathy or *enthesitis* is the term used to describe inflammation at the site of tendinous or ligamentous insertion into bone. This type of inflammation is seen most frequently in patients with seronegative spondyloarthropathies and various infections, especially viral infections. The other definitions apply to other terms used in the orthopedic and rheumatic examination. *Subluxation* is the alteration of joint alignment so that articulating surfaces incompletely approximate each other. *Synovitis* refers to inflammation at the site of tendinous or ligamentous insertion into bone. Inflammation of a saclike cavity near a joint that decreases friction is the definition of *bursitis*. Finally, *crepitus* is a palpable vibratory or crackling sensation elicited with joint motion.

29. The answer is C.
(Chaps. 9 and 21) This patient complains of symptoms consistent with a diagnosis of fibromyalgia. These patients frequently complain of diffuse body pain, stiffness, paresthesias, disturbed sleep, easy fatigability, and headache. The prevalence of fibromyalgia is approximately 3.4% of females and 0.5% of males. This disorder is thought to represent a disturbance of pain perception. Disturbed sleep with a loss of stage 4 sleep has been implicated as a factor in the pathogenesis of the disease. Serotonin levels in the cerebrospinal fluid have also commonly been seen and may play a role in

the pathogenesis. A diagnosis of fibromyalgia is based on the American College of Rheumatology criteria, which combine symptoms and physical examination. The patient must exhibit diffuse pain in all areas of the body with tenderness to palpation at 11 of 18 designated tender point sites. These sites include the occiput, trapezius, cervical spine, lateral epicondyles, supraspinatus muscle, second rib, gluteus, greater trochanter, and knee. Digital palpation should be performed with a moderate degree of pressure. Examination of the joints shows no evidence of inflammatory arthropathy. There are no laboratory tests that are specific for the diagnosis. Positive antinuclear antibodies may be seen, but at the same frequency as in the normal population. HLA-B27 is found in 7% of the white population, but only 1–6% of people with HLA-B27 will develop ankylosing spondylitis. Radiograms are normal in these patients.

30. The answer is A.

(Chap. 21) The first step in the treatment of fibromyalgia is to improve the quality of the patient's sleep. This has been shown to improve quality of life and reduce symptoms. Improving sleep hygiene through nonpharmacologic methods should be encouraged, though tricyclic antidepressants are also recommended. Tricyclic antidepressants improve stage 4 sleep, resulting in clinical improvement. Other treatments that have shown improvement in sleep or symptoms independent of depressive disorder include trazodone, zolpidem, and duloxetine. All patients should be reassured that their condition is not degenerative nor life threatening, and that a variety of treatments are available. Mind-body therapies such as acupuncture, meditation, and yoga have shown benefit in some patients with fibromyalgia and should also be considered.

31. The answer is C.

(Chap. 9) Ankylosing spondylitis is a chronic disease that progresses to complete ankylosis over the course of several decades in a minority of individuals with this disease. Poor prognostic factors that are associated with an increased risk of progression include earlier onset of disease, male sex, and involvement of the hip joints. Spinal fracture is the most serious complication, with even minor trauma increasing the risk of fracture in the rigid spine. Spinal cord injury is a dreaded complication of spinal fracture. The estimated lifetime risk of spinal fracture in AS is >10%. An important component to prevent disability is to maintain a healthy weight and an exercise program with the goal of maintaining posture and range of motion in the spine. In addition to an exercise program, use of NSAIDs reduces pain and tenderness and increases mobility. When individuals who used NSAIDs daily regardless of pain symptoms were compared to a group of individuals who used NSAIDs only when pain was more severe, those with daily use of NSAIDs had less radiographic progression of their disease. Anti–TNF-α therapy (infliximab, etanercept, adalimumab) has a rapid and dramatic effect in AS, but these drugs are not first-line therapy at the present time because the effects of long-term use are unknown. However, there can be remarkable improvement in mobility and bone mineral density once TNF-α inhibitors are initiated.

32. The answer is A.

(Chap. 4) SLE is a chronic disease that has relapses and remissions, but is without cure. In individuals without major organ involvement, therapy can be directed at suppression of symptoms. This patient's limiting symptoms are due to articular involvement of SLE. Hydroxychloroquine was developed as an antimalarial drug and has been demonstrated to result in significant improvement in arthritis, dermatitis, and fatigue in SLE. Further, there is evidence that hydroxychloroquine reduces the number of disease flares, and this drug is often first-line therapy for treatment of joint and skin symptoms in SLE. Acetaminophen may be prescribed to control joint pain but is often less effective. While nonsteroidal anti-inflammatory drugs (NSAIDs) are often effective, caution should be used when prescribing these medications because there is an increased risk of NSAID-induced aseptic meningitis in SLE patients. Further, NSAIDs may also worsen hypertension and cause renal disease. Quinacrine is another antimalarial drug that may be substituted for hydroxychloroquine, but it is considered second-line therapy due to its side effect of causing diffuse yellowish skin discoloration. Physical therapy may be appropriate in combination with anti-inflammatory medications but is not expected to significantly improve the patient's functioning without control of the underlying disease. Prednisone is a potent anti-inflammatory medication that would be effective in suppressing the patient's symptoms. However, high-dose therapy (0.5–1.0 mg/kg daily) is not indicated in mild disease unless the patient is refractory to conservative therapies or develops major organ involvement, as the benefits in this situation would not outweigh the side effects. Methotrexate is often useful for joint symptoms as well as systemic manifestations, if prednisone therapy cannot be safely decreased or if the patient develops intolerable side effects of less toxic medications.

33. The answer is E.

(Chap. 10) This patient most likely has polyarteritis nodosa with a symptom complex consisting of abdominal pain, weight loss, hypertension, and mononeuritis. Polyarteritis nodosa (PAN) is an uncommon vasculitis that affects primarily medium-sized arteries without the involvement of venules. There are no diagnostic serologic tests for PAN. Up to 30% of patients with PAN are positive for hepatitis B surface antigen. In cases of PAN associated with hepatitis B, the virus, IgM, and complement can be demonstrated in vessel walls on biopsy. In light of the patient's past history of injection drug use, the presence of hepatitis B should be evaluated. However, demonstration of hepatitis B surface antigen is not diagnostic of PAN. ANCA is rarely positive in PAN patients, and hepatitis C is associated with cryoglobulinemic vasculitis but not with PAN. With the patient's abdominal pain that is worsened with eating, mesenteric ischemia caused by vasculitis should be considered. On mesenteric angiography, one would expect to find aneurysmal dilatation of the arteries. Again, however, this is not pathognomonic for PAN. The most definitive way to diagnose PAN is by finding vasculitis on a biopsy of the affected nerve. Therefore, a radial nerve biopsy should be pursued.

34. The answer is A.

(Chap. 23) This patient has a classic presentation for olecranon bursitis, with warmth, swelling, fluctuance, and tenderness over the posterior aspect of the elbow. Most often this is due to repeated trauma or pressure to the area that can occur through leaning on the elbow or through immobility with continuous pressure. Alternatively, infections, generally with gram-positive organisms, can cause olecranon bursitis, and crystalline disease, especially monosodium urate, can cause this picture. Initial evaluation involves aspiration of the fluid for Gram stain, culture, cell count and differential, and crystal evaluation. Empirical antibiotics would be warranted in this patient because of concern for infection with fevers and systemic illness. Incision and drainage should be reserved for bursitis of infectious etiology that is not responding to antibiotics and repeated aspirations.

35. The answer is A.

(Chap. 10) Cyclophosphamide in combination with glucocorticoids has increased the survival in Wegener's granulomatosis from 5% at 5 years to >70%. However, cyclophosphamide is a cytotoxic alkylating agent that has serious side effects that limit its long-term use. The incidence of cystitis at doses of 2 mg/kg daily is at least 30%, with a concomitant incidence of bladder cancer of at least 6%. For this reason, patients are instructed to take cyclophosphamide in the morning with large volumes of water. Frequent urinalyses are performed to assess for development of microscopic hematuria. In addition, there are significant bone marrow effects including bone marrow suppression and development of chromosomal abnormalities that may lead to myelodysplasia. Most clinicians monitor complete blood counts at least monthly. Infertility with gonadal suppression may occur during treatment, and the effects of cyclophosphamide can result in permanent infertility in both men and women. Other side effects of cyclophosphamide at the usual doses for vasculitis include gastrointestinal intolerance, hypogammaglobulinemia, pulmonary fibrosis, and oncogenesis. Neurotoxicity is not a side effect of cyclophosphamide.

36. The answer is C.

(Chap. 2) The human major histocompatibility complex genes are located on a 4-megabase region on chromosome 6.

The major function of the MHC complex genes is to produce proteins that are important in developing immunologic specificity through their role in binding antigen for presentation to T cells. This process is nonspecific, and the ability of an HLA molecule to bind to a particular protein depends upon the molecular fit between the amino acid sequence of a particular protein and the corresponding domain on the MCH molecule. Once a peptide has bound, the MHC-peptide complex binds to the T-cell receptor, after which the T cell must determine if an immune response should be generated. If an antigen is similar to an endogenous protein, the potential antigen will be recognized as a self-peptide and tolerance to the antigen will be continued. The MHC I and II complexes have been implicated in the development of many autoimmune diseases, which occur when T cells fail to recognize a peptide as a self-peptide and an immune response is allowed to develop. MHC I and II genes also play a major role in tissue compatibility for transplantation and are important in generating immune-mediated rejection. The other options listed as answers refer to functions of immunoglobulins. The variable region of the immunoglobulin is a B cell–specific response to an antigen to promote neutralization of the antigen through agglutination and precipitation. The constant region of the immunoglobulin is able to nonspecifically activate the immune system through complement activation and promotion of phagocytosis by neutrophils and macrophages.

37. The answer is B.

(Chap. 23) Inflammation of the abductor pollicis longus and the extensor pollicis brevis at the radial styloid process tendon sheath is known as De Quervain's tenosynovitis. Repetitive twisting of the wrist can lead to this condition. Pain occurs when grasping with the thumb and can extend radially along the wrist to the radial styloid process. Mothers often develop this tenosynovitis by holding their babies with the thumb outstretched. The Finkelstein sign is positive in De Quervain's tenosynovitis. It is positive if the patient develops pain by placing the thumb in the palm, closing the fingers around the thumb and deviating the wrist in the ulnar direction. Management of De Quervain's tenosynovitis includes nonsteroidal anti-inflammatory drugs and splinting. Glucocorticoid injections can be effective. A Phalen maneuver is used to diagnose carpal tunnel syndrome and does not elicit pain. The wrists are flexed for 60 s to compress the median nerve to elicit numbness, burning, or tingling. Gouty arthritis will present with an acutely inflamed joint with crystal-laden fluid. Rheumatoid arthritis is a systemic illness with characteristic joint synovitis and radiographic features.

38. The answer is C.

(Chap. 10) Microscopic polyangiitis (MPA) is a small-vessel vasculitis associated with antineutrophil cytoplasmic antibodies (ANCA) of the perinuclear type. MPA was recognized as

a discrete entity in 1992, when it was distinguished from polyarteritis nodosa because of the involvement primarily of small vessels. Twelve percent of cases present primarily with diffuse alveolar hemorrhage. MPA is distinct from Wegener's granulomatosis because it does not induce granulomatous inflammation. The glomerulonephritis associated with MPA is pauci-immune, showing a lack of immunoglobulin deposition. pANCA staining is positive in 75% of patients with MPA, with anti-myeloperoxidase antibodies being the target of the immunofluorescent staining pattern of the pANCA. Therapy begins with high-dose steroids and often requires the addition of cytotoxic therapy with cyclophosphamide. The 5-year survival rate is 74%; however, the disease tends to be chronic, with at least a 34% relapse rate.

39. The answer is B.

(Chaps. 17 and 18) This patient has osteoarthritis. His obesity predisposes him to degenerative joint disease that will be worse in the large weight-bearing joints. The physical examination findings of decreased range of motion, crepitus, and varus deformity that is exacerbated on weight bearing are consistent with this diagnosis. The radiogram of the knee demonstrates narrowing of the joint space with osteophyte formation. Occasional effusions may be seen, especially after overuse injuries. The joint fluid analysis in patients with osteoarthritis reveals a clear, viscous fluid with a white blood cell count <2000/µL. Positively birefringent crystals on polarizing light microscopy will be seen in pseudogout that most commonly affects the knee, whereas negatively birefringent crystals are characteristic of gout. Joint fluid in these inflammatory conditions would generally have a white blood cell count of <50,000/mm^3 and is yellow and turbid in character. Septic arthritis presents with fevers and a very warm and tender joint. The joint fluid can have the appearance of frank pus and is opaque. The white blood cell count is usually higher than 50,000/mm^3 and can have a positive Gram stain for organisms.

40. and 41. The answers are A and B.

(Chap. 11) Behçet's syndrome is a multisystem disorder of uncertain cause that is marked by oral and genital ulcerations and ocular involvement. This disorder affects males and females equally and is more common in persons of Mediterranean, Middle Eastern, and Far Eastern descent. Approximately 50% of these persons have circulating autoantibodies to human oral mucosa. The clinical features are quite varied. The presence of recurrent aphthous ulcerations is essential for the diagnosis. Most of these patients have primarily oral ulcerations, although genital ulcerations are more specific for the diagnosis. The ulcers are generally painful, can be shallow or deep, and last for 1 or 2 weeks. Other skin involvement may occur, including folliculitis, erythema nodosum, and vasculitis. Eye involvement is the most dreaded complication because it may progress rapidly to blindness. It often presents as panuveitis,

iritis, retinal vessel occlusion, or optic neuritis. This patient also presents with superficial venous thrombosis. Superficial and deep venous thromboses are present in one-fourth of these patients. Neurologic involvement occurs in up to 10%. Laboratory findings are nonspecific with elevations in the erythrocyte sedimentation rate and the white blood cell count. Treatment varies with the extent of the disease. Patients with mucous membrane involvement alone may respond to topical steroids. In more serious or refractory cases, thalidomide is effective. Other options for mucocutaneous disease include colchicines and intralesional interferon α. Ophthalmologic or neurologic involvement requires systemic glucocorticoids and azathioprine or cyclosporine. Life span is usually normal unless neurologic disease is present. Ophthalmic disease frequently progresses to blindness.

42. The answer is D.

(Chap. 23) Rotator cuff tendonitis is the most common cause of shoulder pain. The rotator cuff consists of the tendons of the supraspinatus, infraspinatus, subscapularis, and teres minor muscles. It inserts on the humeral tuberosities. The supraspinatus tendon is most frequently involved, likely due to the impingement that can occur between the humeral head and the acromion and coracoacromial ligament. Abduction of the arm causes a decrease in blood supply to this tendon, likely increasing the supraspinatus tendon's susceptibility to inflammation as well. Patients over 40 are particularly susceptible to rotator cuff injury, and pain is often worse at night. Nonsteroidal anti-inflammatory drugs, glucocorticoid injection, and physical therapy are all first-line management strategies for rotator cuff tendonitis. Bicipital tendonitis is produced by friction on the tendon of the long head of the biceps as it passes through the bicipital groove. Patients experience anterior shoulder pain that radiates down the biceps to the forearm. The bicipital groove is painful to palpation.

43. The answer is D.

(Chap. 9) This patient shows the typical features of psoriatic arthritis. Five to ten percent of patients with psoriasis will develop an arthritis associated with the rash. In 60–70% of cases, the rash precedes the diagnosis. However, another 15–20% of patients will have joint complaints as the presenting symptom of their psoriasis. The disease typically begins in the fourth or fifth decade of life. Psoriatic arthritis has varied joint presentations with five commonly described patterns of joint involvement: (1) arthritis of the distal interphalangeal (DIP) joints, (2) asymmetric oligoarthritis, (3) symmetric polyarthritis similar to rheumatoid arthritis (RA), (4) axial involvement, and (5) arthritis mutilans with the typical "pencil in cup" deformity seen on hand radiography. Erosive joint disease ultimately develops in almost all these patients, and most of them become disabled. Nail changes are prominent

in 90% of patients with psoriatic arthritis. Changes that are frequently seen include pitting, horizontal ridging, onycholysis, yellowish discoloration of the nail margins, and dystrophic hyperkeratosis. The diagnosis of psoriatic arthritis is primarily clinical. Thus, in patients with joint symptoms that precede the onset of rash, the diagnosis is frequently missed until dermatologic or nail changes develop. A family history of psoriasis is important to ascertain in any patient with an undiagnosed inflammatory polyarthropathy. The differential diagnosis of DIP arthritis is short; only osteoarthritis and gout are commonly seen in these joints. Radiography may show typical changes, particularly in patients with arthritis mutilans. Treatment is directed at both the rash and the joint disease simultaneously. Anti–TNF-α therapy has recently been shown to be helpful for both dermatologic and joint manifestations of disease. Other treatments include methotrexate, sulfasalazine, cyclosporine, retinoic acid derivatives, and psoralen plus ultraviolet light.

44. The answer is C.
(Chap. 12) Relapsing polychondritis is frequently a disease of abrupt onset with inflammation of one or more cartilaginous sites. Systemic symptoms such as fever and fatigue may precede the overt inflammation. The peak age of onset is in the forties to fifties, but it may occur at all ages. Approximately 30% of patients will have another rheumatologic disorder, most commonly systemic vasculitis. Auricular chondritis is the most common clinical manifestation of relapsing polychondritis, occurring 43% of the time as the presenting complaint, and with 89% cumulative frequency. Reduced hearing can occur in up to 40% of patients. Arthritis is a presenting complaint in 32% of patients. Saddle nose deformity, perhaps a well-known, or "classic," sign associated with relapsing polychondritis, is a presenting complaint of only 11% of patients and has a cumulative frequency of 25%. Aortic regurgitation, due to dilation of the aortic ring or destruction of the cusps, is an uncommon finding in this illness, occurring in ≤5% of cases. The diagnosis of relapsing polychondritis is based on recognition of the characteristic clinical features, including two or more separate sites of cartilaginous inflammation that responded to treatment with prednisone or dapsone. Biopsy can confirm the diagnosis but may not be necessary if the clinical features are typical.

45. The answer is B.
(Chap. 8) Sjögren's syndrome is associated with a lifetime risk of non-Hodgkin's lymphoma of 5% that usually presents later in the illness. The primary non-Hodgkin's lymphoma associated with Sjögren's syndrome is a low-grade, marginal zone B-cell lymphoma that usually presents extranodally. Many instances are found incidentally on labial biopsy. Persistent parotid enlargement, leukopenia, cryoglobulinemia, and presence of rheumatoid factor should prompt evaluation for possible lymphoma. Treatment for Sjögren's syndrome should be the same as that for other B-cell non-Hodgkin's lymphomas. Factors that influence survival include size >7 cm, presence of B symptoms, and high or intermediate histologic grade. Adenoid cystic carcinoma is the second most common malignant tumor of the salivary glands after mucoepidermoid carcinoma, but it does not occur more commonly in Sjögren's syndrome. An impacted sialolith could cause unilateral enlargement of the parotid gland but should present with pain with palpation. A sialolith may be complicated by bacterial sialadenitis. Pain is worse with eating or the anticipation of eating, which would stimulate saliva production. Mumps is unusual in the United States today due to immunization. Mumps most commonly presents with associated fever and systemic symptoms. Recurrent vasculitis would also be likely to present with systemic symptoms. Salivary glands are unlikely to be affected by vasculitis.

46. The answer is B.
(Chap. 11) Behçet's syndrome is a multisystem inflammatory disease of unknown etiology that presents with recurrent oral and genital ulcerations. The ulcerations are generally painful, occur in groups, and subside spontaneously in 1–2 weeks without leaving scars. Diagnosis of Behçet's syndrome is made based on clinical characteristics. The diagnosis requires the presence of recurrent oral ulcers plus two of the following criteria: recurrent genital ulcers, eye lesions, skin lesions (including erythema nodosum), or positive pathergy test. A pathergy test is considered positive when nonspecific skin inflammation develops 2–3 days after a scratch or injection of sterile saline. This is manifested as a small 2- to 3-mm papule at the site of injection. Other clinical manifestations of Behçet's syndrome include nonerosive arthritis, gastrointestinal ulcerations, and neurologic involvement. In addition, individuals with Behçet's syndrome are at increased risk of venous thromboembolic disease. The cause of Behçet's syndrome is unknown. It is more common in individuals from the Mediterranean region, Middle East, and Far East. In advanced disease, antibodies to α-enolase of endothelial cells and *Saccharomyces cerevisiae* have been shown. The pathologic lesion is perivasculitis with neutrophilic infiltration, endothelial swelling, and fibrinoid necrosis. Oral and genital lesions can usually be treated with topical glucocorticoids alone. Other treatments that are effective include thalidomide, colchicine, and systemic glucocorticoids. For central nervous system disease, azathioprine is added to systemic glucocorticoids. The severity of the disease tends to abate over time, and lifespan in Behçet's disease is normal. Development of 10 mm of dermal induration with overlying erythema occurring 49–72 h after injection of an antigenic protein is typical of a type IV hypersensitivity reaction. The most common use of this reaction is to assess for infection with tuberculosis

after injection of a purified protein derivative to *Mycobacterium tuberculosis*. The Kveim reaction refers to the development of granulomatous inflammation 4–6 weeks after injection of a protein derived from the lesion of sarcoidosis. An urticarial reaction demonstrates immediate hypersensitivity reaction and is typical of allergy phenomena.

47. The answer is C.

(*Chap. 4*) This patient is presenting with acute lupus nephritis with evidence of hematuria, proteinuria, and an acute rise in creatinine. Together with infection, nephritis is the most common cause of mortality in the first decade after diagnosis of SLE and warrants prompt immunosuppressive therapy. It is important to assess for other potentially reversible causes of acute renal insufficiency, but this patient is not otherwise acutely ill and is taking no medications that would cause renal failure. The urinalysis shows evidence of active nephritis with hematuria and proteinuria. Even in the absence of RBC casts, therapy should not be withheld to await biopsy results in someone with a known diagnosis of SLE with consistent clinical presentation and urinary findings. This patient also has other risk factors known to predict the development of lupus nephritis, including high titers of anti-dsDNA and African-American race. The mainstay of treatment for any life-threatening or organ-threatening manifestation of SLE is high-dose systemic glucocorticoids. Addition of cytotoxic or other immunosuppressive agents (cyclophosphamide, azathioprine, mycophenolate mofetil) is recommended to treat serious complications of SLE, but their effects are delayed for 3–6 weeks after initiation of therapy, whereas the effects of glucocorticoids begin within 24 h. Thus, these agents alone should not be used to treat acute serious manifestations of SLE. The choice of cytotoxic agent is at the discretion of the treating physician. Cyclophosphamide in combination with steroid therapy has been demonstrated to prevent development of end-stage renal disease better than steroids alone. Likewise, mycophenolate also prevents development of end-stage renal disease in combination with glucocorticoids, and some studies suggest that African Americans have a greater response to mycophenolate than to cyclophosphamide. Plasmapheresis is not indicated in the treatment of lupus nephritis but is useful in cases of severe hemolytic anemia or thrombotic thrombocytopenic purpura associated with SLE. Finally, this patient has no acute indication for hemodialysis and, with treatment, may recover renal function.

48. The answer is D.

(*Chap. 5*) Rheumatoid arthritis (RA) is a multisystem disease without a known etiology. Genetic factors appear to explain ~60% of disease susceptibility. The hallmark, or characteristic feature, of RA is persistent, inflammatory synovitis. The prevalence of RA is 0.8% in the general population, and women are affected three times more often than men. About 10% of patients will have a first-degree relative with the disease. 80% of patients will develop the disease between the ages of 35 and 50. The disease course can be variable between patients; some patients experience minimal joint damage, while others have a relentless and debilitating polyarthritis.

49. The answer is D.

(*Chap. 5*) Felty's syndrome is a syndrome of chronic RA, splenomegaly, and neutropenia. Anemia and thrombocytopenia are also sometimes related. Patients who develop Felty's syndrome most commonly have more active disease with high titers of rheumatoid factor, subcutaneous nodules, and other systemic manifestations of disease. However, Felty's syndrome can develop when joint inflammation has regressed. The leukopenia is a selective neutropenia with polymorphonuclear leukocytes below 1500/mm³. Bone marrow biopsy reveals hypercellularity with a lack of mature neutrophils. Hypersplenism has been proposed as a cause of Felty's syndrome, but splenectomy does not consistently correct the abnormality. Excessive margination of granulocytes caused by antibodies to these cells, complement activation, or binding of immune complexes may contribute to neutropenia.

50. The answer is A.

(*Chap. 9*) Anterior uveitis occurs in up to 30% of AS patients and may antedate the onset of the spondylitis. Attacks usually occur unilaterally with pain, photophobia, and blurred vision. Recurrent attacks are common, and ultimately cataracts may result. Other commonly seen problems include inflammation in the colon and ileum in up to 60% of AS patients, but only rarely do these patients develop inflammatory bowel disease. Cardiac disease is present in only a few percent of these patients and most commonly presents as aortic regurgitation. Other cardiac manifestations include complete heart block and congestive heart failure. Rare complications are upper lobe pulmonary fibrosis and retroperitoneal fibrosis.

51. The answer is C.

(*Chap. 16*) This patient presents with the classic symptoms, signs, and laboratory findings of polymyositis (PM) with antisynthetase antibodies. The differential diagnosis for a patient with proximal muscle weakness includes inclusion-body myositis, viral infections, denervating conditions such as amyotrophic lateral sclerosis (ALS), metabolic myopathies such as acid maltase deficiency, endocrine myopathies such as hypothyroidism, paraneoplastic myopathy, and drug-induced myopathies such as D-penicillamine, procainamide, statins, and glucocorticoids. PM is associated with an elevated creatine kinase, electromyography (EMG) showing irritability, and biopsy showing T-cell infiltrates primarily in the muscle fascicles. Many patients with PM have autoantibodies targeted against the ribonucleoproteins involved in protein synthesis (antisynthetases). The antibody directed against histidyl-transfer RNA synthetase or anti–Jo-1 identifies a group of patients with PM who have a high likelihood (80%) of having interstitial lung disease. Antiglomerular antibodies are found in patients with Goodpasture's syndrome, antihistone antibodies in those with drug-induced lupus, and antimicrosomal antibodies in those with autoimmune hepatitis.

52. The answer is E.
(Chap. 18) Osteoarthritis (OA) is a disease of joint failure due to joint stress and vulnerability. As the primary driving force of the disease is mechanical, first-line therapy should be nonpharmacologic. Avoiding activities that cause pain and overload the joint, strengthening and conditioning the adjacent muscle groups, and supporting or unloading the joint with a brace or crutch are all examples of fundamental treatments aimed at reversing the pathophysiology of OA. In the case above, weight loss should be the primary goal of therapy. Each pound of weight increases loading across a weight-bearing joint three- to six-fold. This patient would benefit from a daily minimal-weight-bearing exercise regimen combined with nutritional goals aimed at slow, consistent weight loss. Avoidance of walking is impractical; a cane or supportive device to lessen the joint load can be offered. Steroids and narcotics are not indicated in this case.

53. The answer is E.
(Chap. 21) Fibromyalgia is characterized by chronic widespread musculoskeletal pain, stiffness, paresthesia, disturbed sleep, and easy fatigability. It occurs in a 9:1 female-to-male ratio. It is not confined to any particular region, ethnicity, or climate. While the pathogenesis is not clear, there are associations with disturbed sleep (disruption of stage 4 sleep) and abnormal pain perception. Fibromyalgia is diagnosed by the presence of widespread pain, a history of widespread musculoskeletal pain that has been present for >3 months, and pain on palpation at 11 of 18 tender point sites. Besides pain on palpation, the neurologic and musculoskeletal examinations are normal in patients with fibromyalgia. Psychiatric illnesses, particularly depression and anxiety disorders, are common comorbidities in these patients but do not help satisfy any diagnostic criteria.

54. The answer is B.
(Chap. 8) Sjögren's syndrome may present in patients as a primary disease or as a secondary disease in association with other autoimmune disorders, such as rheumatoid arthritis, systemic lupus erythematosus, scleroderma, mixed connective tissue disease, and primary biliary cirrhosis. This patient is typical in that most persons affected by this disorder are middle-aged females with a female-to-male ratio of 9:1. Symptoms are related to diminished

lacrimal and salivary gland function. Oral dryness, or xerostomia, is very common. Parotid enlargement occurs in 66% of these patients. Ocular involvement resulting in symptoms of a sandy or gritty feeling under the eyelids, burning, redness, itching, decreased tearing, and photosensitivity is due to destruction of corneal and bulbar conjunctival epithelium, defined as keratoconjunctivitis sicca. Diagnostic evaluation includes the measurement of tear flow by Schirmer's test. Slit-lamp examination of the cornea after rose Bengal staining may show punctate corneal ulcerations and attached filaments of corneal epithelium. The most common extranodal manifestation of Sjögren's syndrome is arthralgias or arthritis (up to 60% of patients). Autoantibodies to Ro/SSA or La/SSB are very suggestive of this syndrome and are part of the classification criteria. Rheumatoid arthritis may be considered; however, the examination did not demonstrate inflammation, and the diffuse joint complaints without persistent morning stiffness make this less likely. Vitamin A deficiency may lead to dry eye but does not explain the patient's other symptoms.

55. The answer is D.
(Chap. 5) There are no blood tests that are specific for diagnosing rheumatoid arthritis (RA). Rheumatoid factors, which are autoantibodies to the Fc portion of IgG, have been used to help with diagnosis, and can be found in two-thirds of patients with RA. In the general population, rheumatoid factors become more prevalent with age, and 10–20% of patients older than 65 will have them. In unselected individuals, the predictive value of a positive rheumatoid factor is poor; no more than one-third of those with rheumatoid factors will have RA. False-positive results can occur in patients with systemic lupus erythematosus, Sjögren's syndrome, chronic liver disease, sarcoidosis, hepatitis B, mononucleosis, tuberculosis, malaria, and a host of other conditions. Recently, antibodies to cyclic citrullinated polypeptides (anti-CCP) have been shown to be helpful in diagnosing RA. In early RA, anti-CCP has been shown to be more predictive of disease than rheumatoid factor. Anti-CCP is felt to be a more specific test, and is positive in 1.5% of healthy individuals. The ESR has been used for decades as a nonspecific marker of inflammation. It is elevated in virtually all patients with active RA. In the patient above, radiographs would not add anything to the diagnostic evaluation. In early disease they are no more revealing of active synovitis than a careful physical examination. (See Table 5-1.)

56. The answer is C.
(Chap. 5) Rheumatoid arthritis is chronic, symmetric inflammatory polyarthritis. In two-thirds of patients, an initial clinical presentation of fatigue, anorexia, and weakness precedes joint complaints. In established RA (i.e., in a patient known to be diagnosed with this disorder), the